BETTER ENERGY

Paperback ISBN: 979-8-9850961-1-8
Hardback ISBN: 979-8-9850961-2-5

BETTER ENERGY

WHY HEALTH, HORMONES, AND METABOLISM DEPEND ON HOW WELL YOU TURN YOUR FOOD INTO ENERGY

KATE DEERING

Holistic and Lifestyle Coach, CNC, PT

The Science-backed companion to *How to Heal Your Metabolism*

DISCLAIMER

The information in this book is provided for educational purposes only and is not intended as medical advice, diagnosis, or treatment of any condition. Readers should not take action based solely on the content of this book and are encouraged to consult qualified healthcare professionals regarding any health-related concerns.

The information and opinions presented are based on the author's research and professional judgment and are believed to be accurate at the time of publication. However, this material is not a substitute for individualized medical care. Any application of the information contained in this book is undertaken at the reader's own discretion and risk.

The author and publisher assume no responsibility for any injury, loss, or damage resulting from the use or misuse of the information provided.

GET YOUR FREE MONTHLY NEWSLETTER

Continued education matters when it comes to your health, metabolism, and energy. Join Kate's community of thousands of curious, independent thinkers and receive a FREE monthly newsletter featuring up-to-date, science-based insights on nutrition, hormones, and energy production.

You'll find information on:

- Why carbohydrates are essential for optimal energy production
- Why estrogen is not a "female hormone," but a stress hormone
- Why fat burning is not always a good thing
- What most health practitioners are missing when it comes to true healing
- How to improve menopause symptoms without hormone therapy

To join the community of out-of-the-box, nutritionally minded readers, visit **www.KateDeering.com** and enter your name and email.

For daily insights on metabolism, hormones, and energy, please follow Kate on social media: Instagram & Facebook: **@KateDeeringFitness**

ABOUT THE AUTHOR

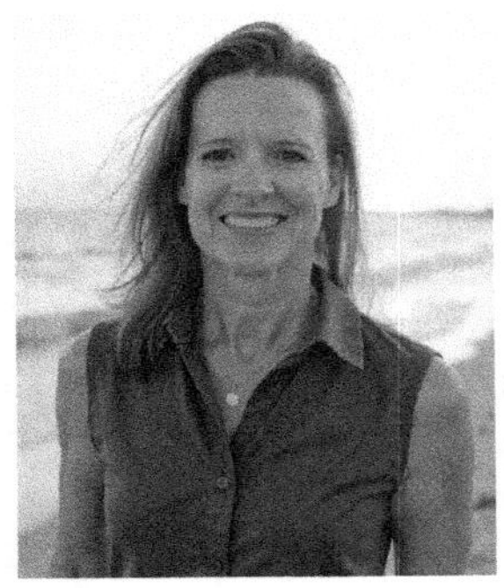 Kate Deering is a respected health educator, author, and metabolic researcher with over 30 years of experience in the health and fitness industry. Known for her evidence-based, out-of-the-box approach, Kate challenges conventional nutrition and exercise paradigms by focusing on cellular energy production as the foundation of lasting health.

Her work is grounded in the understanding that health is not built through chronic dieting, excessive exercise, or willpower, but through supporting metabolism, hormonal balance, and the body's ability to efficiently produce energy. Kate's own health journey led her to question mainstream advice and ultimately shaped her philosophy that better health is often achieved by eating more, resting more, and training smarter—not harder.

Through ongoing research and clinical application, Kate emphasizes the central role of cellular energy in metabolism, hormone health, longevity, and overall well-being. As an author, mentor, consultant, and educator, she works with individuals worldwide to improve metabolic health using real food, restorative sleep, appropriate exercise, and stress reduction.

Kate holds degrees in psychology and exercise science, is a Certified Nutritional Coach, and is a Holistic Exercise and Lifestyle Coach through the CHEK Institute. Her writing and teaching continue to bridge scientific research with practical, real-world application.

Kate lives in Del Mar, California, with her small but mighty dog, Ginger.

For more information, visit **www.KateDeering.com.**

ACKNOWLEDGMENTS

This book is dedicated to the late Dr. Ray Peat. His decades of independent research, intellectual rigor, and commitment to questioning conventional healthcare laid the groundwork for much of the thinking and researching that made this book possible. Without his work, books like this would not exist.

Thank you to Peyton Berg for sharing time and insight, and for helping refine the grammar, content, and overall flow of this book.

I am deeply grateful to Donna Kozik—my coach and editor—for keeping me focused, grounded, and helping me translate the last 10 years of learning into clear, coherent ideas on the page.

Thank you to Kitty Blomfield, Craig McDonald, and Jay Feldman for taking time out of their very busy lives to read and review this book. Your thoughtful feedback and perspective were greatly appreciated.

And finally, thank you to my clients, who trusted me to guide them through their health journeys. Your curiosity, feedback, and willingness to challenge conventional wisdom continue to shape my work.

CONTENTS

Everything has a beginning and that beginning starts with Energy!!

FOREWORD

Being asked to write the foreword for this book feels pretty special. Kate's work has shaped how I understand metabolism more than anything else I've ever read and it's a privilege to share what her work has meant in my own life.

I still remember discovering Dr Raymond Peat back in 2014. Coming from the fitness industry, dieting culture and the rather surface level understanding of human physiology his ideas were a complete eye-opener... To that end (if I'm honest) I kept most of it to myself in the beginning— not because I didn't believe it, but because I couldn't quite articulate why this bioenergetic model made more sense than everything I had been taught.

It was around this time that I discovered Kate's first book, *How to Heal Your Metabolism*. That book became the resource that finally pieced everything together. It clarified the concepts, grounded the principles and gave me a framework I could use. To this day, it remains the only book I recommend to clients, coaches, and anyone genuinely curious about improving their health.

As the years passed and as I continued working within the bioenergetic model, there was a natural inclination to go deeper. Whether through my own personal health challenges or through helping clients navigate theirs; I found myself peeling the layers back repeatedly and asking the questions:

- Why did this happen?
- How did this happen?

- What mechanism is driving this?
- Where are the gaps in my understanding?

Anyone who has gone down this path knows that this kind of curiosity becomes part of the journey. You don't just want answers. You want to understand the "why" behind the answers.

And that's exactly where this new book comes in.

Kate gives readers a clearer view into the body's deepest operating system - the part most people feel, but never fully understand. She breaks down how energy is created, how stress disrupts that process, why thyroid hormone is central, why oxygen and CO_2 matter, and why digestion and hormones begin to fall apart the moment your cells can't produce enough energy to stay safe.

She brings clarity to the things people experience every day:
- Why certain foods stabilize you while others drain you.
- Why digestion collapses under metabolic pressure.
- Why women struggle with estrogen "YES...ESTROGEN" issues they can't explain.
- Why iron, PUFA, and endotoxin quietly sabotage cellular energy.
- And, above all, why you can't separate metabolism from your nervous system.

In a world overflowing with noise and confusion, guru's and biohackers Kate has a rare ability to translate the complexities of mitochondrial function, thyroid conversion, gut permeability, bile recycling, estrogen clearance, and oxidative stress into something anyone can understand without diluting the science. This book reveals the deeper mechanisms behind the principles she introduced in her first book, making this — the natural next step once you've grasped the basics and want the full picture.

"Better Energy" is a major milestone in the bioenergetic world and a testament to her dedication, intelligence, and the way she thinks. It's truly something to celebrate.

I'm genuinely excited for you to read this, and remember—"There is no health without Energy"

Craig McDonald
Co-founder - NuStrength

INTRODUCTION

WHAT'S HAPPENED SINCE *HOW TO HEAL YOUR METABOLISM*

It has been quite a ride since my last book came out in 2015. My initial goal with *How to Heal Your Metabolism* was to make it easier for my own clients to understand how optimal nutrition and metabolism worked hand in hand. Yet, what ended up happening was something I never dreamed—the book went mainstream.

I'm deeply proud of what that first book accomplished. Since 2015, *How to Heal Your Metabolism* has sold nearly 100,000 copies in hardcover, paperback, digital, and audio. Readers have written to me about better digestion, clearer skin, stronger hair and nails, warmer bodies, deeper sleep, pain-free periods, improved sex drive, and boosted fertility (there are so many "Bioenergetic babies" out there now!). They've reported fewer hot flashes (without hormones), leaner body composition, brighter moods, sharper thinking, more motivation, and healthier relationships with food, finally breaking free from the restrict-binge cycle. I've even heard stories of recovery from PCOS, Lyme, IBS, SIBO, pre-diabetes, and even full-blown diabetes.

In the last decade, an entirely new world of nutrition has emerged, or at least, it's finally gotten to the masses. People call this world of nutrition *pro-metabolic, bioenergetic,* or even the "Ray Peat diet," since so much of it draws inspiration from the late, great Dr. Ray Peat. But none of those labels really capture what it's about. As Dr. Peat himself said countless times, he wasn't prescribing a specific diet. His focus was always on discovering what works for the individual. And I couldn't agree more.

Similar to *How to Heal Your Metabolism*, this book is meant to be a guide, not gospel. It's not a rigid blueprint, but rather a framework to help you navigate your unique path.

For many people, simply understanding their physiology and the needs of their metabolism sheds light on mysteries no doctor could solve. I'd like to think *How to Heal Your Metabolism* played a part in that by offering a simple roadmap for how your body works and what it needs.

My Own Rollercoaster: The Crash that Nearly Broke Me

On a personal note, I wish I could tell you my health has been "perfect" since that first book. But life has a way of throwing curveballs just when you think you're rounding third base.

In 2016, just as *How to Heal Your Metabolism* was taking off, I ended a toxic relationship. Feeling vulnerable and insecure, I made a choice I'd later regret; I decided Botox might help me feel better about myself. (If you don't know, Botox is literally a neurotoxin injected into facial muscles to temporarily smooth wrinkles.)

Within 24 hours of receiving 40 units, my life flipped upside down. I woke with a vice-like headache, eye pressure, blurry vision, a feeling of pins and needles everywhere, racing heart, anxiety, muscle weakness, and bone-deep fatigue. I thought maybe I'd caught a virus, but this was unlike anything I'd ever felt.

When I nervously asked my doctor if Botox could cause this, her response was; *"I've never heard of that, so I don't think so. Maybe you're just stressed. Want something for anxiety?"*

Um, no. I knew this wasn't "just stress." I needed someone to listen and investigate. If you've ever had that dismissed, helpless feeling in a doctor's office, I see you.

Eventually, a neurologist confirmed what others brushed off. A skin biopsy revealed I'd developed small fiber neuropathy (SFN), damage to the tiny nerves that regulate pain, temperature, heart rate, and gut function. SFN is often linked to diabetes, autoimmune disease, chemotherapy, or some sort of toxin exposure. In my case, the trigger was Botox. There was no magic pill, just time, nourishment, and hope. Some women recover in weeks, some in years, and some never fully do.

The Missing Puzzle Piece: It Wasn't Just Botox

What took me years to realize, and why this story belongs in a book about metabolism, is that Botox wasn't the only cause. It was just the final blow. My body was already vulnerable.

For years, I'd been chasing "anemia." My labs always showed low iron, so I loaded up on iron supplements. I didn't realize that I was also low in copper, the mineral your body needs to recycle iron safely through the reticuloendothelial system. Without copper (and without enough vitamin A and zinc), iron doesn't fuel your mitochondria, it stockpiles in tissues instead. I was literally storing iron in my skin (age spots), joints (stiffness, aches), and likely even in my pancreas and nerves, all while still feeling "anemic."

It's called functional iron deficiency; plenty of iron stored in the body but trapped where it can't help you make energy. My mitochondria were already under oxidative assault. My detox systems were strained. My nervous system was over-stressed. Botox was simply the tipping point.

Recovery meant stopping the iron, leaning into nutrient-dense foods like beef liver (to restore copper, vitamin A, and more), and slowly rebuilding. Even then, it wasn't just about food, I had to retrain my brain, calm my nervous system, and completely rethink stress.

What I Learned in the Dark

Through this process, I learned a few truths that shape this book:

- Your nervous system and metabolism are inseparable. If your nervous system is stuck in overdrive, healing stalls.

- The nervous system sits at the top of the energy hierarchy. Fix this first, and everything else starts to fall into place.

- There's a world of difference between burning calories under stress and producing energy under healthy thyroid function.

- You need multiple ingredients to make energy: thyroid hormone, oxygen, glucose, key minerals, and cofactors. Missing any one of them produces "low energy" symptoms.

- There are six main energy blocks that can cripple metabolism, and unless they're addressed, you won't restore full energy.

It took crawling through a very dark hole to fully understand, at both a cellular and soul-deep level, the fear, pain, loneliness, and exhaustion so many of you feel when your health collapses. This book will honor that.

I believe deeply that when life knocks you down, it's also inviting you to grow. You can let misfortune break you, or you can let it shape you into someone stronger, wiser, and more compassionate. Instead of sitting in my mess, I chose to go deeper, to learn more, and eventually, to share it all with you.

What You'll Find in This Book

This book isn't just about food, though food matters enormously. It's about everything that shapes energy production: fuel, nutrition, thyroid, oxygen. And everything that blocks it; stress, digestion, hormones, excess iron and estrogen, and yes, those pesky polyunsaturated fats (seed oils) everyone's still talking about.

This book is divided into three main parts:

1. Everything that supports energy production.
2. Everything that blocks energy production.
3. *Better Energy* in action: Fat loss and how to utilize this information.

My goal is for this book to give you the tools and confidence to become your own health practitioner. But let me be clear, I won't hand you a strict protocol. Your path will never look exactly like someone else's. What it will give you is frameworks, science, research, stories, suggestions, and reminders to help you stay the expert on your body.

If there's one thing I've learned from my own research, trial and error, and plenty of mistakes, it's this; the real magic happens when you start to understand your physiology, learn to trust yourself, work through your mess, and come out stronger on the other side.

So, pour yourself a big glass of orange juice (brain fuel) and let's discover why your cell's ability to make energy is the secret to a long, healthy, energy-filled life.

PART 1

SUPPORTING ENERGY PRODUCTION (METABOLISM)

Let's talk about energy production. It's the core of your metabolism; the more energy you produce—healthfully—the higher your metabolic power. The less you produce, the lower it runs. If you read my first book, you know all about this. But don't worry, if this is your first book, you will become educated within these chapters.

The truth is that most people don't know how energy production works. How do your cells make energy? Why does it matter? What do they need, and what happens when any piece is missing? Over the next five chapters, you'll see why energy is the true currency of health. You'll learn what cells require to produce it—supportive fuel, essential nutrients and protein, oxygen (and its partner, carbon dioxide), and a responsive thyroid. You'll get practical steps you can start using today to become a better energy maker.

Use this first part as your foundation. When fuel is supportive, nutrients are abundant, oxygen is well-used, and thyroid is responsive, ATP flows. With those four ingredients in place, everything gets easier; sleep deepens, digestion smooths out, mood steadies, recovery improves, and yes, fat loss becomes safer and more sustainable. Nail the basics here, then move on to Part 2 to clear the not-as-fun energy blocks.

CHAPTER 1

THERE IS NO HEALTH WITHOUT ENERGY

When most people think of energy, they think of feeling awake after coffee or having enough gas in the tank to get through the day. But in biology, energy is much more literal. It's the force that makes every single process in your body possible. Breathing, thinking, pumping blood, repairing cells, digesting food, moving, laughing, even smiling, all of it requires energy.

However, the energy your body runs on doesn't come directly from the calories in your food. Calories are a measurement of potential energy—raw material your cells must convert. To be usable, every calorie you eat must be converted into a molecule called ATP, or adenosine triphosphate. ATP is the spendable form of energy your cells use.

ATP is the true energy currency of life. Think of every cell in your body as a factory, and ATP is the payment that keeps the workers, which includes your enzymes, hormones, and muscles, on the job. It also keeps critical systems operating, including your gut, brain, liver, kidneys, heart, blood, lymph, pancreas, and sex organs.

Without ATP nothing gets done. You can eat all the food you want, but if you can't convert it into ATP, that "currency" either gets wasted or locked away in storage, making it harder to access when you need it.

This is why metabolism is more than calories in vs. calories out. Health depends on how efficiently your body turns calories into ATP, and how well that ATP production keeps up with life's demands. When production is high, your body works like a well-oiled machine: sharp brain, smooth digestion, balanced hormones, steady warmth and energy. When ATP falls short, your body cuts corners, choosing which systems to fuel and which ones to sacrifice. That's when symptoms begin to show.

Understanding Energy Balance

From a bioenergetic perspective, energy balance is when the energy your cells produce keeps up with the energy your body demands (see below for all your demands). When production matches demand, you feel energized, warm, clear-headed, resilient, and symptom-free. Sleep, digestion, hormones, skin, hair, mood, and performance all benefit.

Mainstream health circles often define energy balance as *calories in = calories out.* That equation may work for simple weight math, but it doesn't explain metabolism. We don't run on "calories," we run on ATP. Every calorie you eat must first be converted into ATP before your cells can use it.

Think of it like money. If you fly to Europe with U.S. dollars, you can't buy a coffee until you exchange those dollars for euros. In the same way, your body can't "spend" calories directly; it must convert them into ATP. That's why the better formula is:

Energy Balance: ATP Production (Calories in x How well your body converts them) =ATP Demands (Energy needed to run all your demands).

How You Make Energy: The Production Side

Your health comes down to one thing, how well your cells can turn food (fuel) into energy. And just like baking sourdough bread, you need the right ingredients, and the right conditions, for it to rise. Miss one piece, and the whole thing falls flat.

To make ATP efficiently, four main ingredients must come together; adequate fuel, nutrients, oxygen, and thyroid hormone.

Think of this as a recipe for health. Leave out one ingredient (or a reduced amount) and your health will fall short.

Fuel

Your primary fuels are carbohydrates and fats. Protein *can* be burned for energy, but that's not its main job. Protein is the builder of your muscles, bones, hormones, and enzymes. Carbs and fats, on the other hand, are like logs for your metabolic fire. Carbs (glucose) are the quick, clean-burning logs, especially important if you're active or stressed, because your nervous system runs best on glucose. Fats are slower burning, traveling through your lymph system before reaching circulation. Both are important. Your cells often use some fat and some glucose at the same time, but certain hormones and enzymes can tilt the mix so one usually dominates in that single moment.

Nutrients

Even the best fuel won't ignite without spark plugs, and that's where nutrients come in. Your mitochondria, the power plants of your cells, are nutrient-hungry. They need a constant stream of B vitamins (B1, B2, B3, B6, B12, folate, biotin) and minerals like magnesium, potassium, calcium, zinc, copper, manganese, and iron to turn food into ATP.

Without them, your cellular factories slow down. This is why nutrient-dense foods like dairy, liver, shellfish, grass-fed meats, fruits, and cooked vegetables, are so essential. They supply the spark plugs that keep your engines firing. Deficits often show up as low energy, constipation, poor sleep, cold body, hair loss, weight gain, brain fog, and feeling like sh#t.

Oxygen

Oxygen is an obvious need, without it, we're done in a matter of minutes. But oxygen is not just about breathing, it's also about O_2 delivery. If you have airway issues, anemia, or low carbon dioxide (CO_2 helps hemoglobin release oxygen into tissues), then even if you're "breathing fine," your cells can suffocate. Sometimes, just improving how you breathe, by nasal breathing, better posture, and improving CO_2 production, can upgrade energy levels dramatically. I'll go much deeper into this in Chapter 4, but for now; no oxygen, very little ATP.

Thyroid Hormone

Finally, the thyroid is your body's thermostat, the switch that turns energy production up or down. When thyroid hormone is active (T3), it speeds up how quickly your body can turn food into ATP. When it's low, that whole process drags. Some people don't make enough thyroid hormone (hypothyroidism). While others make plenty of T4 (the storage form) but due to stress, illness, low nutrients, or liver and kidney issues, can't convert it into T3, the active form. That's why you can have "normal" labs yet still feel cold, tired, and sluggish. I'll talk more about this later, because thyroid touches every part of energy production.

Ultimately, when fuel, nutrients, oxygen, and thyroid are all in place, ATP flows, and every system in your body runs smoothly. When one or more are missing, energy production slows, and your body adapts, cutting corners, down-regulating systems, and leaving you with symptoms.(Each of these energy ingredients is so essential, I've dedicated a full chapter to them later in this book.)

But here's the deal, it's not always as simple as having enough fuel, nutrients, oxygen, and thyroid hormone. Many people check those boxes and still feel fatigued, cold, or anxious. Does this resonate with you?

This happens because there are powerful energy blocks that interfere with healthy ATP production.

The big ones I've seen repeatedly are:

- Chronic stress: shifts healthy metabolism toward survival mode.
- Poor digestion and absorption: fewer nutrients in, less ATP out.
- Endotoxins: slow mitochondria function.
- Excess iron stored in tissues: drives oxidative stress and slows down energy production.
- Excess estrogen: can inhibit thyroid and increase stress signals.
- Polyunsaturated fats (PUFAs): prone to oxidation and gumming up mitochondrial efficiency.

These blocks explain why someone can eat a seemingly perfect diet yet still feel stuck. Something deeper is getting in the way of efficient energy production.

This realization is what motivated me to write this second book. I kept meeting people who were "doing everything right," me included, yet weren't getting better. That told me there had to be hidden barriers keeping their metabolism from thriving. My goal here is to help you identify and dismantle those blocks so your body can finally produce energy robustly.

Understanding Energy Demands: How You Use Energy

Your body's energy needs come from two main places:

- Internal demands (inside the body): breathing, detoxification, hormone production, nervous system function, digestion, and the constant repair of muscle, bone, and tissue.

- External demands (outside the body): movement, work, exercise, shopping, cooking, basically anything you physically do in the world.

When you produce enough energy to cover both, your body runs smoothly. You feel energized, warm, and symptom-free. You sleep well, think clearly, maintain healthy hair, skin, and nails, and keep a stable body size without excessive dieting or punishing workouts. In short, you can meet life's demands with ease and still have energy left for the things you *want* to do.

Your Total Daily Energy Expenditure (TDEE) is the energy your body needs to run both internal and external tasks.

Here is where I give you the lowdown of your metabolic needs—stick with me.

TDEE is made up of:

BMR + NEAT + Exercise + TEF = TDEE

Internal Demands

BMR (basal metabolic rate) : Energy needed at rest to run your brain, nervous system, liver, kidneys, immune system, hormones, and tissue repair. This is your biggest demand—often 60–70% of total energy needs.

TEF (thermic effect of food): The energy cost of digesting and processing food, about 10% of intake, varies by macronutrient (protein ~20–30%, carbs ~5–10%, fat ~0–3%) (1).

External Demands

NEAT (non-exercise activity thermogenesis): All your non-exercise movement—working, errands, chores, fidgeting, even singing in the car. Highly variable and can take 20–30% of energy needs.

Exercise: Formal workouts—lifting, running, sports, yoga. Energy-hungry while you do it, but usually only 5–10% of daily needs because it's such a small slice of the day.

When fuel is limited, the body prioritizes external demands (NEAT and exercise) over internal demands (BMR and digestion). That's why eating less during busy, stressful periods often shows up as constipation, poor sleep, and hormonal turbulence.

What Happens when Production Falls Short?

When you don't have the resources to make enough energy, or when energy production gets blocked while demands stay high, your body prioritizes what it can. It will try to keep up with external demands (work, stress, movement) but cut back on internal demands (digestion, sleep, hormones).

Most have felt this. Digestion slows, sleep gets disrupted, sex hormones tank, the "energy" initially felt from stress hormones eventually collapses, and you feel fatigued and exhausted.

We know this happens thanks to a famous study: the Minnesota Starvation Experiment of the 1940s. Dr. Ancel Keys recruited 32 healthy men and cut their calorie intake by 55% (from 3,492 kcal to 1,570 kcal) for 24 weeks. Each participant lost about 24% of their body weight, and their resting metabolism fell almost 40% (2).

Let me repeat that; the men reported an almost 40% lower metabolism in just 24 weeks.

Much of this was explained by lost lean and fat mass, but about a third was pure *metabolic adaptation*, meaning their bodies simply learned to use less energy, thus, symptoms appeared (3).

The symptoms were anemia, edema, bradycardia, fatigue, depression, excessive urination, low libido, constipation, anxiety, GI distress, dizziness, headaches, sleep problems, hair loss, and cold intolerance.

Basically, when you cut calories hard, your body goes on an energy production strike, which means many of your systems slow down.

Think of it like a city budget. You're the mayor and need $10 million in tax revenue (food) to run your city (your body). You need $4 million for safety, $2 million for roads, $2 million for government workers, and $2 million for schools. But this year, you only get $9 million in revenue (you went on a diet), and a surprise bridge repair adds another million in costs (you have additional stress).

You're forced to slash 10% of the budget (less fuel), while also using some of the budget for "other" expenditures (stress). Safety, schools, and infrastructure all take a hit. Over time, potholes spread, classrooms overflow, and the city declines. In metabolic terms, this could mean slower digestion, dysregulated hormones, poor sleep, fatigue, brain fog, etc.

That's how metabolic adaptation works. It will keep a city working, or someone alive when there is less energy available, yet these adaptations come at a price. An increase in symptoms and health issues—or, by using our example above, less safety, fewer teachers, and more potholes.

Signs of Energy Balance vs. Imbalance

So how do you know if your body is in energy balance? Well, the signs will show up throughout your body—in body temperature, pulse, digestion, sleep, mood, even how your hair and skin behave.

When metabolism is strong (balance):

- Warm body temp (97.8–98.6°F)
- Pulse 75–90 bpm
- Warm hands, feet, nose
- 1–3 easy bowel movements daily
- Clear thinking, stable mood, deep sleep
- Healthy libido, fertility, strong hair/skin/nails

- Steady energy, easy weight maintenance

When metabolism is sluggish (imbalance):

- Low temp/pulse, cold extremities
- Constipation or diarrhea
- PMS, heavy bleeding, low libido
- Hair loss, thin nails, aged skin
- Fatigue, depression, anxiety, poor sleep
- Resistant weight gain/loss
- Migraines, menopausal symptoms
- Frequent urination (>10x daily)
- Higher risk of chronic issues (MCAS, fibromyalgia, diabetes, autoimmune disease, high BP, high cholesterol, cancer, etc.)

Why This All Matters

Healthy energy balance isn't just "calories in = calories out." It's about:

ATP Production (fuel, nutrients, O_2, thyroid ± blocks) = Total Demands (BMR + NEAT + Exercise + TEF).

When production meets demand, your body thrives. But when demand outweighs production, the body shifts into an adaptive stress mode; slower internal functions, adrenaline and cortisol rise, free fatty acids flood the bloodstream, and the system burns reserves (glycogen, fat, muscle, organs, and even bone).

In a robust body, a short-term deficit may just mean fat loss. But in a stressed system, these same deficits drive symptoms, thyroid suppression, and long-term metabolic slowdown. Which means over time, weight loss becomes harder, sleep gets worse, hormones get trashed, and your energy plummets.

Remember the city budget analogy? When tax revenue falls short, the mayor cuts funding from schools, safety, and infrastructure to keep the city functioning at the most basic level. Your body does the same cutting back on digestion, reproduction, and repair to keep you alive. The result? More "potholes" in your health.

Now that you understand what real energy balance means, here's where we're headed. In the chapters ahead, I will walk you step by step through everything that powers your metabolism, and everything that can block it.

You will:

- Discover your best fuel sources and why excessive fat oxidation can backfire.

- Understand what your cells need nutritionally and the exact foods that supply those nutrients.

- Learn why oxygen and carbon dioxide are partners in cellular respiration.

- See how thyroid hormone ties into every single metabolic process in your body, and what happens when production or conversion falters.

- Identify and fix the major energy blocks: stress hormones, digestive issues, endotoxins, excess iron, excess estrogen, and PUFA.

By the end, you'll not only understand how your body really works, but you'll have a roadmap to fixing your energy roadblocks, all the while working to optimize your cells' ability to produce energy.

As a bonus, once your foundation is strong, fat loss becomes safe, strategic, and sustainable. I will discuss this at the end of the book, for those looking for fat loss without crushing their metabolism.

To start us off, let's discuss our first ingredient for optimal energy production—the fuel (food) you put into your body.

CHAPTER 1

THE BOTTOM LINE

There Is No Health Without Energy

1. ATP, not calories, runs the show. Calories are just raw material; your body must convert them into ATP before they're usable. ATP is the true "currency of life," powering every cell, organ, and process. Without it, nothing works.

2. Real energy balance isn't "calories in = calories out." It's whether your ATP production can meet your body's total demands (internal + external). When they match, you thrive; when they don't, symptoms and breakdown follow.

3. The four ingredients of energy production include:
    - Fuel (carbs + fats, with glucose as the preferred clean burner)
    - Nutrients (B-vitamins, minerals, nutrient-dense foods)
    - Oxygen (and CO_2 balance for proper delivery)
    - Thyroid Hormone (the "thermostat" that sets your metabolic rate)

3. The biggest blocks: chronic stress, poor digestion, endotoxins, excess iron, excess estrogen, and polyunsaturated fats (PUFAs).

4. Your body prioritizes survival tasks over "luxuries" like reproduction, digestion, and repair. The result is fatigue, hormone disruption, poor sleep, gut issues, and chronic symptoms.

5. Signs of balance vs. imbalance: Balanced: warm temps, steady energy, strong digestion, deep sleep, fertility, resilient mood. Imbalanced: cold hands/feet, constipation, PMS, hair loss, fatigue, anxiety, resistant weight changes.

CHAPTER 2

SUPPORTIVE FUEL FOR OPTIMIZING ENERGY PRODUCTION

When it comes to a well running metabolism, quality fuel and nutrition are essential to optimize energy production. And where do you get your best fuel and nutrition?

Quality food, of course!

Optimizing energy production goes hand-in-hand with quality food. I define quality food as whole food, less processed, minimal additives, nutrient rich, low in polyunsaturated fats, and well tolerated by the digestive system. Without enough of the right, quality food, energy production (ATP) can become hindered, and metabolic adaptations can occur.

Explaining this was the catalyst in writing my first book, *How to Heal Your Metabolism*. Foods that support the body are essential to a well running metabolism, or how well you produce energy (ATP) from your food.

When it comes to energy production, you want your body to be able to extract what it needs from food (macro and micronutrients) without a lot of wasteful byproducts or gut irritants. When your food is filled with tons of additives, preservatives, anti-nutrients, and cheap oils, it tends to hinder energy production, while also supporting energy storage (fat gain).

You also want your food to be filled with high quality, bioavailable nutrients, as your body needs numerous vitamins and minerals to produce energy effectively. When it comes to optimal energy production, B1, B2, B3, biotin, B6, B12, Vitamin C, folic acid, calcium, phosphorus, iron, magnesium, zinc, copper, manganese, and chromium, are all vital as they are all needed at different times during cellular respiration (1). This means a deficiency of any one of these could slow down the production of ATP. Sure, you could go the supplement route to make this happen, but rather than ingesting a dozen or more supplements to get adequate amounts of all these nutrients, wouldn't it be nice to get all your daily nutrients from food?

I think so.

On a side note, I am not saying all supplements are "bad," as there are some very useful supplements in the right situations. In addition, there are people who might have to rely on certain nutrient supplements due to their current health situation or diet. These people include those who have gone through bariatric surgery, those with IBS or absorption issues, severe anemia, the elderly, vegans, or those who live in areas that lack sunlight.

It is also true that our soils have become less nutrient rich due to industrialized farming practices, herbicides, pesticides, soil erosion and a loss of biodiversity in soils (2, 3, 4).

Which could mean that those eating a calorie restrictive diet would also need to supplement, due to an even lower amount of nutrients in their reduced calorie diet. If you're taking a bunch of supplements but not paying attention to what you're eating, you're going to be disappointed–supplements alone cannot fix everything.

Food should always be addressed first, supplements should be there to fill in the cracks, not build the roads.

In this chapter, I discuss your different fuel sources, and why one may be better than the other when it comes to optimizing energy production. I will dive into the fat vs. carb debate, and why low-carb diets may not be the best for energy production. And finally, I will give you a quick overview of the pro-metabolic foods that are the most supportive in maintaining a well-running metabolism.

Fats, Carbohydrates, or Proteins, Which Fuel Is Best?

When it comes to energy production, you have three possible types of fuel: carbohydrates, fats, and proteins. Carbohydrates are broken down into glucose, fats are broken down into fatty acids, and proteins are broken down into amino acids. Each of these molecules can then be taken through numerous metabolic processes to produce energy (ATP).

Despite being able to use all your macronutrients as energy, carbohydrates and fats are your primary fuel sources. Protein is normally reserved for building your structure. Bones, muscles, skin, nails, hair, hormones, and enzymes are all created from protein. However, under certain conditions, like starvation or on a high-protein diet, your body will break down protein and use it to create energy. This can be a normal and safe process, at least for short periods of time, but for reasons I will later explain, living off protein is not an ideal situation if you want to support optimal energy production.

Before we discuss protein as potential energy, let's talk about our two biggest players: fat and carbs. There is a constant debate going on in the health space on which one of these macronutrients is the better source of energy. People on low carb, ketogenic or carnivore type diets will argue fat is the ideal source of energy, and carbs are not needed, or at least needed in much smaller amounts. Vegans and plant-based advocates will argue that carbs are your ideal source of fuel, and that fat, at least animal fat, is not needed. And then there are people in the bioenergetic community, like me, who will argue that carbohydrates are your preferred fuel source, yet fat is still a needed fuel, and can be the preferred fuel in certain situations—like sleep and rest.

Why do I believe carbohydrates are the preferred energy source?

Well, before we discuss the above million-dollar question, let me first give you a quick overview of carbs, glucose, and how carbohydrates convert into energy.

There are simple carbohydrates (monosaccharides and disaccharides) which have 1-2 sugars, and complex carbohydrates (polysaccharides), which contain many sugars. Complex carbohydrates consist of fiber, starch, and glycogen (foods that contain complex carbs are rice, potatoes, and all vegetables and fruits with fiber). Simple carbohydrates consist of sugars, the most common being sucrose, lactose, and fructose. Simple carbs are found in foods like fruit, milk, sugar, and honey.

Almost all carbohydrates (besides fiber) are eventually converted into glucose, as it is glucose that enters the cell to be used as energy. Yes, even the evil fructose (it is not evil, this is my sarcasm in full effect), converts into glucose (about 50% of it), while 25% converts into lactate, another 20% is stored as liver glycogen, while a measly 1% is converted into triglycerides (fat) via de novo lipogenesis (DNL). DNL is a metabolic process in which the body synthesizes fatty acids from carbohydrates (5), something that humans do at a very low rate.

Ok. Back to carbs (aka glucose) being king as a fuel source.

When it comes to energy production, glucose is the ideal source of fuel, for numerous reasons.

The four main reasons carbs are king as a fuel source:

Thyroid production. First, glucose is needed to convert your inactive thyroid (T4) to active thyroid (T3) (read more in the chapter on thyroid) (7). T3, also known as triiodothyronine, is needed at the cell levels to produce energy. Remember that thyroid active hormone is the switch that turns energy production up. Without enough active thyroid, energy production slows, resulting in your system getting less ATP to run properly and you feeling more fatigued. I have an entire chapter dedicated to thyroid, so I will chat more about this later in Chapter 5.

Carbon dioxide. Second, glucose oxidation produces 50% more carbon dioxide than fat oxidation. Carbon dioxide (CO_2) is a byproduct produced during cellular respiration. Many medical professionals consider it a waste product of energy production, yet it is so much more. CO_2 is needed to help oxygen get into the cell to produce energy Without enough CO_2; the tissues will become less oxygenated (8). Less oxygenated tissues will result in less energy production. Interested in this? Flip to Chapter 4, where I go into the importance of CO_2, O_2, and energy production.

Nervous system function. Third, glucose is the preferred source of energy for the nervous system (it can also use ketones under stress or if you are on a ketogenic diet) (9). Your brain and nerves cannot use fat or protein as fuel; thus, glucose must be available. Under stress, your body will require more glucose, and if it is not provided, a stress response will occur, telling your body to break down your structure in order to produce additional glucose. Yes, glucose is so important to energy production, that your body will make its own via gluconeogenesis by breaking down muscle, tissue, and organs to make the needed glucose.

You produce energy faster and more efficiently. I am going to dive into the biochemistry of cellular metabolism again. Another reason to use glucose over fat as fuel is that glucose oxidation is a more efficient way to produce energy, producing more energy over time. This is due to the higher ratio of nicotinamide adenine dinucleotide (NADH) to flavin adenine dinucleotide ($FADH_2$) over fat oxidation (10).

Say what? What are NADH and $FADH_2$? I know, I know—let me explain.

If you are not into biochemistry, you can skip this next part, as it can be a bit complex. If you are a science nerd like me, and you really want to understand cellular respiration, you will find this incredibly interesting.

NADH and FADH$_2$ are both coenzymes that play critical roles in energy production. They are both electron carriers, where the energy from these electrons is used to produce ATP. Each NADH molecule has the capacity to help produce 2.5 ATP molecules, while each FADH$_2$ can support the production of 1.5 ATP molecules.

Think of it this way.

Imagine a factory (the cell) where the primary product is energy, packaged as ATP. The raw materials for making these energy packages come from various sources like glucose and fat.

NADH and FADH$_2$ are like full delivery trucks that transport these energy-rich packages (electrons) from the production sites, glycolysis, and pyruvate oxidations (glucose), beta oxidation (fat), and the Krebs cycle (both fat and carbs) to the power plant (the electron transport chain) (both fat and carbs). Refer to the sidebar for a complete explanation.

How Carbohydrates Are Converted into Energy

First, it is important to remember that almost all carbohydrates (fruits, vegetables, starch, grains, honey, sugar) are broken down into glucose during digestion. Once the glucose enters the blood it travels to all your cells to be converted into energy.

Once glucose arrives at your cell, it is converted into ATP (energy) through a process called cellular respiration. Cellular respiration is a multi-step metabolic pathway that involves several key stages:

The Production Sites:
STEP 1 Glycolysis: Glycolysis occurs in the cytoplasm of the cell and involves breaking one molecule of glucose into two molecules of pyruvate. This process generates a net gain

of 2 ATP (energy) and 2 nicotinamide adenine dinucleotide (NADH) molecules.

STEP 2 Pyruvate Oxidation: The two pyruvate molecules produced in glycolysis are transported into the cell's mitochondria (where you produce most of your energy), where each pyruvate is converted into acetyl-CoA. This step produces 2 more NADH (one per pyruvate) and releases Carbon Dioxide.

It should be noted that once you get to the Krebs cycle, fats, carbs, and proteins are all metabolized the same. It is what happens *before* the citric acid cycle that causes these molecules to be metabolized differently.

STEP 3 Krebs Cycle (citric acid cycle): The acetyl-CoA enters the citric acid cycle and goes through a series of metabolic changes. This process produces another 2 ATP (1 per acetyl-CoA), as well as additional NADH and $FADH_2$ molecules. Carbon dioxide is also released in the citric acid cycle.

The Power Plant:
STEP 4 Electron Transport Chain (ETC): The ETC occurs in the inner mitochondrial membrane. The ETC is where the high energy electron carriers, NADH and flavin adenine dinucleotide ($FADH_2$), donate their electrons to oxygen through a series of redox reactions that occur in series of structural proteins, referred to as complex I, II, III, and IV. The energy released from the electron transfer is used to pump protons across the inner mitochondrial membrane creating a proton gradient. The ETC does not directly produce energy, but rather just transfers the electrons through the protein complexes.

The Results of the Actions of the ETC:
STEP 5 Oxidative Phosphorylation: It is the *process* by which Adenosine triphosphate (ATP) is synthesized from adenosine diphosphate (ADP), at complex V, because of the ETC. Phosphorylation is when you add a phosphate group

to an ADP molecule. Oxidative phosphorylation is tightly connected to the ETC, as the proton gradient created by the ETC drives the synthesis of ATP. During this process anywhere from 29-36 ATP molecules are created (6).

I will give a little more understanding of the importance of all this below.

The ETC is a place in the cell's mitochondria where you produce most of your energy. This happens no matter the fuel source; it could be coming from fat, carbs, or protein.

Once the delivery trucks arrive at the power plant, the energy packages are unloaded and processed to generate energy (ATP).

The NADH truck drops its energy packages off at the place in the ETC called complex 1. We will refer to the complexes as "drop off sites." Complex 1 can push more energy packages through the production process; thus, it generates about 2.5 ATP per NADH molecule. On the other hand, $FADH_2$ drops its packages off at complex 2 in the ETC. This complex pushes fewer energy packages through the production process, generating less ATP, only 1.5 ATP per molecule.

Essentially, NADH trucks become more efficient at producing energy, as they will produce more energy per delivery "drop off."

You see, while carbs and fats are both converted into energy (ATP), the metabolic processes to produce energy are a little bit different, or should I say, the beginning stages are different, while the middle and end stages are the same.

The Beginning Stages of Glucose Oxidation

Through the process of glycolysis, one molecule of glucose is converted into two molecules of pyruvate. Each pyruvate is then converted into one acetyl-CoA, through pyruvate oxidation, producing one NADH, 1 molecule of CO_2 per pyruvate.

This means that from one molecule of glucose, you get two acetyl-CoA, two NADH molecules, and two CO_2 molecules from this stage of metabolism. Essentially, from glucose, the conversion of acetyl-CoA provides two NADH 'trucks' ready to deliver electrons to the next energy producing steps.

The Beginning Stages of Fat Oxidation

Through a process called beta-oxidation, fatty acids are broken down in steps, and each step removes two carbons at a time to form acetyl-CoA. Every beta-oxidation cycle produces 1 NADH and 1 $FADH_2$, but it doesn't produce CO_2 or ATP directly. Once formed, acetyl-CoA from fat enters the citric acid cycle, where it produces 3 NADH, 1 $FADH_2$, and 2 CO_2—the same as acetyl-CoA from glucose.

The key difference happens *before* acetyl-CoA. When glucose is converted to acetyl-CoA, it generates an additional NADH that fat metabolism does not. Fat metabolism, on the other hand, tends to generate relatively more $FADH_2$. A higher NADH supply generally drives cellular respiration faster and more efficiently, while excess reliance on $FADH_2$ can slow energy flow and increase reactive oxygen species (ROS). Over time, excessive ROS contributes to oxidative stress, cellular damage, and aging-related disease processes.

I will discuss this more in the fat loss chapter, but what you should know for now is glucose, with its higher NADH/$FADH_2$ ratio, can produce more energy over time, producing fewer ROS (11).

The bottom line:

Glucose is a more efficient energy source that produces less ROS than fat. Glucose also mitigates the stress response, keeping the body from going through metabolic adaptations. Finally, glucose also plays a role in other areas of energy production, supporting active thyroid production and oxygenation of the tissue. No other macronutrient has the power to support optimal energy production in so many ways!

Best Sources of Carbohydrates

What are your best sources of carbohydrates for energy production?

Ultimately this depends on you—your health, your preferences, your digestion, and your blood sugar responses will all play a role in determining which carbs work best for you.

Ideally, you should eat a variety of simple and complex carbohydrates that taste good to you and you can tolerate. These include fruits, roots like white and sweet potatoes, fruit juices, cooked vegetables, honey, milk, sourdough bread, masa harina, and even white table sugar.

For many, specifically those who have energy production and digestive issues, simple carbohydrates can be preferred over complex carbs, since they are easier to digest. Easy to digest carbohydrates place less burden on your digestive tract, leading to improved nutrient and energy absorption. Foods that contain simple carbohydrates are fruits, honey, milk, fruit juices, well cooked vegetables, and white sugar. The caveat with simple sugars is due to their faster digestion, they can be less satiating and can increase blood sugar levels faster. This is why I advise my clients to combine them with some fat and protein and eat them slowly.

If you can handle them (good digestion), additional complex carbohydrates, like white potatoes, oats, white rice, sourdough bread and masa harina can also be consumed. Although these carbohydrates are harder for your body to digest, if they are prepared properly (soaked, cooked, nixtamalized), many digestive systems can handle them just fine. Yet, for some people, specifically those with a compromised, under-functioning digestive system, many, if not all, complex carbohydrates may need to be reduced or even avoided—at least until metabolism starts to improve. (Jump to Chapters 7 and 8 for more information on digestion.)

Think about this, when a baby is born, their digestive system is not fully developed, thus, parents feed them cooked, pureed, and soft foods. Feeding them this way helps them digest, absorb, and utilize their food until their digestive system can handle more challenging foods. When your body is compromised, eating like a baby will help you with digesting and absorbing food too.

How many carbs should you eat?

Well, that is going to depend on you, your health, how much energy you currently need (what your energy demands are), your stress, and what dietary approach you may be on now.

Ideally, your diet should be anywhere from 30-60% carbohydrates. If you are less tolerant to carbohydrates, coming off a low carb diet, sedentary, have blood sugar issues, then keeping carbs on the lower side may work best for you. If you are active, already eating a significant amount of carbohydrates (plant-based or vegan), have a lot of stress in your life, sleep issues, or significant "sugar" cravings, then you might need more carbs in your diet. It is very important to account for total calories (energy intake), when adding in carbohydrates. Adding in too many carbs, too quickly, will lead to a calorie surplus. If you are unable to metabolize this surplus, it will lead to excess weight gain.

Which makes you ask the question:

Will carbs make you fat?

I can't tell you how many people have messaged me telling me every time they eat carbs they gain weight. In fact, many people are fearful of eating carbs for this very reason.

First, we must address, what does weight gain mean? Weight gain can come from glycogen storage, water weight, intestinal food waste, and fat weight. If you have been avoiding carbs for months or years, once you start consuming carbs, you will increase muscle and liver glycogen stores. For every gram of glycogen you store, you will hold an additional 3 grams of intermuscular water weight. Thus, for most people who claim to gain weight eating carbs, this is coming from muscle glycogen and water storage. This is why overall body composition and how you feel should be a better metric for health than your body weight.

Which brings back the question, are carbs actually fattening? Or when you are increasing your carbs, are you also eating additional calories? Most people who gain fat when adding in additional carbs, are normally just eating more calories. Suddenly, they are adding in more fruit, milk, and/or a sweet treat like custard or ice cream. Yet, they are not taking into consideration total fuel intake. It is a lot easier to eat less when you are avoiding carbs altogether.

FUN FACT: Did you know that for every gram of stored glucose (glycogen), you will store approximately 2-3 grams of water? So, just because you gain scale-weight when consuming carbs, does not mean you are gaining fat. It just means your body is holding onto more glycogen and water, which does increase scale weight, but is very different from fat weight.

When you start adding in carbs, I would advise food logging and considering your current fuel intake. When you start adding in more carbs, you might have to decrease your fat and protein intake, at least initially, until you are able to improve energy production. Lowering fat or protein, while slowly adding in carbs will keep total fuel intake the same, preventing any weight gain. Of course, over time, you should be able to increase your total fuel intake as energy production increases.

The truth is carbohydrate consumption is less fattening than fat consumption due to de novo lipogenesis (DNL) (12). DNL is the process by which the liver converts carbohydrates into fats. DNL only happens after all glycogen (stored glucose) stores are full, meaning, carbohydrates will get stored as glycogen first before they ever get stored as fat. Excess fat will always get stored as fat.

A study published in the American Journal of Clinical Nutrition studied nine lean and seven obese men and over-fed them an isoenergetic diet with a 50% increase above energy requirements of either fat or carbs. "Carbohydrate overfeeding produced progressive increase in carbohydrate oxidation and total energy expenditure resulting in 75-85% of excess energy being stored. Alternatively, fat overfeeding had minimal effects of fat oxidation and total energy expenditure, leading to a storage of 90-95% of excess energy" (13). They concluded that excess dietary fat leads to greater fat accumulation than does excess carbohydrates.

FUN FACT: When people say carbs are fattening, this is normally ONLY the case when the carbs are consumed with fats. Thus, foods like cookies, cakes and other highly palatable sugary-fat foods are not just "sweets," they are high calorie foods that also provide a considerable amount of fat—fat that is consumed in excess, is getting stored on you.

Like I said above, when adding carbs back into your diet, make sure to do slowly. It is imperative to remove the metabolic blocks (polyunsaturated fats, poor digestion and endotoxins, excess estrogen and iron, high stressed state and blood sugar issues, low nutrient diet) before adding in too many carbohydrates, as all of these may contribute to your body's inability to utilize this fuel source. Yes, I am aware I just threw these "metabolic blocks" at you, don't worry, I am going to go into a deeper explanation later in this book, so stay with me.

To sum it up, carbohydrates are your best source of energy due to supporting thyroid conversion, increased carbon dioxide production, supporting your nervous system and helping mitigate the stress response, while increasing how quickly energy is produced with NADH to FADH$_2$ ratio. The best sources of carbohydrates are the ones that work best for you, they can include fruits, roots, milk, cooked vegetables, honey, and even white sugar. And finally, carbohydrates are not fattening, in fact, carbs turn to fat at a very low rate. However, eating excess carbohydrates with excess fat can be very fattening, but mostly because the excess fat will turn to fat quickly.

Next, let's talk about fat as fuel.

What about using fat to produce energy?

Now, just because carbohydrates are your preferred fuel, does not mean using fat as fuel is bad. You see, you are still using fat as fuel all day long. Sitting down right now, as you are reading this book, you are using fat and carbs as fuel. In fact, you are using both fat and carbs as fuel, all day long, all the time.

Fat is your preferred energy source while resting and sleeping. Remember fat takes longer to produce energy, so it makes sense to use it when you need less energy. On the other hand, carbohydrates are your preferred energy source while you are thinking, doing anything, exercising, moving, etc.

Under stress and in activity, your body will require more quick energy, so the need for carbohydrates goes up during this time. While sleeping, your brain and muscles will primarily use fat as fuel, bringing down your need for glucose. During sleep, the body's energy needs drop, so fat becomes the preferred, slower-burning fuel source. Of course, glucose is still needed while you sleep, and if the liver is unable to store enough glycogen to get you through the night a stress response will occur, waking you up in the middle of the night.

To be clear, there is nothing wrong with fat oxidation. A healthy person is burning fat all day long, along with producing energy from carbohydrates. The issues can occur when there is an excessive forced oxidation of fat over glucose oxidation for an extended period. This can happen under starvation, excessive dieting, excessive exercise, or some sort of low carb/high fat diet (ketogenic diet).

Why is excessive "forced" fat oxidation a problem?

By "forced fat oxidation," I mean pushing the body to rely on fat over glucose—through dieting, chronic low-carb intake, or stress, rather than letting fuel usage follow normal needs. This can be a problem for the exact same reasons carbohydrates work as the most efficient day to day fuel. Excess fat oxidation tends to lower CO_2 production, which can reduce O_2 delivery to tissues. Fat oxidation decreases the NADH to $FADH_2$ ratio making energy production less efficient and raises ROS. It is often driven by higher stress hormones, including glucagon, but also cortisol and adrenaline. And finally, sustained reliance on fat can lower the conversion of inactive thyroid to active thyroid, producing less peripheral T3. Lower T3 production can also affect the production of your steroidal hormones, including testosterone (14, 15).

When there is a lack of glucose, due to dieting, low carb-based diets, or starvation, you will force the body to use more fat as fuel. Over time, there's a cost. Anytime you promote fat oxidation over glucose oxidation, you can elicit a stress response (16).

When glucose is scarce, the body makes more via gluconeogenesis, a process under the direction of stress hormones. So, when someone lacks enough glucose and becomes fat adapted (relies on fat as primary fuel), their stress hormones will elevate—these include glucagon, adrenaline, and cortisol, while also showing a decrease in active thyroid and testosterone. Lower active thyroid levels make sense in this case, since we know glucose is needed for thyroid conversion.

Those on a low carb ketogenic diet are using fat and ketones as fuel. Keto diets restrict carbohydrates to 5-10% and protein consumption to 10-20%. Fat consumption is around 70-80% of calories. In addition, when there is not enough glucose available your liver will break down fat and make ketones, so that certain vital systems of your body, specifically your nervous system—have enough fuel to survive. Ketones are the backup, brain-friendly fuel used when carbohydrate intake is very low. Like fat, there is nothing wrong with using ketones as fuel. Ketones are a very safe fuel source. The trade-off is that getting and staying in a ketogenic state usually involves some degree of physiological stress, which can become even worse in a high-stress life.

I am very aware that ketogenic diets have shown numerous health benefits, including weight loss, improved gut issues, improved autoimmune issues, improved allergies, and even a solution for diabetes. Most positive trials run shorter than 12 months; longer-term evidence is limited. And while the evidence suggests keto diets can offer significant short-term benefits, maintaining both adherence and benefits can be challenging over time.

The bottom line is, unless you enjoy eating fatty meat, cream, and eggs with a side of butter for every meal, then this might not be the diet for you, even if it temporarily fixes your gut and glucose markers. Yes, it's very possible that a ketogenic diet is better than the Standard American Diet. However, we don't yet have strong evidence that low carb, high-fat eating extends longevity—in fact, numerous studies suggest the opposite (17, 18).

Ok, I know I went off on a little tangent, but I think it is important to mention the ketogenic diet, as it is super popular in the nutrition/health world. I will also say, if you are on a keto diet, and it is working for you, then do what works for you. Yet, you should know the ketogenic diet has many limitations, including the ones above.

However, I am going to guess that if you are reading this book, and you have tried keto, you are more than likely looking for another way.

Lastly, in addition to a low-carb diet being more stressful on your body, using fat as fuel over glucose will produce less carbon dioxide and an increase of $FADH_2$ over NADH. Remember this ratio is important, because more $FADH_2$ over NADH can make energy production less efficient and produce additional ROS. These negative effects seem to be more prevalent under stress when we force our body to run on fat due to the lack of glucose.

With that said, I don't want you to think eating fat, or using fat as fuel, is "bad," at least in the right context. At rest, heart and skeletal muscle often prefer fatty acids, which is not the same as forcing fat use during stress or low-glucose states. When the body is sleeping or at rest, you can use fat as fuel, with less ROS, as these are times you do not need fuel at a quick rate.

So yes—fat belongs in a healthy diet. The key is context and quality. Choose fats that come with nutrients, support digestion, and make real food taste great.

When it comes to fat intake, which fats are best?

For cooking and stability, saturated fats work best.

Saturated fats (SFA) are fatty acids with chains of carbon, hydrogen and oxygen molecules that are held together by single bonds. These single bonds are strong and stable, which helps prevent saturated fats from going rancid or breaking down. This is one reason why saturated fats are ideal for cooking.

Foods that are rich in saturated fat, like butter, ghee, dairy fat, and egg yolks, come with fat-soluble vitamin A, D, and K2, which support energy production. Saturated fats can protect against endotoxins (19), and protecting the cells against these toxins will help your body produce more energy (don't worry, I talk more about endotoxins in Chapter 8).

The best saturated fats for cooking, sautéing, and baking are coconut oil, ghee, butter, cacao, and tallow. You can also find healthy saturated fats in dairy, eggs, grass-fed meats, and dark chocolate. I discuss saturated fats in far more detail in my first book, *How to Heal Your Metabolism*, so if you want more information, give that book a re-read.

What about monounsaturated fats?

Like saturated fats, monounsaturated fats (MUFA), like olive oil, are fatty acids containing carbon, hydrogen, and oxygen molecules. The difference is MUFA's contain one double bond. That single double bond makes them less stable than saturated fats. Used at low-moderate heat or as dressings, MUFA's are quite safe.

If you are going to use a MUFA oil, I suggest using an extra virgin olive oil over the newer, en vogue, avocado oil, as the research of avocado oil seems to be less than stellar. According to a 2020 UC Davis study, out of the 29 refined avocado oils studied only three met both quality and purity standards. They found that most retail avocado oils were poor quality, rancid, mislabeled, or tainted with other oils (20).

And finally, what about polyunsaturated fats?

Well, if you read my first book, you know I have a lot to say about polyunsaturated fats (PUFA). And since I wrote an entire chapter on PUFAs at the end of this book, I will spare you the extended explanation here. Yet, I think a quick overview is helpful, as PUFA fats can become an issue in energy production.

The basic difference between PUFA fats, and SFA and MUFAs, is PUFAs have multiple double carbon bonds, which makes them more prone to oxidation. Their lack of several hydrogen bonds makes them not fully saturated, which is why they are referred to as "unsaturated." Like I said above, a single double bond is more reactive to oxygen and less stable than a fully saturated fat, which means a fat with many double bonds is even less stable.

High PUFA exposure has been reported to impair aspects of cellular respiration (21), alter membrane permeability (22), and raise oxidative stress (23, 24), effects that can interfere with efficient energy production. Yes, PUFA fats are one of those energy-blocks I was discussing in the beginning of this book. Since PUFAs can interfere with cellular respiration, they can back up the entire energy producing system, leading to a slower metabolism and less energy! See Chapter 12 for the full PUFA deep-dive.

Essentially, it is best to limit foods and oils that are high in PUFAs. These include most nuts and seeds, and vegetable, seed, and nut oils.

These oils consist of sunflower oil, safflower oil, soy oil, canola oil, vegetable oil, walnut oil, peanut oil, grapeseed oil and even fish oils.

When it comes to using fat for optimal energy production and reduced oxidative stress, it is best to use saturated and monounsaturated fats. These fats include coconut oil, ghee, butter, cocoa butter, beef tallow, cacao (chocolate), and olive oil. Limit high-PUFA nut, seed, and vegetable oils.

Protein as Fuel?

What about protein as a usable fuel source? The main reason you do not want to use protein as fuel is because it has a bigger purpose, a purpose that neither fat nor carbs can carry out.

Protein's main job isn't day-to-day energy. It's structure and repair: muscle and collagen, organs and skin, nails and hair. It also makes movement possible (muscle contraction) and builds hormones, transport proteins, enzymes, and antibodies. Yes, your body can burn protein for fuel, but that isn't ideal. Turning protein into ATP creates more waste and costs more energy than using carbs.

Why is protein more energy expensive? Protein has a higher thermic effect, about 20–30% of its calories are spent just to digest, absorb, and process it, compared with ~5–10% for carbohydrates. Which means protein uses 3x more energy to digest and absorb, a plus if you are in a fat loss phase, but negative if you are trying to improve energy production. Essentially, when you use protein as fuel, you spend more energy to get energy.

How the Body Uses Protein for Energy

When carbs are limited (very low-carb diets, fasting, heavy stress), the body leans more on protein as fuel. This happens in two different ways:

Gluconeogenesis (Turning Amino Acids into Glucose)
Many amino acids are glucogenic. Your liver can turn them into glucose, which then runs through glycolysis and the Krebs cycle just

like glucose from food. Gluconeogenesis happens at a background level all the time, but it ramps up when carbs are low or stress is high. It works, but it's less efficient than using carbohydrates you eat.

Deamination and Direct Entry (Using Amino Acids as Fuel)

Amino acids can be deaminated (the nitrogen is removed), leaving carbon skeletons. Glucogenic skeletons feed into pyruvate or TCA intermediates; ketogenic ones form acetyl-CoA or acetoacetate. These can then be oxidized for ATP. Useful in a pinch, but not the most economical way to power your day.

This is why carbohydrates are called protein-sparing; eating enough carbs protects your structural protein from being burned for fuel.

Other Issues with Using Protein as Energy

Breaking down more protein creates more ammonia, a nitrogen waste product. In healthy people, the liver and kidneys usually clear this without trouble. But excess ammonia (hyperammonemia) can be dangerous (25), and people with compromised liver or kidney function should avoid excessive protein breakdown or extremely high protein loads (26, 27).

In addition, excess protein intake and breakdown may interfere with healthy thyroid physiology. Thyroid peroxidase (TPO) is an enzyme in your thyroid gland required to make thyroid hormone. It helps add iodine to tyrosine and form thyroid hormones like T4 and T3. However, when large amounts of certain amino acids such as cysteine, methionine, and tryptophan are released through muscle breakdown or consumed in high-protein diets without enough carbohydrate, they may exert inhibitory effects on TPO activity. Over time, this can contribute to less efficient thyroid hormone production and a slowdown in metabolic function (28).

Put simply; when carbs are too low and the body burns more protein, you can see more nitrogen waste, higher processing costs, and lower T3—none of which helps energy production.

Bottom line: Protein is precious. We want it building and repairing, not fueling your metabolic engine all day. Eat enough protein to meet structural needs but rely on carbohydrates (with supportive fats) as your efficient, daily fuel. This allows you to spare protein, support thyroid, and keep energy production running smoothly.

What about high protein diets, like the carnivore?

The carnivore diet centers on animal foods, including meat, fish, eggs, organs, and depending on the carnivore influencer you listen to, some add whole milk and hard cheese. It's high in protein and fat, and extremely low in carbohydrates. The carnivore diet can overlap with keto since they are both lower carb, higher fat. Yet, due to the higher protein, carnivore dieters do not produce ketones (but, some people are keto-carnivores). Increased protein intake will inhibit someone from going into ketosis. Instead of producing ketones, they break down some of their ingested protein via gluconeogenesis, turning it into glucose. The produced glucose will meet their "quick energy" needs.

Client Story

Shelly—From Vegan to Carnivore to Bioenergetic

When I met Shelly, she was tired, had a painful menstrual cycle, and was dealing with debilitating migraines. Shelly, a 37-year-old homemaker and mother of two, had been dieting for the last 10 years to help with her gut issues. The last 10 years consisted of vegan, raw vegan, intermittent fasting, and when these stopped working, she shifted to a carnivore diet.

She informed me that she felt pretty good doing a vegan diet, but over time she started to have bad gut issues. She then shifted to a carnivore diet, removing all carbs and fibers, and finally her gut felt amazing. Yet, after a few months on the carnivore diet (no carbs), she started to feel exhausted, her period became heavy, and she had terrible migraines. This is when I met Shelly.

Shelly was frustrated because she wanted to lose some weight and feel like herself again after her second child, but was finding every time she restricted either animal foods or carbs, she would fix one thing, while making another thing worse. Shelly was also pushing herself in her workouts, yet was finding they were becoming more challenging, and were only making her feel worse.

I explained to Shelly that while removing all fibers can help the gut feel better, as there is a reduction in gut irritants, the removal of her most efficient energy source (carbs), was going to slow down energy production, which, for a busy mom, was going to make her feel worse. Busy moms, who are also attempting to workout, need quick energy.

I also explained that for her to feel better, we needed to establish some level of energy balance. We needed to make sure she was producing enough energy to keep up with daily demands, which, if she was fatigued, I knew was not happening.

I asked Shelly to take a break from her intense workouts for a month. Instead, I asked her to take enjoyable walks, outside in the sun, if possible. I had her, slowly but consistently, add carbohydrates back into her diet. We started with simple, low fibrous carbohydrates (cooked fruits, sweet fruits, juices, sugar, milk), until I could make sure Shelly's gut could handle the fibers. Over the next three months we went from almost zero carbs/day to over 225g/day. This was a slow and steady process, adding in about 20 grams each week. We also removed some of her daily fat, so that her total energy intake would not exceed what she was previously eating.

In the first few weeks, Shelly's energy started to return. Yes, once your body has its quick energy resources again, energy production will return, and your energy will return.

By the end of month six, Shelly's migraines were gone, her cycle became more regular, and she started to lose some weight. Shelly was also back in the gym—her workouts were finally feeling energizing, and she was feeling strong.

What I loved about Shelly's journey is that she became good at understanding her limits. When she ate well and slept well, she pushed herself in the gym. When life happened, kids woke her up, or her food wasn't great, she would be gentler in her training.

This is the ultimate lesson in energy balance. Always meeting your body where it is at and respecting its daily limits, as they can change.

Carnivore advocates will argue that there is no need for ingesting carbs/glucose because your body will make its own. That is true in principle, but the upregulation of gluconeogenesis is driven by glucagon and often accompanies higher adrenaline and cortisol when carbs are low. And, as I have already said many times, this breakdown will come with metabolic cost, like reduced T4 to T3 conversion, lower testosterone, and a more stress-dependent energy supply (29, 30, 31).

Many people do report improvements with autoimmune issues, gut issues, skin issues, blood sugar issues, and weight loss. However, long-term evidence is limited, so long-term health outcomes are uncertain. In my personal practice, I have worked with several people who had great results on a carnivore diet for a year or two. Then suddenly, usually after a stressful period, they hit an energetic wall, at least until carbohydrates were slowly reintroduced.

Now, this does not mean protein is "bad" as it is not, it is incredibly important. Yet, what it does mean is most of your ingested protein should be used for structure, function, and nutrient bioavailability, not fuel.

This is why I have listed protein as an essential nutrient first, rather than a primary fuel source. And why I will discuss the benefits of protein in the next chapter. (It should be noted that fats, carbs, and protein are all macro nutrients).

In summary, when it comes to fuel sources, carbohydrates are king, fats are the queen, and protein is running a different kingdom, the nutrient kingdom. Carbohydrates are the preferred fuel due to their role in thyroid conversion, increased production of CO_2, direct mitigation of the stress response, ability to produce more energy over time, and their energy efficiency.

Fat, your secondary fuel source, is still used to produce energy all day, but it is not the preferred fuel during intense activity or under stress. Fat oxidation takes more time to produce energy; thus, it is preferred in times of low activity, rest, and sleep.

When carbohydrate-driven metabolism rises, total energy turnover rises, so fat oxidation rises overall, too. This means when you become a better carb burner, you will also become a better fat burner.

And finally, protein can be burned as fuel, but it's not preferred because it increases nitrogen waste (ammonia), leans more on stress hormones, and can inhibit thyroid conversion in certain contexts. Protein belongs at the construction site, not in the furnace. Your body can use all three macronutrients as fuel, and none of these pathways are "bad." The context is what matters. For producing high amounts of ATP day to day, your body usually prefers glucose first, then fat, while protein stays busy building you. When we get to fat loss later, you'll see why being a strong carb burner often leads to better fat burning, too.

Alright, next stop, are you ready to zoom into nutrients and how they work directly with energy production?

CHAPTER 2

THE BOTTOM LINE

Supportive Fuel for Optimizing Energy Production

1. Your body can use carbohydrates, fats, and protein as a fuel source. Under stress, your body can also use your structure (glycogen, fat, muscle, skin, and tissue) as a fuel source.

2. Carbohydrates are your best fuel source due to their thyroid support, increased CO_2 production, ability to mitigate the stress response, and their high NADH to $FADH_2$ ratio. The best carbohydrates are fruits, roots, well prepared grains like sour dough and masa harina, honey, milk, and even white table sugar.

3. Fats can also be used to produce energy yet are preferred in times of rest and sleep. Saturated fats are preferred over polyunsaturated fats due to being less prone to oxidative damage. The best fats are coconut oil, butter, tallow, ghee, coconut butter, cacao, and olive oil.

4. Protein, although it can be used as a fuel, is inefficient, producing excess ammonia, increasing the stress response, and decreasing thyroid conversion.

5. A healthy person should be able to utilize all macronutrients as fuel sources, depending on the circumstances.

CHAPTER 3

ESSENTIAL NUTRIENTS FOR
ENERGY PRODUCTION

Now that you know all about your best fuel sources for energy production, let's talk about the other nutrients that help you turn fuel into energy. Protein, vitamins, and minerals don't act as fuel themselves.

Before I get started, I want to be clear about one thing. Carbohydrates and fats are nutrients and, like protein, they are considered macronutrients. Macronutrients are nutrients that are needed in large amounts. When it comes to understanding energy production, I separate carbs and fat from protein because their main role is to serve as the body's fuel sources, while protein is primarily used for structure and repair. I placed the other macronutrient, protein, with the micronutrients, which are nutrients required in smaller amounts consisting of vitamins and minerals, as they all play more of a functional and structural purpose rather than being used as actual fuel. Protein and micronutrients are more of the "where and how" energy is being made, vs. just the fuel that is turned into energy.

Make sense?

Think of carbs and fat as the gas and oil to run your power plant, while the additional nutrients (protein, vitamin, and minerals) are the engine, cylinders, workers, and assistants. The fuel turns into energy to make the power plant function, just as your food turns into ATP to make you go. The engine parts and workers are needed to produce energy in your power plant, just like your mitochondria, enzymes, and coenzymes/cofactors are needed to produce ATP (energy) in your cell. These nutrients help you make energy, even though they aren't the fuel.

In addition, when you run your power plant long and hard, and put crappy fuel and gas into the engine, the longevity of your machinery shortens. The same is true for your body. When you don't take care of yourself, and you eat crappy food with little nutrition, the longevity of your body will shorten—at least the longevity of a healthy body. Sadly, modern medicine has not managed to make us healthier, yet it has managed to keep sick people living longer (1, 2, 3).

Of course, there will always be "unicorns" when it comes to nutrition and longevity. I can already hear someone tell me their Uncle Bill consumed Snicker bars every day, yet lived to be 100. Unicorns do happen, but they are not the norm, and I would rather bet the odds (nutritious food and healthy lifestyle habits) when it comes to my health and longevity.

Essentially, the fuel you consume, along with enough of the right nutrients (protein, vitamins, and minerals) are all needed to work together to produce optimal energy. An inefficient amount of any of these could hinder energy production.

In many scenarios, improving the quality and quantity of various nutrients (improving the functioning engine) can be the missing link to your low energy production.

Ever heard of someone being iron anemic, and then all of a sudden, they consume iron-rich foods, and they magically feel more energized? Well, it is not actually magic, as iron is a vital nutrient needed in a cell's mitochondria to produce energy. Iron is also vital for hemoglobin production, which is needed to carry oxygen to the tissue, and without adequate oxygen, energy production is limited. (Jump to Chapter 4 and 11 for more information on oxygen and iron).

This is why high-quality foods that can give you both adequate fuel and nutrition are recommended for optimal energy production. And since we have already talked about the best foods for fuel, let's talk about the best foods for the delivery of vital nutrients.

In this chapter, I am going to discuss the importance of the nutrient protein and how protein is used for optimal energy production. I will tell you which protein sources are best and which ones should be limited. In addition, I am going to give you some insight into the specific micronutrients (vitamins and minerals) that are needed to produce ATP, and what can happen if any of them are lacking. And finally, I will go over the foods that can hinder nutrient digestion and absorption, so you know what to avoid or limit.

As Taylor Swift would say, "Are you ready for it?" (Yep, more cheesiness.)

The Role of Protein in Energy Production

Like I discussed in the last chapter, protein's main role is to create structure. Bone, skin, hair, organs, muscle, and nails are all made of protein. In addition, protein is needed for muscle contraction, and is used to produce hormones, antibodies, transport proteins, and enzymes. While your body *can* burn protein for fuel, that's not ideal. Still, protein is essential for energy production because the "workers" and "tools" that make ATP are proteins.

Cellular respiration (how you produce energy) is a complex, multi-step process that converts your fuel into adenosine triphosphate (ATP), the energy currency for the human body. Central to this amazing process are proteins, which perform various essential roles. Proteins are needed to catalyze numerous biochemical reactions (enzymes), provide the structure to facilitate the transportation of molecules, and they help regulate numerous metabolic pathways to produce energy.

Referring to my analogy in the last chapter, imagine that the production of ATP is like a busy factory (the cell). In this factory (cell), protein provides the workers (enzymes), the factory and power plant (the structure), the shuttles (transport proteins) and the managers (regulatory proteins). Together, all the functions of protein ensure the factory operates efficiently, producing enough energy to sustain your health and life.

Enzymes (The Workers)—Biological Catalyst

At the heart of energy production are enzymes. Enzymes act as catalysts that accelerate biochemical reactions without being consumed in the process. Glycolysis (breakdown of glucose to pyruvate), pyruvate oxidation (break down of pyruvate to acetyl-CoA), beta oxidation (breakdown of fat to acetyl-CoA), the Krebs cycle, and oxidative phosphorylation (electron transport chain and ATP synthesis) rely heavily on enzymatic activity.

FUN FACT: Most enzymes end in "ase," so when you hear words like lactase, sucrase or dehydrogenase, you know they are enzymes, due to the "ase."

Considering there are dozens of different enzymes needed to produce energy, whether from carbs or fat, I am only going to go over a few in each stage to make your life a little less complicated. Even medical doctors can't remember all the enzymes needed for energy production—at least none whom I have met.

The Breakdown of Glucose to Acetyl-CoA

Glycolysis involves enzymes such as hexokinase, phosphofructokinase 1, and pyruvate kinase. Each enzyme in this pathway plays a specific role, breaking down glucose into pyruvate and producing a small amount of ATP and NADH.

Pyruvate oxidation relies on the pyruvate dehydrogenase complex, which consists of pyruvate dehydrogenase, dihydrolipoamide acetyltransferase, and dihydrolipoamide dehydrogenase. These enzymes help convert pyruvate into acetyl-CoA.

The Breakdown of Fat to Acetyl-CoA

The key enzymes to beta oxidation are acyl-CoA dehydrogenase, enoyl-CoA hydratase, B-Hydroxyacyl-CaA dehydrogenase, and acyl-CoA acetyltransferase. Together these enzymes break down fatty acids into acetyl-CoA. And remember, after you produce acetyl-CoA, regardless of how the acetyl-CoA was produced, it enters the Krebs cycle.

The Krebs cycle, the initial stage of aerobic (requiring oxygen) respiration, features enzymes like citrate synthase, aconitase, and succinate dehydrogenase. These enzymes facilitate the complete oxidation of acetyl-CoA, generating NADH, $FADH_2$, and ATP.

The electron transport chain (ETC) and oxidative phosphorylation, which ends up producing most of your ATP, relies on a series of enzyme complexes in the ETC, including NADH dehydrogenase (Complex I), succinate dehydrogenase (complex II) cytochrome bc1 (Complex III), and cytochrome c oxidase (Complex IV). These enzymes help transfer electrons from NADH and $FADH_2$ (remember our delivery truck analogy in the last chapter) to oxygen, driving the production of ATP.

If you can think of enzymes as the highly specialized workers along an assembly line, you can imagine that each one has its own specific job. Each worker has a unique task that contributes to the final product. Without these workers, the assembly line would grind to a halt, and no products would be made.

Structural Proteins (The Factory)

Proteins also provide structural support crucial for where energy is being made. The inner and outer mitochondrial membranes (the power plant), where most of the energy production occurs, are reinforced by various proteins. Mitochondria are often referred to as the powerhouses of the cell, as this is where ATP is produced.

Within the cell, the mitochondrial membranes are rich in proteins that help maintain their structure and functionality. The inner membrane forms cristae (folds in the membrane) to increase the surface area for energy production. Proteins stabilize these cristae, ensuring efficient ATP production.

In addition, the electron transport chain (the power grid), is composed of a series of protein complexes (where electrons get dropped off and transferred through the ETC), that facilitate electrons being moved through the proton gradient to produce energy.

And finally, at the end of the ETC is the final complex V, also known as ATP synthase. This is the location where the majority of ATP is created. This process is referred to as oxidative phosphorylation.

Think of the structural proteins as where your product (energy) is being made. These proteins provide the necessary framework that supports the drop off and transfer sights, the warehouse, and the power plant, allowing other systems to function within it.

Transport Proteins (The Shuttle)

Transport proteins play a vital role in moving molecules across the mitochondrial membranes, ensuring that substrates and products of energy production are efficiently managed. Since these proteins oversee transportation, try to think of them as a shuttle within the factory (cell).

The transport protein ADP/ATP translocase exchanges ATP and ADP across the inner mitochondrial membrane at complex V, ensuring a continuous supply of ADP for phosphorylation and the export of newly synthesized ATP to the cytoplasm. Phosphate carrier proteins transport inorganic phosphate into the mitochondria, which is necessary for ATP synthesis. In addition, carnitine palmitoyl transferases I and II facilitate the transport of fatty acids into the mitochondria for beta-oxidation, converting them into acetyl-CoA for use in the Krebs cycle.

Regulatory Proteins (The Managers)

Proteins also serve as regulators for energy production, ensuring that metabolic pathways operate smoothly and efficiently. Think of regulatory proteins as the factory's managers, making sure everything is working properly.

In glycolysis and the Krebs cycle, there are allosteric enzymes such as phosphofructokinase-1 and pyruvate dehydrogenase, which are regulated by other molecules to increase or decrease their activity based on the cell's energy needs. In addition, transcription factors are proteins that regulate the expression of genes encoding enzymes and other proteins involved in energy production. By controlling gene expression, they ensure that the cell produces the right amount of metabolic machinery.

The bottom line is proteins are essential for energy production, as they make up the enzymes (workers), structural components (factory), the transporters (shuttle), and the regulators (managers). Without enough protein, the framework of where you produce energy and the workers needed to produce energy will suffer. Knowing all this you can see why it makes far more sense to use protein for these reasons, vs. breaking it down and using it for energy.

Whew! Who knew protein was so vital for energy production? I think most people just think of protein as muscle, skin, hair, and nails, never taking into consideration how important it is for your cells to produce energy!

Now that you understand the importance of protein when it comes to energy production, I am sure you are wondering what proteins are best.

It's those that contain the most bioavailable nutrients of course!

Animal Proteins vs. Plant Proteins

Just like carbohydrates, the ability to digest and absorb the energy, amino acids and nutrients in the protein is pretty darn important. Most individuals need anywhere from 0.8 grams protein/kg of body weight to 2 grams of protein/kg of body weight. How much you need will depend on your size, age, sex, health, and goals, such as muscle building or weight loss.

Due to their increased nutrient and protein bioavailability, animal proteins are recommended over plant proteins (4). Dairy, shellfish (like oysters, shrimp, mussels, clams, and lobster), white fishes, organs (like beef liver, heart, and kidneys), pastured eggs, grass-fed meats, and bone broth (collagen and gelatin) are all generally recommended.

For vegans or vegetarians, or anyone with a severely compromised digestive system, potato juice can serve as high quality protein due to its keto acids.

Of course, this does not mean you can never eat other plant proteins like beans and legumes, yet it does mean you should prepare them properly (like soak and sprout), so their protein and nutrients become more bioavailable.

Protein can be used to increase satiety in a meal, slowing down the absorption of carbohydrates. Increasing protein in your diet can increase the thermic effect of the meal, as it takes more energy to convert protein into fuel, yet like I discussed in the previous chapter, this can come at a price.

Bottom line: The best proteins for energy production are animal proteins including dairy, eggs, shellfish, white fish, organs, grass-fed meats and bone broth, collagen, and gelatin. If you want to learn more about these specific foods, check out my first book, *How to Heal Your Metabolism*.

Alright, now that we know how important carbs and fat (fuel) and protein are for your cells to produce energy, I want to go over some specific nutrients that are vital for your cells to produce ample energy. While I move through this list, I want you to keep in mind that when I am discussing each nutrient, I am discussing their roles in energy metabolism only. Many of these nutrients may be needed in other biological functions, but to keep me from going off into 99 tangents, discussing their role in ATP production will be the goal of this chapter.

Here are the primary nutrients involved in cellular energy production.

The Magic of B Vitamins

I am sure at some time in your life; someone has told you to take one or all eight of the B vitamins. There is a reason for this, every B vitamin has a role in energy production. Most of the B vitamins serve as coenzymes to support the numerous enzymes used during energy production. Coenzymes are organic molecules that enhance the catalytic functions of an enzyme and are often derived from vitamins—like B vitamins. In our power plant analogy, think of the B vitamins as assistants to the workers (enzymes). Some of the B vitamins will play a direct role (assistant) in energy production, while others will play a secondary role, or indirect role (assistant to the assistant) in producing energy. I will go over each B vitamin briefly, so you gain a better understanding of their specific importance in energy production.

B1, B2, B3 and B5 all have direct roles in energy production. Each of these nutrients directly participates in the biochemical pathways that generate energy (ATP).

B1 (Thiamine) - Thiamine is converted into thiamine pyrophosphate (TPP), a coenzyme needed for the activity of two key enzymes in cellular respiration. The enzyme pyruvate dehydrogenase (PD) is needed during the breakdown of glucose to convert pyruvate into acetyl-CoA (5). Thiamine is also needed by alpha-ketoglutarate dehydrogenase, which is needed during the Krebs cycle to convert alpha-ketoglutarate to succinyl-CoA.

Remember that you will require more B1 if you are consuming more carbohydrates, due to the pyruvate dehydrogenase enzyme. If someone has deficiency of B1, the oxidation of carbohydrates can slow, backing up pyruvate, slowing down the production of energy (6). This means if you are having a hard time tolerating carbohydrates, adding in foods high in B1 might be a smart decision.

Best food sources of B1: pork chops, mussels, salmon, acorn squash, asparagus, and brewer's and nutritional yeast.

B2 (Riboflavin) - Riboflavin is converted into the coenzymes flavin adenine dinucleotide (FAD) and flavin mononucleotide (FMN), which are both involved in redox reactions. Redox reactions are reactions involving the transfer of electrons*. These coenzymes are needed by succinate dehydrogenase in the Krebs cycle and in the ETC, at complex II, to help break down fatty acids and glucose. B2 is also needed to help activate the acyl-CoA dehydrogenase enzyme, which is involved in beta oxidation of fatty acids (7).

Without enough B2, the breakdown of fats, carbs, and proteins can be inhibited, leading to, you guessed it, less energy production. In addition, a deficiency of B2 can alter iron absorption, leading to anemia and even more fatigue. As I will show you later in this chapter, iron is another nutrient that is vital for energy production.

Best food sources of B2: beef liver, beef, milk, salmon, mushrooms, pork chops, well-cooked spinach, eggs, nutritional and brewer's yeast.

B3 (Niacin and niacinamide) - Niacin and niacinamide are forms of B3. Niacin is found in food but can convert into niacinamide in the body. Both forms are used to synthesize the coenzyme nicotinamide adenine dinucleotide (NAD$^+$). This coenzyme is crucial for redox reactions (the transfer of electrons) (8).

Remember our NADH "delivery trucks" from Chapter 1? NAD$^+$ can accept electrons and can be reduced to NADH. NADH is an electron carrier (delivery truck) that drops off the electrons at the ETC to produce ATP!

This means B3 is very important for energy production, as it is needed to help transport the electrons through the mitochondria (power plant). Best food sources of B3 are beef liver, chicken liver, chicken breast, tuna, turkey, salmon, anchovies, pork, beef, mushrooms, and potatoes. If you opt to take a B3 supplement, niacinamide is often recommended, due to niacin creating a flushing effect.

B5 (Pantothenic Acid) - B5 is essential for the synthesis of coenzyme A (CoA). CoA is essential in several metabolic processes when you generate energy. These include the conversion of pyruvate into acetyl-CoA, the acetyl-CoA then combines with oxaloacetate to form citrate to start the Krebs cycle, and the beginning stages of beta oxidation (fat oxidation). Without CoA, glucose and fat oxidation would be hindered and your body would produce a fraction of the ATP your cells would need to function (9).

So, yes, vitamin B5 is important for optimal energy production.

Best food sources of B5 include beef, beef liver, poultry, seafood, milk, eggs, and other organ meats (10). You can also get B5 in vegetarian sources like mushrooms, potatoes, and avocados. Like other B vitamins, B5 bioavailability is going to be much higher in animal sources (4).

B6, B7, B9, and B12 are all needed indirectly to help produce energy. Each of these nutrients supports or facilitates the metabolic pathways that directly lead to energy (ATP) production.

B6 (Pyridoxine) - B6 plays several indirect roles in supporting energy production (11). B6 is essential for transaminase enzymes, which facilitates the interconversion of amino acids. These amino acids are involved in specific metabolic pathways needed to produce energy.

B6 is needed during gluconeogenesis (making glucose out of non-carbohydrate sources) and glycogenolysis (breaking down glycogen to produce glucose). Both processes will help produce energy when food is not available.

B6 is involved in heme synthesis. Heme is involved in producing hemoglobin to help with oxygen transportation (refer to Chapter 4) and to produce energy in the ETC.

The best food sources of B6 are beef liver, pork, chicken, turkey, and tuna. Vegetarian sources of B6 are potatoes, banana, squash, and soaked and sprouted chickpeas. Like other B vitamins, the naturally occurring B6 in plant sources exhibits reduced bioavailability (12).

B7 (Biotin) - Like B6, Biotin plays several indirect roles in energy production.

B7 acts as a coenzyme for carboxylation reactions. Carboxylation reactions add a carboxyl group (COOH) to a molecule, modifying it in a way that enhances its function and enables it to carry out specialized roles within the cell. Carboxylation is like upgrading your standard tool with a new attachment that allows it to perform more specialized tasks. These biotin-dependent carboxylases catalyze reactions are essential for gluconeogenesis (the breakdown of non-carbon molecules into glucose), glucose oxidation, fatty acid synthesis, and amino acid metabolism (13).

If someone has a biotin deficiency, carboxylase enzymes cannot function optimally. This will lead to a decreased ability to convert glucose, fat, and proteins into forms that can be used for energy production, and for the ability to produce certain structural components needed to produce energy.

The best food sources for biotin are egg yolks, beef liver, beef heart, and beef kidney. Other sources are nutritional and brewer's yeast, sweet potatoes, bananas, avocados, and mushrooms. Biotin is more bioavailable in animal-based foods (4).

B9 (Folate) - Like B6 and biotin, folate indirectly helps convert fats and carbs into energy (ATP). Yet, folate is involved in numerous metabolic pathways that support maintaining cellular function, enabling cells to grow, divide, and perform necessary biochemical reactions—like DNA synthesis, repair, and methylation. These processes are essential for rapid cell division, which is why folate is so vital to fetal development in pregnant women.

Folate also helps in the production of red blood cells. Red blood cells contain hemoglobin, which binds oxygen molecules and transports them throughout the body. If someone is deficient in folate, you can have fewer and less effective RBC, called megaloblastic anemia. Megaloblastic anemia lowers the blood's capacity to carry oxygen, which directly impacts the amount of oxygen transported, hindering energy production.

The best food sources of folate are beef liver, chicken liver, egg yolks, lamb liver, well cooked spinach, asparagus, and avocados.

B12 (Cobalamin) - B12, like B6, biotin, and folate, is indirectly involved in the oxidation of glucose and fats. B12 is a cofactor for methylmalonyl-CoA mutase, an enzyme that converts methylmalonyl-CoA to succinyl-CoA, a critical step in the breakdown of fatty acids and some amino acids. Succinyl-CoA then enters the Krebs cycle, where it is further metabolized to produce ATP. Without sufficient B12, the conversion process is hindered, leading to a reduction in ATP production (14).

Like folate, B12 is needed for the proper formation and maturation of red blood cells. Thus, a deficiency in B12 can also lead to megaloblastic anemia. A B12-driven anemia will reduce the oxygen-carrying capacity of the blood, which will ultimately reduce energy production.

The most common reasons for a B12 deficiency are a low B12 diet, IBD, gastrectomy (part of stomach is removed), and pernicious anemia. Pernicious anemia is an autoimmune issue that attacks the parietal cells in the stomach. These cells produce a glycoprotein called intrinsic factor. Intrinsic factor binds to B12, allowing it to be absorbed properly. Without intrinsic factor, your body will be unable to absorb adequate B12.

The best food sources of B12 are beef liver, beef, sardines, clams, and dairy products. B12 is only found in animal products, so all those eating a plant-based or vegan diet, would need to supplement.

Whew! Does it make sense why B vitamins are so vital to energy production? Before I continue with the additional nutrients needed to support glucose and fat oxidation, I want to take a second to give a big shout out to beef liver! Beef liver is an amazing food source of all the B vitamins, except B1. Back in my parents' generation, beef liver was a weekly staple—now, most families avoid organ meats, as they are less desirable in taste.

Is the avoidance of this super food contributing to our growing epidemic of energy production issues? It is quite possible. I cannot tell you how many people I finally get to eat liver regularly and notice an increase in energy levels. It only takes a 2-3 ounce serving/week to get a big dose of bioavailable B vitamins. And no, more is not better. This one super food could be the answer to many of your energy issues.

As Nike says, "Just do it"! Yep, I am very cheesy, I mean livery! Ok. I will stop.

Now that you know all about the vitamins (B vitamins) that are needed for optimal ATP production, let's review all the minerals you need for your cells to produce energy effectively.

Here is a list of all the minerals needed for optimal energy production:

Iron (Fe) - Iron is a trace mineral needed by your body in numerous ways to produce energy. Iron plays a crucial role in how the ETC functions and how ATP is transported through the ETC. In addition, iron plays a vital role in oxygen transportation and thyroid production, both of which are essential for energy production.

To start with, the conversion of pyruvate to acetyl-CoA involves the enzyme pyruvate dehydrogenase, which requires an iron-sulfur (Fe-S) cluster (a grouping of related elements) to function properly. Fe-S clusters are also needed in the Krebs cycle, but most importantly they are needed in the ETC.

Think of these clusters as short-distance electrical connectors in our power plant analogy. Just like these connectors carry electricity within a machine in the power plant, Fe-S clusters carry electrons *within* complexes I, II, and III in the ETC.

In addition, iron helps make up a heme-containing protein called cytochromes. Cytochromes are in Complex III and IV, as well as freely moving between all complexes. Think of cytochromes like long-distance power lines that carry electrical energy across different areas of the power plant. These cytochromes carry electrons *between* each complex.

Without Fe-S clusters and cytochromes, the NADH and $FADH_2$ (delivery trucks carrying electrons) would be unable to transfer the electron to complex I and complex II, while also failing to drop off the final electrons to create water in the ETC. Essentially, the entire energy system would get backed up and ATP production would be inhibited (15, 16).

In addition to being needed to create ATP directly, iron is essential for hemoglobin production. Hemoglobin is a protein found in your red blood cells that is responsible for transporting oxygen from your lungs to your tissues. Without enough iron, you can become iron anemic. Anemia is when you have low red blood cells or hemoglobin, which produces a state where less oxygen is getting to your tissues. Less oxygen to the tissues will inhibit energy production. I will go into this in more detail in Chapter 4, as it is important to understand iron's role in oxygenation of your tissue (17).

And finally, iron has a role in thyroid hormone production and thyroid (T4-T3) conversion. Iron is a cofactor for the enzyme thyroid peroxidase, which is needed to form both thyroxine (T4) and triiodothyronine (T3). In addition, iron is required as a cofactor for the deiodinase enzymes. These enzymes are needed to convert inactive (T4) to active (T3). Thus, low iron can lead to both low thyroid production and conversion. And since we need ample thyroid for optimal energy production, lower thyroid will lead to less ATP. More on this in Chapter 5.

As you can see, iron is vital for energy production. You need it in the cell to help transport electrons through the ETC. You need it to make hemoglobin to transport oxygen. And finally, you need iron to produce and convert enough active thyroid hormone. Essentially, iron is a super star when it comes to energy production.

But let me stop for a minute before you start thinking you need to down iron pills to fix all your energy issues.

Iron metabolism is complex. Even though it is essential for energy production, too much iron can be detrimental to your health. Like most things in health the dose makes the poison, and with iron this is especially true. This is why I have designated an entire chapter on why iron is a double-edge-sword, while it is vital, too much can be detrimental.

I KNOW! Why can't things be black and white? Well, welcome to your health, where everything is a little (or a lot) bit gray!

The best food sources of iron-rich foods are beef liver (another win for beef liver), beef, kidney, oysters, clams, mussels, eggs, sardines, and tuna. Vegetarian sources are well-cooked greens, dried fruits, and blackstrap molasses. Like so many other nutrients, animal-based foods that contain heme-iron are far more bioavailable than vegetable (non-heme iron) sources.

Ok. On to our next mineral.

Magnesium (Mg) - Magnesium is another essential mineral needed for energy production. Magnesium is needed for the synthesis and utilization of ATP in glycolysis, the Krebs cycle and the ETC. In fact, magnesium is involved in hundreds of enzymatic functions and various physiological processes.

In the first stage of glucose oxidation (glycolysis), magnesium is required by the enzyme's hexokinase and phosphofructokinase, which catalyze the first steps in the breakdown of glucose into pyruvate.

Magnesium is also needed by the enzyme pyruvate dehydrogenase to break down pyruvate into acetyl-CoA, and isocitrate dehydrogenase needed in the Krebs cycle.

In addition, magnesium is essential for the function of ATP synthase, an enzyme complex at the end of the ETC. ATP synthase produces ATP from ADP, during oxidative phosphorylation. Essential ATP synthase helps add a phosphate molecule to ADP, creating the energy we run off (ATP). You can think of ATP synthase as the motor or generator in our power plant. It used the energy generated through the ETC to convert ADP and inorganic phosphate into ATP (18, 19).

Insufficient magnesium can disrupt glycolysis, Krebs cycle, and oxidative phosphorylation, reducing energy production. Which means a magnesium deficiency can impair ATP synthesis and utilization, leading to fatigue, sleep issues, decreased performance, and a low energy state. It also means that increasing your magnesium levels can improve energy, mood, sleep, and overall well-being.

FUN FACT: Although magnesium is sold as a relaxing mineral, it can be quite stimulating if you are deficient, due to it activating energy production. This is one reason I suggest trying a magnesium supplement early in the day (at least initially)—to ensure it does not keep you up at night.

Your body holds about 25 grams of magnesium. Your body's magnesium is in your bones (50-60%), and your soft tissue (39-49%), while less than 1% is in your blood serum. Magnesium homeostasis is mostly controlled by your kidneys, excreting about 120 mg of magnesium into your urine each day.

If you consume an excessive amount of magnesium, you will excrete more magnesium. If your magnesium status is low, you will excrete less magnesium. In addition, under stress you tend to use more magnesium, while also excreting more magnesium (20). So, if you are stressed, additional magnesium may make sense.

The best food sources of magnesium are well-cooked greens, dark chocolate, cacao powder, oatmeal, coffee, soaked beans, and avocados. Magnesium supplements can be a safe source of additional magnesium. Jump to Chapter 6, where I discuss all my favorites.

Copper (Cu) - Copper is another trace mineral that is needed for energy production. Copper plays roles in several key enzymatic functions in energy production, as well as playing an important role in iron metabolism—which is essential for oxygenation of tissue and thyroid production, both needed for optimal energy production.

Copper is a vital component to cytochrome c oxidase (remember, cytochromes are heme-containing proteins that help electrons move through the ETC). Cytochrome c oxidase, located at complex IV at the ETC, is responsible for the final electron transfer to oxygen, reducing it to water. Copper is also a part of an enzyme called copper-zinc superoxide dismutase (SOD1), which protects the cells against oxidative damage from the byproducts of the ETC. SOD1 is found in the cytoplasm, nucleus, and peroxisomes of the cell. This enzyme helps maintain cellular health during energy production.

In addition, copper plays a role in iron metabolism. Ceruloplasmin and hephaestin are two copper-containing enzymes that help iron oxidize from ferrous iron to ferric iron, so it can be bound to transferrin and be transported in the blood. Transferrin-bound iron can then be transported to various tissues, including bone marrow, where it can help synthesize hemoglobin. And finally, copper is involved in the mobilization of stored iron from the liver, spleen, or bone marrow, making it available for energy production, hemoglobin synthesis and thyroid production.

Essentially, without enough copper, iron becomes dysregulated. From the outside (or in a blood lab) it may look like iron anemia. Yet, what it may truly be is low copper, as iron needs copper to be regulated. Either way, the result will be lower energy production, which will present as sleep issues, colder body, and fatigue. Although copper deficiency is rare in the US, it can and does happen. Those with celiac disease or absorption issues can become low in copper.

In addition, those who consume excessive iron and zinc (normally from supplements) can become copper deficient, as each of these can impair copper absorption. (21, 22). I talk about this a bit more in Chapters 4 and 11.

You will never guess what food is highest in copper. You guessed it—beef liver. Other food sources of copper are oysters, crab, and turkey. Vegetarian copper sources are from baking chocolate, dark chocolate, potatoes, mushrooms, well-cooked spinach, and soaked and sprouted cashews (23). The RDA of copper is around 1mg/day.

Zinc (Zn) - The trace mineral zinc plays several crucial roles in energy production within the cell. Although zinc is not directly involved in the primary pathways of ATP production, it serves as a cofactor for numerous enzymes and proteins that are required for optimal cellular energy production.

As stated above, zinc, along with copper, make up the enzyme superoxide dismutase (SOD1). SOD1 protects the cell's mitochondria from oxidative stress by neutralizing reactive oxygen species (ROS). Oxidative stress can damage mitochondrial membranes and proteins involved in the ETC, reducing the efficiency of ATP synthesis. Essentially, the zinc-copper SOD1 is like a security guard in our power plant analogy, protecting the power plant from vandals (oxidative damage) (24).

Another important zinc-containing enzyme is carbonic anhydrase. Carbonic anhydrase helps maintain pH balance (in the blood) by catalyzing the conversion of CO_2 to carbonic acid and back again to CO_2 to be released by the lungs (more on this in Chapter 4). Carbonic acid also helps carbon dioxide (CO_2) transport from the lung tissue to the alveoli, which in turn helps respiration (breathing). Proper pH balance is essential for the optimal function of enzymes involved in cellular respiration. Enzymes have a preferred pH range in which they function most efficiently, and any type of deviation can reduce their activity, slowing certain steps in ATP production (25).

Think of carbonic anhydrase as the ventilation system in our power plant analogy. Carbonic anhydrase ensures the power plant's internal environment (your body and blood) remains stable, so that the workers (enzymatic reactions) can work properly.

It should be noted that increased carbonic anhydrase activity can be harmful to the body, as it can lead to excessive carbon dioxide breakdown, leading to a decrease in tissue oxygenation (as oxygen needs CO_2 to get into your tissue). I'll talk more about this in Chapter 4, but it's just another example of how too much of a good thing can be bad.

In addition, zinc influences the production of hepcidin, a hormone needed to regulate iron absorption. Dysregulation of hepcidin production can lead to iron-related disorders, such as iron overload or iron anemia—both of which can inhibit energy production.

And finally, zinc is essential for the synthesis of various proteins involved in the production of red blood cells. A zinc deficiency can impair red blood cell production, leading to anemia, and a decrease in energy production (26).

Although zinc is not used directly in cellular energy production, it is still an essential nutrient for optimal energy production. A deficiency in zinc can lead to an increase in oxidative stress, blood pH imbalances, iron dysregulation, anemia, and reduced oxygenation of your tissue—all of which will negatively impact energy production.

The best food sources of zinc-rich foods are oysters, beef, crab, pork, turkey, shrimp, mussels, cheese, milk, and beef liver. Oysters are the star when it comes to zinc content, as they contain about 32 mg per 3-ounce serving. To put this into perspective, the second highest foods, beef and crab, give you only about 3.5 mg/3-ounce serving. Of course, not everyone loves oysters, thus eating a variety of other meats and dairy sources can be the ticket to meeting your daily zinc requirements. The RDA is around 10mg/day (27).

Phosphorus (P) - Phosphorus plays a crucial role in energy production, primarily through its role in the structure of AT (adenosine triphosphate)—the body's main energy currency.

ATP is made of adenine, ribose (a sugar), and three phosphate groups (that is the triphosphate part). The high-energy bonds between these phosphate groups store energy that can be released and used by cells whenever it's needed.

Phosphorus also participates in phosphorylation reactions—the process of transferring a phosphate group from ATP to another molecule. This transfer can activate or deactivate enzymes, switch metabolic pathways on or off, or modify a protein's function. Essentially, phosphorylation is one of the key ways your cells regulate energy production and signal when it's time to make or use energy.

Another key process involving phosphorus is oxidative phosphorylation. Although the terms sound similar, they are quite different. Phosphorylation is when ATP donates a phosphate group to another molecule. Oxidative phosphorylation is how ATP itself is made—from ADP—during energy production in the mitochondria's ETC.

So, phosphorus is needed for both the structure of ATP and the process that creates it. A deficiency in phosphorus, although rare, can limit ATP production and lower overall cellular energy availability.

As always in nutrition, nothing is black and white. Too much phosphorus can be just as harmful as too little. Excess intake can impair kidney function, weaken bones, or create vascular and soft tissue calcification. It can also lead to secondary hyperparathyroidism, a condition where the body produces excess parathyroid hormone to try and rebalance calcium and phosphorus levels.

Most people today consume too much phosphorus, not too little. This happens largely due to phosphate additives being added to foods, especially processed foods, as a food preservative. Of course, there are always exceptions to this. Those on a very low-calorie diet, who have malabsorption issues, hyperparathyroidism, or who consume an excessive amount of alcohol could create a phosphorus deficiency.

The RDA for most adults is around 700 mg/day.

The best whole food sources of phosphorus are dairy products, meats, poultry, fish, and eggs. Vegetarian sources are soaked and sprouted nuts, legumes, vegetables, and well-prepared grains.

Calcium (Ca) - Although most people think of calcium as the major bone mineral (and it is), it is also an essential nutrient for optimal energy production and cellular respiration. Calcium contributes to energy production in several ways.

First, calcium acts as a cofactor for several key enzymes involved in ATP production. A cofactor is similar to a coenzyme in that it helps speed up enzyme activity, but a cofactor is typically derived from a metal ion, whereas a coenzyme is derived from a vitamin.

Calcium activates the pyruvate dehydrogenase complex, as stated before in this chapter, this enzyme converts pyruvate into acetyl-CoA in glucose oxidation. Calcium also regulates the enzymes isocitrate dehydrogenase and a-Ketoglutarate dehydrogenase, which influence the production of NADH and $FADH_2$ (the delivery trucks) for ATP production.

Second, calcium can influence the activity of ATP synthase, this is the enzyme responsible for synthesizing ATP from ADP during oxidative phosphorylation. Without calcium, the activity of ATP synthase would be hindered, and ATP production would slow.

FUN FACT: All dehydrogenase enzymes are similar because they all facilitate redox reactions (transfer of electrons) during cellular respiration. In our power plant analogy, dehydrogenases can be seen as specialized converters that transform raw material (glucose, fatty acids, amino acids) into energy intermediates (NADH, FADH2) by transferring energy (electrons).

And finally, calcium acts as a secondary messenger in various cellular signaling that regulates energy metabolism. Calcium signaling is involved in the actions of both insulin and glucagon, which are regulators of glucose metabolism. In addition, calcium release from the sarcoplasmic reticulum triggers muscle contraction, which requires ATP. The energy demand during muscle activity stimulates increased ATP production. *This is a big reason why you should want to build more muscle; you will produce more ATP.

Although 99% of your calcium is stored in your bones and teeth, the other 1% is busy doing numerous metabolic functions. Due to the importance of these functions, your bones act as a reservoir for calcium, releasing it into the bloodstream as needed. A diet rich in calcium can help replenish and restore bone calcium levels, keeping bones healthy and strong. However, if the diet is deficient in calcium or contains excessive phosphorus compared to calcium*, then more calcium will be pulled from the bones, and bone strength can decrease.

*When it comes to bone health, the phosphorus to calcium ratio is very important. Too much phosphorus to calcium can lead to bone fractures and osteoporosis. Ideally you should be getting a ratio between 1:1 or 2:1 CA:P. If you want to understand the importance of the calcium to phosphorus ratio, I go into a much deeper explanation in *How to Heal Your Metabolism* (28).

The best food sources of calcium are milk, cheese, yogurt, and sardines. Vegetarian sources of calcium are well-cooked greens, like spinach, collard greens, and kale. Like so many other nutrients, animal sources of calcium are far more bioavailable than the plant sources (29).

Manganese (Mn) - Manganese is another trace mineral that is involved in energy production. Manganese acts as a cofactor for numerous enzymes, protects against oxidative stress, and supports various metabolic pathways.

Manganese acts as a cofactor for the enzyme manganese-superoxide dismutase (SOD2). Like the zinc-copper superoxide dismutase (SOD1), SOD2 protects the cell against oxidative damage. SOD2 works within the mitochondria of the cell, and ensures the mitochondria can continue to produce ATP, without being damaged by ROS.

Manganese is also a cofactor for the enzyme pyruvate carboxylase. Pyruvate carboxylase converts pyruvate into oxaloacetate, a key intermediate in the Krebs cycle (where NADH, $FADH_2$, and ATP are produced). Essentially, pyruvate carboxylase helps produce a specific "fuel" needed to run our power plant. Proper function of this enzyme ensures there is a sufficient supply of intermediates (things that make up the fuel) for energy production.

And finally, manganese is a cofactor in the enzyme arginase. Arginase is involved in the urea cycle. The urea cycle is responsible for removing ammonia, a byproduct of protein metabolism, from the body. Excess ammonia in the body can lead to liver disease, neurological disorders, increase acidity in the body, and cellular damage.

A deficiency in manganese can increase oxidative stress on the cell, while impairing the activity of numerous enzymes needed for ATP production.

The best food sources for manganese are blue mussels, oysters, and clams. Vegetarian sources are soaked and sprouted hazelnuts, boiled spinach, pineapple, and oatmeal. The RDA for adults is 1.8mg - 2.3 mg per day. This could be obtained in about one ounce of hazelnuts or one ounce of mussels.

Alright, are you ready for a little breather? I know this chapter has been dense with biochemistry and became a little bit technical. What I can say is, if you can continue to see your cells as factories, your mitochondria as power plants, and see how each individual worker (enzyme-proteins), assistant (coenzyme and cofactors—vitamin and minerals), are helping the power plant produce energy, then you are right where you need to be. It is not necessary to know each individual enzyme and coenzyme, yet it does help to see where each of these nutrients is needed along the path to produce ATP.

Now, before I wrap up this chapter, I want to take a few minutes to go over the foods that can interfere or inhibit nutrient digestion and absorption. Where you can get individual nutrients is just as important as knowing that things could interfere with the absorption of these same nutrients. You must understand that just because a food contains a significant amount of nutrients, doesn't mean you are going to digest and absorb all those nutrients, particularly if that food contains antinutrients.

What Are Antinutrients?

Antinutrients are built-in defense mechanisms used to protect seeds, nuts, legumes, raw vegetables, and unripe fruits from being consumed by an animal. They "defend" the food by disrupting the animal's digestive system when consumed. Not only do antinutrients affect digestion, but they can also inhibit nutrient and protein digestion and absorption. And yes, these same antinutrients can negatively affect how well YOU digest and absorb the protein and nutrients in that food.

Antinutrients Affecting Protein and Nutrient Absorption:

Here is a list of antinutrients that can interfere with nutrient and protein digestion and absorption

Oxalates: Inhibit calcium, iron, and magnesium absorption. Found in grains and leafy greens, seeds, chocolate.

Phytates: Inhibit zinc, iron, copper, calcium, and magnesium absorption. Found in soy, grains, seeds, beans, and nuts.

Trypsin Inhibitors: Inhibit protein digestion. Found in soy and legumes.

Goitrogens: Can inhibit iodine uptake, affecting thyroid production and conversion.

Protease Inhibitors: Inhibits protein digestion. Found in legumes, grains, potatoes, and some seeds.

Tannins: Inhibit iron absorption. Tannins are found in plums, berries, grapes, peaches, pears, nuts, beans, buckwheat, wine, tea, and cacao beans.

Saponins. Inhibits iron absorption and protein digestion. Found in legumes, soy, spinach, grains, potato skins.

Lectins. Binds to the gut lining, causing digestive issues and interfering with nutrient uptake. Found in legumes, grains, nightshades.

In the context of energy production and a need for certain nutrients in our power plant analogy, we can think of antinutrients as contaminants in the fuel supply that reduce the quality or quantity of our fuel needed to run the power plant. This poor fuel supply (lack of nutrients, protein) can cause wear and tear on our machinery (body), while reducing efficiency and output.

Remember, a nutrient-rich food is only as good as its ability to be digested and absorbed. Thus, a nutrient-rich food that is unable to be broken down and absorbed, is nutrient-deficient.

Foods that are high in antinutrients and are harder for the human body to digest and absorb nutrients from, are seeds, nuts, most grains, corn, soy, beans, spinach, kale, lettuce, and cruciferous vegetables like broccoli, cauliflower, Bok choy, chocolate, unripe fruits, and coffee.

Now, before you panic because your favorite food was just listed, it should be noted that preparing these foods properly can significantly reduce the antinutrients.

Here Are Five Ways You Can Reduce Antinutrients.

1. Soaking and sprouting foods, like beans, grains, and seeds can reduce the levels of phytates, lectins, tannins, and protease inhibitors.

2. Cooking foods, like beans, vegetables, nuts and seeds, can reduce the goitrogenic compounds, phytates, oxalates, tannins, protease inhibitors, saponins, and lectins.

3. Fermenting foods, like sourdough bread, can reduce phytates and tannins. It can also improve protease activity and increase the breakdown of gluten, which can improve protein digestion.

4. Nixtamalization (treated with lime) of corn (masa harina), reduces phytates, improves the digestibility and availability of protein, and increases nutrient bioavailability.

5. Roasting coffee and chocolate beans can reduce the phytates, tannins, and oxalates.

Raw, GMO, or canned versions of these foods will have the most impact on nutrient absorption, while also creating the most digestive issues. Soaking, sprouting, cooking, fermenting, nixtamalization, and roasting can all decrease the antinutrients, while improving the digestibility and absorption of nutrients in your foods.

Yet, they are not 100% effective.

Which means, if you have energy production issues, and your digestive system is already compromised, you might want to consider limiting or even avoiding most of these foods, at least until your health starts to improve. My advice is to experiment on yourself; your first step might be to just prepare the foods properly and see how your body tolerates them. If you continue to have digestive issues, then I would significantly reduce foods high in antinutrients, all the while focusing on animal-based foods and easy to digest carbohydrates, as explained in the last chapter.

Personally, I am not nearly as strict with my food as I was ten years ago when I wrote my first book. I give myself a lot more leeway with my food choices, especially when the food is prepared properly. My belief is you should be able to consume a wide variety of foods, when your body is healthy. Of course, this means a wide variety of different properly prepared carbs, fats, and proteins—not a wide variety of fast and ultra-processed foods (although even these foods are fine if you eat them sparingly).

Most of us want to be able to eat a diverse diet and stay healthy, this makes food and life more enjoyable and less stressful. Yet, we must know our own personal limits. If you are trying to gain your health back, then it is going to help you the most to consume the foods suggested. If you are like me and want to keep your health while also enjoying a few non-recommended treats, then go for it—just know your limits. I feel best when 90% of my diet consists of dairy, eggs, fruit, organs, gelatin, grass-fed meats, coffee, rice, potatoes, and well-cooked vegetables. This gives me space for an occasional pizza, sushi, and a few peanut butter cookies (I do love a good peanut butter cookie).

Well, there you have it, you now have a decent understanding of cellular energy production and how certain nutrients can support this process, while others can hinder this process. You now know how essential protein is for energy production, as it makes up the structure of the cell (the power plant), the transport proteins (the shuttle), the regulators (managers) and the enzymes (the workers). Of course, these enzymes (workers) do not work alone, they need coenzymes—vitamins (assistants), and cofactors—minerals (assistant of assistants).

As you can see, when we consume a wide variety of supportive, nutrient-rich foods, we can supply our cell (power plant) with all the resources it needs to function optimally. Of course, if our body is overridden with anti-nutrients and ultra-processed foods (contaminants), these metabolic processes will be negatively affected, and energy production will be impaired.

We have now discussed our best fuel sources and essential nutrients for energy production. But we are not done with how you produce optimal ATP, there are two other essential substances that are required for healthy energy production, and the first has to do with the band The Police.

"Every Breath You Take"...yep, you know it—oxygen!

Please excuse my ongoing cheesiness, after 20 hours of writing, a girl must entertain herself somehow.

CHAPTER 3

THE BOTTOM LINE

Essential Nutrients for Energy Production

1. Fuel powers. Nutrients build. Carbs and fats are the fuel. Protein, vitamins, and minerals are the engine, wiring, and crew that turn that fuel into ATP. If the "machinery" is underbuilt or underfed, even perfect fuel sputters with ATP production.

2. Protein is infrastructure, not gasoline. Protein supplies the enzymes, transporters, scaffolding, and regulators that run glycolysis, the Krebs cycle, and the ETC. Use it to build and maintain the plant, not to burn for heat.

3. B vitamins are the enzyme assistants. Direct drivers: B1, B2, B3, B5 feed pyruvate dehydrogenase, redox carriers (NAD^+/FAD), beta-oxidation, and CoA synthesis. Support crew: B6, B7, B9, B12 backstop glucose/fat handling, red blood cell formation, and methylation so oxygen delivery and ATP output stay high.

4. Minerals make ATP production happen. The primary minerals for cellular energy production are iron, magnesium, copper, zinc, phosphorus, calcium, and manganese. With vitamins and minerals, quality food beats mega doses.

5. Digestion is half the battle, absorption is the other.

6. Anti-nutrients in seeds, nuts, grains, legumes, certain greens, and raw forms can block protein and mineral absorption. Soak, sprout, cook, ferment, nixtamalize, or roast to lower their impact. If digestion is fragile, lean on animal foods and easy-to-digest carbs while you heal.

7. Build plates that build ATP. Center meals on nutrient-dense, bioavailable foods: dairy, eggs, fruit, shellfish, white fish, organs, gelatin, quality meats, potatoes/rice, and well-cooked vegetables. These deliver fuel and the co-factors convert that fuel.

CHAPTER 4

WHY DO WE BREATHE—THE IMPORTANCE OF OXYGEN (AND CO$_2$)

I am sure you know how important oxygen is to life, without oxygen there is no life. Yet do you understand how important oxygen is for energy production? Oxygen is vital for energy production. In fact, when you understand that energy production is the foundation of life, without oxygen there is no life or energy production.

You need oxygen to take that sunset run on the beach without collapsing. You need oxygen to binge watch an entire season of Friends without passing out. You need oxygen to create that billion-dollar idea that is going to change the world. Without oxygen your body's ability to move, think, talk, detox, digest, sleep, and pretty much do anything would come to a screeching halt.

So yes, oxygen is important!

We breathe and take in oxygen, because our cells require oxygen for optimal energy production. And without enough energy (ATP) being produced, well, we get sick, diseased, and die. Essentially, we would die without oxygen, because without oxygen we can't produce enough energy to stay alive.

The common theme throughout this book is all about optimizing your energy (ATP) production. When you produce ample ATP healthfully (fuel, nutrients, oxygen, and thyroid), your body has enough energy to run all its systems properly.

Having enough oxygen is essential for all of this to happen. Yet, there is far more to oxygen and energy production than just the air you breathe. How well your body can take in, transport, and then use oxygen is essential for energy production. Each one of these factors is going to affect how oxygen gets into your tissue, and how well you produce energy.

On a side note, it is true that you can produce energy without oxygen. This process is called anaerobic respiration or glycolysis. While some of your cells function this way (like red blood cells) all the time, most of your cells can only function without oxygen for a very short time (seconds to several minutes). You might use anaerobic respiration when you are sprinting or doing some sort of very intense exercise—yet you can normally only sustain this intensity briefly.

Overall, anaerobic respiration (without oxygen) is a very inefficient process, producing only 2 ATP per glucose molecule, while also producing lactate. On the other hand, cellular respiration (aerobic respiration) will produce a total of 36-38 ATP—an almost 1800% increase. So yes, if you want more energy, oxygen is pretty darn important!

In this chapter, I am first going to share where and why oxygen is needed for energy production. I am then going to talk about the most important gas, other than oxygen, that is essential for the oxygenation of your tissue and optimal energy production. I'll then help you understand the physiology of breathing and what nutrients are needed for optimal oxygen transportation. And finally, I am going to discuss how you can improve your energy production by just improving the way you breathe.

So, get comfy, grab a tall glass of orange juice, and take a long deep breath as you are about to become energized with a deeper understanding of breathing, oxygen, and energy production!

First, How Is Oxygen Used for Energy Production?

Oxygen is needed for energy production, as it is the final electron acceptor in the electron transport chain ETC.

To understand how important this is, let's go back to our factory analogy. For the electron transport chain (power grid) to keep producing energy, the electrons (energy packs) moving through each complex need to be removed and then recycled. Think of oxygen as a big recycle bin waiting at the end of the production line. Once the electrons reach the final step in the ETC (at complex IV), they need to be removed to keep the production line moving.

Oxygen combines with these electrons (and removes them), along with hydrogen ions to form water (H_2O). Without this step, the electrons would get backed up, halting the entire electron transport chain. This would halt energy production and well, you would halt living. I know it's a bit morbid, but it's the truth!

Essentially, without oxygen, the ETC (power grid) cannot generate energy (ATP), which would lead to an energy crisis and system shut down (death).

So, yes, oxygen is essential for life, because oxygen is essential for energy production.

Now, before we talk about how you breathe, I think it is essential to talk about the other very valuable gas that is essential for the oxygenation of your tissue—carbon dioxide.

What is Carbon Dioxide?

Carbon dioxide is colorless gas that along with ATP, heat, and water, is a byproduct of cellular respiration. In the medical world, CO_2 is considered a "waste product," as it is the gas your lungs remove to allow for oxygenation of the blood. From an energy standpoint carbon dioxide is so much more than just waste.

You see, CO_2 is required to help oxygen get into the tissue. Without CO_2, oxygen would stay bound to hemoglobin, making it harder for hemoglobin to release oxygen into the tissues. In conditions where CO_2 is abnormally low, such as hyperventilation (increased rate of breathing), oxygen delivery to the tissues becomes impaired—making it harder for you to breathe. This can occur despite having normal or even elevated oxygen levels in the blood.

FUN FACT: Have you ever wondered why you are told to breathe into a paper bag when you are hyperventilating? It's to increase your CO_2 levels. Your breath contains CO_2, and when you breathe into a bag, you end up inhaling your own CO_2. As you increase your CO_2, your body and breathing will calm, as this will help oxygen get into the tissue. Remember, oxygen cannot oxygenate the tissue, without CO_2.

In addition to its role in helping oxygen get into the tissue, CO_2 has antioxidant-like properties. CO_2 can affect the pH balance of your blood. Certain antioxidant enzymes like superoxide dismutase, are pH-sensitive. Thus, the pH balance supported by CO_2 and its metabolites ensures these protective enzymes function optimally. Of course, any time you improve energy production and decrease glycolysis, which happens when oxygen is more available in the tissue, oxidative stress will decrease.

And finally, carbon dioxide influences the diameter of blood vessels (vasodilation), leading to an increase in blood flow. This improvement in blood flow increases the amount of oxygen, nutrients, and fuel to the tissues. By causing vasodilation, CO_2 cannot only improve exercise performance by allowing more oxygen and nutrients to get to the muscles, but it can also influence blood pressure, relax the blood vessels, and reduce blood pressure.

This is one reason why taking deep slow breaths can improve blood pressure—the CO_2 levels increase, allowing for improved vasodilation (1).

Low levels of CO_2 known as hypocapnia (either through decreased production or increased exhalation) can impact both vasodilation and the oxygenation of tissue. Conditions such as chronic obstructive pulmonary disease (COPD), respiratory alkalosis, hyperventilation, asthma, seizures, and cardiovascular problems, such as high blood pressure, can be affected by low CO_2 levels.

If someone is in a low energy state, not consuming enough carbohydrates or nutrients, and/or has numerous energy blocks, then CO_2 production is going to be hindered, as energy production is hindered. Less CO_2 produced means less oxygen arriving in the cell. As you learned above, lower amounts of oxygen back up the entire system, as it is needed for the final electron acceptor (the recycle bin that keeps the ETC moving). When the ETC is backed up, the cell will try to produce energy without oxygen. At this point, cells become inefficient at producing energy (anaerobic glycolysis), which results in less energy and lactate production.

Now, to be clear, anaerobic glycolysis (breakdown of glucose to pyruvate) and lactate production are not bad things. Lactate is produced from pyruvate when there is a lack of oxygen. During this process 2 ATP molecules are produced (vs. 34-38 ATP produced in aerobic respiration), lactate buffers the blood and is then recycled back to glucose in the liver (Cori Cycle).

These are necessary processes that your body goes through when oxygen is scarce. This can happen in times of intense exercise, like when you are lifting weights or sprinting. This allows you to keep going when your body cannot get enough oxygen into the tissue. In addition, some of your cells can only produce energy through anaerobic glycolysis—cells like the retinas of your eyes and your red blood cells (more on this later). So, in some degree, you are producing energy via anaerobic glycolysis all day long

However, for the cells that do have mitochondria and can use oxygen, anaerobic glycolysis should not be their primary way to produce energy—as it is inefficient. Excess lactate or lactic acid can lead to a condition called lactic acidosis. This can occur in numerous diseases like sepsis, shock, heart failure, respiratory failure, liver disease, cancer, diabetes, mitochondrial disease, and as a side effect of numerous drugs.

Essentially, anaerobic glycolysis is a backup system used in times of extreme stress/intensity. You need it so you can keep going. But, like most of our backup systems, you don't want to stay in it for too long.

Unfortunately, increases in lactic acid will oppose CO_2, restricting oxygen even more!

Yes, it can be a total sh#t show!

To restore optimal respiration, adequate oxygen and/or CO_2 are needed to restrain the production of lactate. I will be giving you some insight on how to do this in the context of improving oxygen in the tissues at the end of this book.

The bottom line is CO_2 is far more than just a waste product. It is essential for oxygenation of your tissue and energy production. In fact, Ray Peat, PhD, noted biologist and researcher stated, "Improved carbon dioxide production can help with edema, migraines, brain edema, mountain sickness, osteoporosis, epilepsy, glaucoma, hyperactivity, inflammation, healing wombs and arthritis. Diabetes, cardiomyopathy, obesity, cancer, dementia, and psychosis are also likely to benefit."

Alright, now that you know about the two main gasses in breathing, let's talk about how you breathe.

How Do We Breathe?

Breathing, also known as respiration, refers to the process of inhaling oxygen (O_2) and exhaling carbon dioxide (CO_2) through the lungs. You can also "breathe" in the cells, in a process called cellular respiration, where the cells release CO_2 and take in oxygen. Both processes involve the exchange of two gasses (CO_2 and oxygen) that help facilitate cellular metabolism and energy production.

First, let's discuss breathing and the lungs.

When you breathe, air enters through your nose, where it becomes filtered, warmed, and humidified. The air then travels through the pharynx (throat) and larynx (voice box). The air continues down the trachea (windpipe), into two main bronchi in the lungs (one for each lung). The air then travels through the bronchi into further smaller bronchioles. The bronchioles lead to tiny air sacs called alveoli. Each one of these alveolus (single alveoli) is surrounded by a network of capillaries that is filled with blood. It is at the capillaries where oxygen enters the blood.

In the lungs, hemoglobin drops its CO_2 and binds to oxygen due to a higher affinity for it, making the blood more oxygenated. This process is called the Haldane effect. In the tissue, the opposite occurs, as more CO_2 binds to hemoglobin, its affinity for oxygen decreases, promoting the release of oxygen into the tissue. This effect is essential for CO_2 transportation from tissues to the lungs for exhalation.

It should be noted, if there are low levels of CO_2 at the tissue, less oxygen will be released from hemoglobin. And if there are low levels of CO_2 in the lungs, less oxygen will be picked up. Both scenarios could result in less oxygen reaching the tissues.

Essentially, the Haldane effect optimizes CO_2 transportation. In the lungs, high oxygen levels cause hemoglobin to release CO_2, while in the tissues, low oxygen levels allow hemoglobin to bind and transport more CO_2.

Now, let's talk about breathing at the cell level.

After oxygen is transported to your cells, another form of breathing occurs, referred to as cellular respiration.

Cellular respiration is the process of "breathing" at the cell level. Once oxygen reaches the cell, the exchange between oxygen and CO_2 occurs again, yet in the opposite way. This is where oxygen moves from the blood into the tissue and CO_2 moves from the tissue into the blood.

Along with the Haldane effect, another process occurs that promotes this gas exchange.

This process is called the Bohr effect.

The Bohr effect is when an increase in carbon dioxide concentration and a decrease in pH (more acidic), caused by CO_2 concentrations, reduce hemoglobin's affinity for oxygen. This increase in acidity (due to CO_2) promotes the release of oxygen from hemoglobin, allowing more oxygen to enter the tissues.

Although the Haldane and Bohr effects seem similar, they operate through different physiological principles. The Haldane effect focuses on the interaction between oxygenation and the CO_2 binding capacity of hemoglobin. The Bohr effect focuses on the impact of pH and CO_2 concentrations on the oxygen-binding affinity of hemoglobin.

Due to the Bohr effect, about 70-80% of CO_2 enters the red blood cells and reacts with water to form carbonic acid (catalyzed by the zinc-containing enzyme carbonic anhydrase). Carbonic acid quickly dissociates to bicarbonate and hydrogen ions. CO_2 converts to bicarbonate to maintain the optimal acid-base balance in the blood. Once it gets back to the lungs, with the help of carbonic anhydrase again, the bicarbonate will convert back to CO_2. This occurs so that it can be exhaled out through the lungs.

Due to the Haldane effect, about 20-25% of CO_2 is transported back to the lungs by binding to the transport protein hemoglobin, forming carbaminohemoglobin. Only about 5-10% of CO_2 is transported directly as a gas.

What you need to know is that these gasses work together. Essentially, when carbon dioxide levels are higher (like the tissue), oxygen is displaced from hemoglobin. This will result in more oxygen being available to the cells for energy production. When oxygen levels are higher (like the lungs), carbon dioxide is displaced from hemoglobin, so that it can be exhaled through the lungs.

OK. Do you need a minute to catch your breath? I know I do. Who knew so much was going on in your lungs and cells to coordinate this impressive dance between oxygen and carbon dioxide? Your body is amazing if I do say so myself!

One question you might be asking yourself is, are there simple ways to improve carbon dioxide production, so that your tissues can become more oxygenated?

Well, yes—yes, there are, and I am glad you asked.

Here are 6 ways you can improve oxygenation of your tissues by improving carbon dioxide levels:

1. Consume a diet rich in carbohydrates, as glucose oxidation produces 50% more CO_2 over fat oxidation.

2. Bag breathing. Rebreathing expired air from a paper bag can increase CO_2 in the blood. Doing this several times a day, for around a minute each time, is the suggested dosage.

3. Make a CO_2 bath. Add a cup of baking soda to your warm bath (2).

4. Baking soda. Consuming baking soda in water can increase CO_2 levels. Add ½ -1 teaspoon of baking soda to 10 oz water and drink 1-2 hours away from food. Please consult your health care provider before trying (3).

5. Mouth taping at night. Mouth taping forces you to breathe through your nose vs. your mouth, decreasing hyperventilation and increasing CO_2 retention.

6. Proper, full, deep breaths. Shallow, short breaths encourage hyperventilation and loss of CO_2. Refer to the end of this chapter for breathing practices.

FUN FACT: At high altitudes, the atmospheric pressure is lower, which means there is less oxygen in the air. Initially, this can lead to hypoxia and hyperventilation. Yet over time, as the body adapts to the higher altitudes, CO_2 normalizes, even in a low O_2 environment (4).

*Carbonic anhydrase inhibitors (CAI), like acetazolamide, are taken to cure altitude sickness. They work by inhibiting the enzyme carbonic anhydrase. If you remember from above, carbonic anhydrase is needed to convert CO_2 into carbonic acid. Thus, if you inhibit this process, more CO_2 will stay in the blood, allowing for more oxygenation of your tissue. *Please consult your health care provider before taking any medication.*

Alright, we are not done.

Along with CO_2, there are numerous nutrients that are needed to make sure oxygen is effectively utilized. These nutrients are primarily needed for the transportation of oxygen and include nutrients needed for both hemoglobin and red blood cell production.

Once you breathe in oxygen and it moves through your lungs, into your blood, it must then travel from your lungs to tissues. Like I said at the beginning of this chapter, for oxygen to get from your lungs to your tissue, it must attach itself to hemoglobin—a protein found in your red blood cells.

Red blood cells (RBC) also known as erythrocytes, are produced in your bone marrow (primarily pelvis, sternum, ribs and vertebrae) through a process called erythropoiesis. During this same process, millions of molecules of hemoglobin are produced in each red blood cell.

Hemoglobin is a complex protein made of four heme groups. Each heme group has an iron atom at its center. Each iron atom can bind to one oxygen molecule, allowing for four oxygen molecules to bind to each hemoglobin molecule.

Think of RBCs as tractor trailers in our factory analogy. These tractor trailers are traveling from your lungs (loading docks), picking up oxygen, and then delivering it to trillions of cells (factories). These same red blood cells (trucks) will travel back from your cells to your lungs, to return CO_2 for exhalation. Each red blood cell (tractor trailer) is carrying numerous hemoglobin molecules (cargo containers). These hemoglobin molecules contain oxygen and CO_2 (lifesaving cargo) that are needed for you and your cells' mitochondria (power grids) to operate effectively.

FUN FACT: The average adult has about 5 to 6 liters of blood. Each liter of blood can carry 4-5 trillion red blood cells. And each red blood cell can carry 270 million hemoglobin molecules. Each hemoglobin molecule carries four oxygen molecules. This means your blood can carry a lot of oxygen molecules!

When you do not produce enough RBC or hemoglobin, you are told you have anemia. Anemia results in a reduced ability of the blood to carry oxygen to the body's tissues. This can lead to a low energy state, resulting in numerous symptoms including fatigue, weakness, pale skin, shortness of breath, and dizziness.

All this means is that your RBC and hemoglobin are essential for oxygenation of your tissue, which makes them essential for energy production.

Nutrients Needed To Produce And Maintain
The Transportation Vehicles For Oxygen

As stated above, the transportation vehicles for oxygen are your red blood cells and hemoglobin. Red blood cells and hemoglobin require numerous nutrients for their production and maintenance. These nutrients include glucose (carbohydrates), protein, iron, B12, folate, B6, copper, zinc, and vitamin A!

Let's look at how each of these nutrients plays a role in supporting oxygen in energy production.

Just when you thought I couldn't talk about glucose anymore, I am going to bring it up again in its essentiality to oxygen delivery. As I stated in Chapter 2, glucose is your preferred fuel for energy production for numerous reasons. It is needed for thyroid conversion, increased CO_2 production, nervous system function, quick energy, and it is vital for oxygen transportation.

Why is glucose so important for oxygen transportation?

Glucose is essential for oxygen transportation because red blood cells, which transport oxygen, can only use glucose as energy. And like all living cells, they need energy (ATP) to function. Without it, your RBCs couldn't transport oxygen...and you would die. So yes, pretty damn important.

Every cell in your body needs ATP, but your red blood cells are unique. They do not contain mitochondria—your cell's energy powerhouse (or power plant in our factory analogy). Your mitochondria generate most of a cell's energy through aerobic (oxygen-dependent) respiration. Because your red blood cells lack mitochondria, they rely entirely on anaerobic (without oxygen) respiration, also known as glycolysis, to produce energy.

Glycolysis is the first part of cellular respiration that occurs in the cytoplasm, outside of the mitochondria. As you learned earlier, glycolysis kicks in when energy demands exceed oxygen availability.

But it's also the only option for cells that don't have mitochondria. In other words, without that "power grid," these cells can't burn oxygen for energy.

While glycolysis is a less efficient way to produce energy, it is actually a brilliant design for red blood cells. Why? Because RBCs are in charge of transporting oxygen—not using it. By skipping mitochondria, they avoid consuming the very oxygen they're supposed to transport. Plus, that extra space inside the cell means there is more room for millions of hemoglobin molecules, allowing RBCs to carry even more oxygen to your tissues.

If red blood cells used oxygen for energy, they'd waste part of their own cargo and deliver less to your tissues. This would reduce the efficiency of your entire metabolic system.

The only fuel source that can run glycolysis is glucose! Fats, protein, even ketones cannot be used in anaerobic respiration. Without glucose, your RBCs couldn't make ATP, and like all cells, without energy, they would die.

Just another reason carbohydrates, specifically glucose, are king! And no, that doesn't mean Twinkies, Ding Dongs, or Frappuccinos. It means fruits, roots, juices, honey, and milk—real, whole food sources of carbohydrates.

Of course, glucose isn't the only nutrient your blood cells and hemoglobin depend on. They also require several vitamins and minerals you've already seen throughout this book—nutrients that are equally vital for efficient oxygen transport and energy production. In this next section, we'll look at those supporting nutrients through the lens of oxygen delivery.

Protein and oxygen transportation

Hemoglobin, a transport protein, is essential for oxygen transportation. Remember, hemoglobin is the cargo container that holds (attaches) to your precious cargo (oxygen and CO_2). Hemoglobin is primarily composed of globin, a protein that forms four polypeptide chains (chains of amino acids linked by peptide bonds). These amino acid chains consist of two beta chains and two alpha chains. Without adequate protein consumption, the production of hemoglobin can be reduced, leading to less oxygen transportation, and issues like anemia (5).

Each globin chain is associated with its own iron-rich heme group. The heme group is a ring structure that contains one iron atom in the center. The iron in these heme groups is where oxygen binds, which is why each hemoglobin molecule can bind four oxygen molecules.

The iron-rich hemoglobin is one of the reasons iron is an essential nutrient for oxygen transportation.

Iron and Oxygen Transportation

Like I said above, iron is the binding site in hemoglobin that attaches to oxygen. Think of iron as the hooks or clamps on a cargo container. Just like hooks secure precious freight on a tractor trailer, iron secures oxygen inside the hemoglobin molecule, allowing it to be transported by your red blood cells.

In addition, iron is essential for producing red blood cells (erythropoiesis) in the bone marrow. It's required for immature erythroblasts to mature into fully functional erythrocytes. Without enough iron, hemoglobin synthesis and red blood cell production falter, leading to reduced oxygen delivery, what your doctor would call iron-deficiency anemia.

Iron anemia happens when you have low hemoglobin or low red blood cell counts specifically due to insufficient iron. When oxygen content in the blood drops, less gets delivered to your tissues. This can show up as fatigue, weakness, pale skin, shortness of breath, dizziness, heart palpitations, cold hands and feet, headaches, brittle nails, cravings for non-food items (like dirt, your body's desperate hunt for minerals), and restless leg syndrome.

Many of these symptoms overlap with a general low-energy metabolic state, so just because you have them doesn't automatically mean it's low iron. If you suspect iron is the issue, get a complete blood count (CBC) and a full iron panel to confirm.

Blood Test Lab Results

What Iron Anemia May Look Like (And What it Means)

- **Low hemoglobin (HGB):** Less oxygen-carrying protein in your red blood cells, so less oxygen delivered to your tissues.
  Normal range: 14–18 g/dL (men), 12–16 g/dL (women).

- **Low hematocrit (HCT):** A smaller percentage of your blood is made up of red blood cells.
  Normal range: 40.7–50.3% (men), 36.1–44.3% (women).

- **Low MCV (mean corpuscular volume):** Your red blood cells are too small (microcytic), often from iron shortage.
  Normal range: 80–100 fL.

- **Low MCH (mean corpuscular hemoglobin):** Each red blood cell carries less hemoglobin.
  Normal range: 26–33 pg.

- **Low MCHC (mean corpuscular hemoglobin concentration):** Lower concentration of hemoglobin inside each red cell.
  Normal range: 31–36 g/dL.

- **Low serum iron:** Less circulating iron bound to transferrin in your blood right now.
  Normal range: 50–150 mcg/dL (men), 35–145 mcg/dL (women).

- **Low ferritin:** Your iron storage tank is running low.
  Normal range: 24–336 mcg/L (men), 11–307 mcg/L (women).

- **Low transferrin saturation:** Fewer of your iron transport proteins are loaded up.
  Normal range: 20–50%.

- **High RDW (red cell distribution width):** Wide variation in red blood cell size, indicating uneven production.
  Normal range: 12–15%.

- **High TIBC (total iron-binding capacity):** Your body's capacity to bind more iron is elevated, often meaning it's trying to capture more because it senses a shortage.
  Normal range: 171–505 mcg/dL (men), 149–492 mcg/dL (women).

It's worth noting you may only have a few of these markers and still be iron anemic and sometimes, paradoxically, you might see all of them off, but simply taking more iron to fix the anemia isn't the answer.

Why Do Most People Become Iron Anemic?

Someone can become iron anemic due to:

- **Blood loss:** think monthly periods, external injury, internal bleeding.

- **Increased needs:** like during pregnancy.

- **Poor absorption:** from SIBO, leaky gut, IBD, or celiac (8,9).

- **Deficient diets:** heavy on processed foods or strict vegan.

- **Chronic infections & parasites:** they feed on iron.

- **Cancer:** tumors also thrive on iron.

There's also functional iron deficiency, where iron is stuck in tissues but can't reach your red blood cells, presenting as low iron in labs even though your body is overloaded in the wrong places. I'll talk more about this later in the book, where I take a deeper dive into iron.

For much of my life, I suffered from anemia. For me, this looked like fatigue, cold hands, breathlessness, blurry vision, and a racing heart. Multiple doctors told me, "You're low on iron, take supplements." And I did. Each time, my anemia "fixed" itself. But months later, off iron, the anemia would creep right back. I didn't have heavy periods or hidden internal bleeding. So, what was going on?

Like so many people I've worked with, my anemia had nothing to do with needing more iron.

Wait? What?

Let me explain.

Iron does not regulate iron.

You heard that right. Iron isn't the regulator of iron in your body. That job belongs to a powerful recycling and storage network called the reticuloendothelial system (RES)—yes, it's a mouthful. The RES recycles iron from red blood cells and acts as a major storage reserve for excess iron. About 90% of the iron your body uses each day is recycled; only about 10% typically comes from food. When this system works well, your dietary iron need is actually quite low (6,7).

When the system falters, iron-deficiency anemia can show up—but that doesn't always mean you need more iron.

The health of your gut will impact iron absorption. Conditions like inflammatory bowel disease (IBD) and celiac disease increase anemia risk through poor absorption, inflammation, and blood loss (8,9). In addition, alcohol, phytates, polyphenols found in coffee and tea, calcium, and phosphorus can all inhibit iron absorption (10).

Hepcidin is the master regulator of iron balance. High hepcidin levels block intestinal iron absorption, hindering iron recycling (11). In a healthy system, hepcidin rises when iron is high, in order to lower total iron. It can also rise with inflammation and kidney or liver disorders, all of which can lead to an iron deficiency (12).

And finally, iron is regulated by additional nutrients:

1. Vitamin A increases the utilization of iron; improving vitamin A levels can improve iron anemia without the addition of more iron (13).

2. Copper deficiency impairs the uptake of iron by the mitochondria and reduces heme synthesis; restoring copper can improve iron status.

3. Zinc helps regulate intestinal iron uptake; low zinc levels can impair iron absorption (15).

In other words, your low iron levels may be caused by poor digestion, inflammation, or other nutritional imbalances—not simply low iron intake.

The best way to maintain your iron levels is to eat foods that contain iron and the minerals that help regulate iron. As stated in the last chapter, these foods include beef liver, beef, eggs, oysters, and even well-cooked leafy vegetables.

Luckily for me, once I started to eat beef liver regularly, my iron anemia rectified and has never returned. I likely needed more copper and/or more Vitamin A—nutrients that were missing from my iron supplement. I also suspect years of unnecessary iron pills didn't help my overall health—probably why I suffered so much when numerous stressors hit me like a ton of bricks.

Of course, not everyone's anemia will get fixed by diet alone. Heavy menstrual bleeding may require targeted iron support, at least while you work on why you are bleeding so much in the first place. Malabsorption calls for gut work, while infections, parasites, or cancer need expert care. Beef liver is a smart first step, but if nothing changes in a few months, see your health practitioner.

I have a lot more to say about iron, as wonderful as iron is, it has a very dark side. So dark, that too much is considered one of my energy blocks. This is why I have reserved an entire chapter for the toxic side of iron (jump to Chapter 11 to learn more). For now, all you need to know is that iron is essential for oxygen transport, and just because you appear to be iron deficient doesn't automatically mean you need to take more iron.

Folate and B12 and oxygen transportation

Both folate and B12 are essential for oxygen transportation, as both are needed to produce red blood cells. Vitamin B12 is crucial for proper DNA synthesis in red blood cell production. B12 acts as a coenzyme for methionine synthase, which is necessary for the synthesis of methionine and the metabolism of folate. Methionine and folate are vital for the production and repair of DNA. Without enough B12 and folate, DNA synthesis is impaired, leading to ineffective erythropoiesis (production of RBC) and megaloblastic anemia.

Megaloblastic anemia is characterized by having abnormally large and immature red blood cells called megaloblasts. These large, immature red blood cells are often non-functional, while the ones that are functional contain less hemoglobin than normal cells, and less hemoglobin means less O_2 carrying capacity.

In addition, pernicious anemia occurs when your body is unable to absorb enough B12 from the digestive tract, leading to a deficiency. This condition is specifically caused by a lack of intrinsic factor, a protein normally produced by the stomach's parietal cells. Intrinsic factor binds to B12, allowing it to be absorbed in the small intestine. Without IF, B12 cannot be absorbed, leading to a B12 deficiency. Pernicious anemia will eventually lead to megaloblastic anemia.

B6 (Pyridoxine) and oxygen transportation

Vitamin B6 (pyridoxine) is essential for the synthesis of heme, the iron-containing component of hemoglobin that binds oxygen. B6 serves as a coenzyme for several enzymes involved in heme synthesis. Without sufficient B6, the body cannot produce adequate amounts of heme, leading to impaired hemoglobin production, less oxygenated tissue, and less energy production.

A deficiency of B6 can lead to sideroblastic anemia. Sideroblastic anemia is characterized by the presence of ringed sideroblasts in the bone marrow. Sideroblasts are erythroblasts (immature red blood cells) that contain iron that has accumulated in the mitochondria. Thus, instead of using the iron to make hemoglobin, it gets stuck in the mitochondria. This not only slows down energy production in the cell, but it also leads to less hemoglobin production, allowing for less oxygen transportation, less oxygen delivery—which further slows down energy production. It should be known that a B6 deficiency is only one cause to sideroblastic anemia, low copper, genetic mutations, heavy metal poisoning, and alcoholism are also contributors,

Consuming foods with B6 like milk, pork, chicken, eggs, and beef can improve a B6 deficiency, which can improve hemoglobin production. For those with sideroblastic anemia, and who have iron accumulation, it may be more beneficial to consume a B6 supplement, as pyridoxal phosphate (naturally found in animal foods), as it is the most bioavailable form. 50-200mg of B6 a day has been shown to restore red blood cell production (16).

Copper and oxygen transportation

Copper is involved in the use and transportation of oxygen. As discussed in the last chapter, copper is an essential component of the enzyme cytochrome c oxidase. This enzyme located at complex IV of the ETC is crucial for the final step of cellular respiration, where oxygen is utilized. Cytochrome c oxidase transfers the electrons for cytochrome c to oxygen, the final electron acceptor in the ETC. This reaction reduces O_2 to water and keeps the ETC moving to make more energy.

In addition, copper is a core part of the enzymes ceruloplasmin and hephaestin, which help iron transition from its ferrous (Fe^{2+}) form to ferric (Fe^{3+}). This very important step is essential because only ferric iron can bind to transferrin (your iron delivery trucks), the main transport protein that delivers iron through your blood. Once iron is bound to transferrin, it can be safely escorted to various tissues, including bone marrow, where it's used to synthesize hemoglobin.

And finally, copper is also involved in mobilizing stored iron from places like the liver, spleen, and bone marrow, making it available for new red blood cell production, energy metabolism, and thyroid hormone creation. Without enough copper (and thus without properly functioning ceruloplasmin), iron gets stuck in the gut lining or liver and never makes it into circulation. Thus, it is unable to reach your mitochondria or hemoglobin factories, leaving you with all the signs of anemia, even if your total body iron is technically adequate or even elevated.

In addition to iron, B12, folate, B6, and copper, zinc and magnesium are needed for oxygen utilization and transportation. Zinc is a cofactor for several enzymes that are involved in the synthesis of hemoglobin. Magnesium is a cofactor for numerous enzymes involved in the production of red blood cells. A deficiency in either would hinder the production of our oxygen transportation vehicles and cargo carries, limiting oxygen getting to the tissues.

If you have ever been anemic, like me, you know that when you are deficient in iron, or any of the nutrients that support iron regulation or hemoglobin or red cell production, you feel pretty crappy. Anemia is going to inhibit hemoglobin and red cell production, decreasing the transportation of oxygen, and lowering tissue oxygen. This is going to present as fatigue, blurry vision, increased heart rate, tight neck and shoulder muscles, sleep issues, and possible loss of hair, which are all things I suffered from. The good news is if you eat a diet rich in foods containing iron, copper, zinc, B vitamins, and magnesium, you have a good chance of fixing your issues. And yes, it can be that simple.

I know I have said it many times before, but I think it deserves mentioning again, there are two super foods that can supply you with most of these oxygenating nutrients. Beef liver will give you plenty of B12, B6, iron, copper, and zinc. Oysters are filled with zinc, copper, iron, and B12. These two nutrient-rich foods can contribute to healthy hemoglobin and red blood cell production, while supporting iron regulation and oxygen utilization. Of course, there are other foods that can work, like beef, chicken, lamb, eggs, mussels, clams, dairy, and well-cooked greens—but beef liver and oysters are still the best.

In the final part of this chapter, I want to share a few simple breathing techniques that can help improve oxygen delivery to your tissues. These are practices I've used myself and with clients. They consistently help people relax, sleep more deeply, feel more energized, and release tension in the neck and shoulders.

As you know, when your tissues become less oxygenated, your muscles tighten, your energy drops, your sleep becomes restless, and your nervous system stays stuck in that "tired and wired" state. You've already learned that nutrient deficiencies can lower tissue oxygenation and that a nutrient-rich diet can fix that. But what if the issue isn't nutrition at all? What if it's the way you breathe?

Well, then it's time to learn to breathe better.

For most of us, breathing is something we rarely think about, it just happens. In fact, it happens about 18,000–25,000/day. Yet the way we breathe can have a major impact on how we feel, move, and sleep. For many of us, subtle breathing habits, like shallow chest breathing or mouth breathing, quietly reduce how much oxygen reaches our tissues.

So, for the sake of improving the oxygenation of our tissue, it's worth focusing on a few targeted breathing exercises. Each of the techniques that follow has been shown to improve tissue oxygenation in scientific studies, which will help with things like sleep, energy, happiness, and overall well-being.

Better Breathing Techniques

Here are four breathing exercises that can improve your tissue oxygenation.

1. Diaphragmatic Breathing (Deep Belly Breathing): Diaphragmatic breathing involves deep breathing that engages the diaphragm, the muscle located at the base of the lungs. It focuses on filling the lungs with air by expanding the belly rather than the chest.

This type of breathing increases lung capacity and improves oxygen exchange by allowing more air to reach the lower lobes of the lungs, where blood flow is greatest. It also helps to reduce stress, lower heart rate, and improve overall respiratory efficiency.

A study in the *Indian Journal of Physiology and Pharmacology* examined the effects of diaphragmatic breathing on respiratory strength and oxygen saturation in healthy adults. The study found that participants who practiced deep breathing improved their respiratory rate, chest expansion, and oxygen saturation (17).

How to do it:

1. Sit or lie down in a comfortable position.
2. Place one hand on your chest and the other on your abdomen.
3. Inhale deeply through your nose, allowing your abdomen to rise as you fill your lungs with air.
4. Exhale slowly through your mouth or nose, allowing your abdomen to fall.
5. Repeat for several minutes, focusing on deep, slow breaths.
6. Try this every day for four weeks, and notice if your energy and sleep improve.

2. Box Breathing (Square Breathing): Box breathing involves inhaling, holding the breath, exhaling, and holding the breath again, each for an equal count (usually 4 seconds).

Box breathing helps to regulate the autonomic nervous system, reduce stress, and improve oxygen delivery to tissues by promoting a regular breathing pattern and increasing lung capacity.

A 2003 study in *Applied Psychophysiology and Biofeedback* explored the effects of controlled breathing techniques, including box breathing, on heart rate variability (HRV) and stress reduction. The study found that slow, controlled breathing, such as box breathing, significantly improved HRV and reduced stress levels (18).

How to do it:

1. Inhale slowly through your nose for a count of 4.

2. Hold your breath for a count of 4.

3. Exhale slowly through your mouth for a count of 4.

4. Hold your breath again for a count of 4.

5. Repeat for several cycles, focusing on maintaining a consistent rhythm.

6. Repeat several times a day for about 1-2 minutes each time.

7. Observe your sleep, energy levels, and back and neck tension.

3. Resonance Breathing (Coherent Breathing): Resonance breathing involves slow, rhythmic breathing at a rate of about 5-6 breaths per minute, which is the optimal rate for balancing the autonomic nervous system.

This breathing pattern has been shown to improve heart rate variability (HRV), reduce stress, and enhance oxygen delivery to tissues by optimizing the balance between oxygen intake and carbon dioxide elimination.

A 2014 study in the *International Journal of Psychophysiology* studying the effects of resonant breathing on stress and nervous system regulation, found that resonant breathing improved HRV, reduced stress, and regulated the ANS, all of which contributed to better oxygenation of tissue (19).

How to do it:

1. Inhale slowly through your nose for a count of 5.

2. Exhale slowly through your mouth or nose for a count of 5.

3. Breathe through your belly and expand your chest, not raising your shoulders.

4. Repeat for several minutes, maintaining a calm and steady rhythm.

5. Observe your energy levels, internal stress, sleep, and back and neck tension.

4. Pranayama (Yoga Breathing): Pranayama involves various breathing exercises practiced in yoga that focus on controlling the breath and expanding lung capacity.

Certain pranayama techniques, such as Nadi Shodhana (alternate nostril breathing) are known to enhance oxygenation, improve lung function, and promote relaxation and mental clarity.

A 2004 study in the *Indian Journal of Medical Research* investigated the effects of different pranayama techniques on lung function and oxygenation. The study found that participants who practiced pranayama showed significant improvements in lung function, oxygen saturation, and overall respiratory efficiency (20).

How to do it:

1. Close your right nostril with your thumb, inhale slowly through your left nostril, then close your left nostril with your ring finger and exhale through your right nostril. Inhale through your right nostril, then switch and exhale through your left nostril. Repeat the cycle.

2. Repeat this for about 2-3 minutes daily

3. Observe your energy level, tension in your neck, and sleep levels.

As with most things that improve your health, doing breathing exercises consistently and frequently is what is going to make the most difference. Trying a breathing technique for a single minute, one time, is not going to make any sort of noticeable difference. I suggest trying the breathing technique that feels best to you and that you believe you can perform daily. Give yourself at least 4 weeks of practice before you decide if it is working or not. The benefits of most breathing techniques accumulate over time.

Alright, so there you have it. You now have a good understanding of how important oxygen is for energy production. You now know the main reason for breathing; you need oxygen to be the final electron acceptor (Remember O_2 is the recycle bin). Without O_2 accepting the final electrons, energy production comes to a screeching halt. You also learned how important CO_2 production is for assisting O_2 into the cell, and why if CO_2 production is limited, O_2 in the tissue can also be limited.

In addition, you now know all the nutrients (and foods) that are needed for oxygen delivery and utilization—a vital step in getting oxygen to get where it needs to be—your cells. And finally, you have learned specific breathing techniques that can improve how well your tissues are oxygenated.

You can now take a deep, long, belly breath knowing you now have usable tools and information that can help improve how well your cells breathe. And when your cells breathe better, you live longer, healthier, and happier.

Ok, are you ready for the last and final thing that you absolutely need to produce optimal energy production? The next chapter is all about the amazing, metabolically supportive, CEO of energy production—thyroid hormone.

CHAPTER 4

Why Do We Breathe?
The Importance of Oxygen (and CO_2)

1. You breathe so oxygen can serve as the final electron acceptor in energy production. O_2 clears the last electrons so the electron transport chain keeps moving and ATP keeps flowing.

2. Your cells make carbon dioxide (CO_2) during energy production. CO_2 helps O_2 get into the tissues, supports vasodilation, and has antioxidant-like effects.

3. Red blood cells and hemoglobin carry oxygen. Their production and upkeep requires protein plus iron, copper, zinc, vitamin A, B6, B12, folate, and magnesium.

4. Top foods for healthy RBCs and hemoglobin: beef liver, oysters and other shellfish, beef, lamb, egg yolks, dairy, and well-cooked leafy greens.

5. Simple breathing practices include diaphragmatic (belly) breathing, box breathing, coherent/resonance breathing, and pranayama. Each can improve CO_2 balance and tissue oxygenation.

CHAPTER 5

THYROID HORMONE—YOUR
CELL'S ENERGY DIAL

Now that you know how important optimal fuel, nutrients, and oxygen are for ATP production, it's time to discuss the hormone that oversees this grand energy operation: thyroid hormone.

Yes, let's talk about the CEO of our cell's factories and power plants, the maestro of metabolism, the one hormone that tells your cells to rev things up or take a nap. Think of thyroid hormone as your energy dial on the power grid. Need more power? Crank that dial up, and voilà—more ATP. Feel like conserving energy? Dial it down, and you'll have just enough to keep yourself alive.

Thyroid hormone is the unsung hero behind how you regulate everything from your body temperature to how well you sleep. It's one reason why you can go ski outside in the winter without turning into a popsicle, and why you can muster up enough energy to enjoy the day. Without enough thyroid hormone, you might feel like an old car trying to start on a cold morning—slow, sluggish, and in desperate need of a tune-up. We're talking cold hands, poor digestion, hair that prefers to be on your brush rather than your head, and a sex drive that's more "meh" than "let's go!"

In the medical world, when your thyroid decides to throw a wild party (gets too high), we call it hyperthyroidism. And when it's more of a hibernation situation (goes too low), that's hypothyroidism. The typical response? If you're hypothyroid, here, take some thyroid medication. If you're hyperthyroid, let's calm things down with different meds to slow the party.

Simple, right?

Well, not exactly. As with most things in the body, there's a bit more nuance involved—like whether you need meds or if your body just needs additional (non-hormone) support. You see, sometimes fixing your low thyroid has nothing to do with needing to take an exogenous thyroid hormone, as numerous variables can contribute to a low thyroid state.

How well your thyroid is working will depend on how well YOU are doing. Meaning, your thyroid is responding to the environment in which it is living, which is you. If your body is stressed, undernourished, or restricting carbs, your thyroid will down regulate to conserve energy. If you are well-nourished, healthy, oxygenated, and require more energy, it will upregulate to support your increased energy demands.

In this chapter, I'll dive into the nitty-gritty of thyroid hormone—how it's made, the nutrients it requires, how it gets around the body, and what happens when it finally reaches its destination at the cellular level. I'll talk about all the things that can interfere with thyroid production and conversion. I'll go into why taking a thyroid hormone might not be the first thing you should do if you have low thyroid symptoms. I'll talk about all the things you can do to optimize your thyroid hormone levels. And finally, I'll discuss the different types of exogenous thyroid hormones, which ones work best, and what you should experience when your exogenous thyroid hormone is working properly.

Let's get this thyroid party started!

The HPT-Axis

First up is the Hypothalamus-Pituitary-Thyroid (HPT) Axis. This is the regulatory system for maintaining optimal thyroid hormone levels. The start of thyroid production starts with the hypothalamus, a small, almond-sized structure located at the base of your brain. The hypothalamus can sense a decrease of thyroid hormone in the blood. In response to this decrease, the hypothalamus increases thyrotropin-releasing hormone (TRH). TRH sends a signal to the pituitary gland to secrete thyroid-stimulating hormone (TSH).

The pituitary gland, often referred to as the "master gland," is a small, pea-sized gland located at the base of the brain, just below the hypothalamus. The pituitary gland plays a central role in regulating the endocrine system by releasing hormones that signal other glands to produce their own hormones, one of those being TSH. Most people know of TSH, as it is the hormone most medical doctors take to assess thyroid health, even though it is a pituitary hormone.

TSH prompts the thyroid gland to produce and release thyroid hormones. When enough thyroid hormones are produced, TSH and TRH decrease. However, if the thyroid is unable to produce enough thyroid hormones, TSH and TRH can remain elevated. This elevation can be a sign you have hypothyroidism, or low thyroid production (1).

The Thyroid

The thyroid gland is located in the front of your neck and resembles a butterfly. This is the control center behind your body's energy production (cell's mitochondria or power plants). This gland is responsible for cranking out two important hormones, triiodothyronine (T3) and thyroxine (T4), which keep your metabolism fired up. There's also a third hormone called calcitonin that handles calcium and phosphate metabolism like a true multitasker, but, for now, let's focus on the energy-boosting duo: T3 and T4—the real stars of the thyroid world.

Now, making these thyroid hormones isn't a simple task. It all starts with two fancy (yes, fancy) biochemical reactions: iodination and coupling. Iodination occurs when the residue of the amino acid tyrosine is added to iodine atoms. This happens on a large glycoprotein called thyroglobulin and is facilitated by the enzyme thyroid peroxidase (TPO). TPO adds iodine to the tyrosine residues on thyroglobulin, creating monoiodotyrosine (MIT) and diiodotyrosine (DIT). MIT is one (mono) iodine atom and tyrosine, while DIT is two (di) iodine and tyrosine.

TPO then catalyzes the coupling (the linking) of two iodinated tyrosine residues: One DIT with another DIT, to form thyroxine (T4), or one MIT with one DIT to form triiodothyronine (T3).

Think of tyrosine and the mineral iodine as the raw material making up your thyroid, thyroglobulin as the scaffolding where thyroid hormone is being produced, and the enzyme TPO as the "workers" that are making the thyroid. Essentially, your thyroid is the mini-manufacturing plant that makes your thyroid hormones.

Once these thyroid hormones are made, thyroglobulin takes on a new role as a storage container. It holds onto T3 and T4 until your body sends out a signal (courtesy of thyroid-stimulating hormone, (or TSH) that it's time to release the goods. Then the thyroid cells jump into action, breaking down thyroglobulin and letting your thyroid hormones, T3 and T4, flow into your bloodstream. This very intelligent system ensures that your body always has enough thyroid hormones ready to keep your energy levels balanced and your metabolism running smoothly (2).

Thyroid Hormones

Thyroxine (T4) is the primary thyroid hormone. Approximately 80-90% of your thyroid hormone produced by the thyroid is thyroxine. T4 is made up of a tyrosine backbone and four iodine atoms, that is why it has a "4" in its name. T4 is considered your inactive thyroid hormone, as it needs to be converted (an iodine removed) into T3 to be used by the cell. Essentially, T4 serves as a prohormone (a precursor to a hormone) that can be converted into active T3 if the body needs it.

Triiodothyronine (T3), and yes, it is a mouth full, is referred to as your active thyroid. T3 consists of a tyrosine backbone and three iodine atoms. Only 10-20% of your thyroid hormone produced by your thyroid is in the form of T3. Most of your T3 is produced from your T4 converting into T3 in the peripheral tissues (organs, muscle, glands, brain), rather than the thyroid gland itself. The primary sites of your thyroid conversion are your liver (about 40%) and your kidneys (about 20%). To some degree, your skeletal muscles, brain, fat tissue, and pituitary gland are other sites that support T4 to T3 conversion.

T4 is converted into T3 in the peripheral tissues via the deiodinase enzymes. There are three different deiodinase enzymes—D1, D2, and D3. The job of each deiodinase enzyme is to remove an iodine atom from T4 to make T3.

Type 1 deiodinase (D1) primary role is to work within the liver and kidneys to produce T3 that enters the bloodstream rather than local cellular production. Type 2 deiodinase (D2) converts T4 into T3 in your skeletal muscles, brain, fat tissue, and pituitary (3). D2's primary role is to produce T3 *in the cell* that is to be used locally. About 20% of your T4 to T3 is converted inside the cell and is a big reason why blood levels of T3 are not completely accurate, blood labs only measure what is in the blood, not the cell.

In addition, it is important to mention another hormone related to thyroid health called reverse T3 (rT3). Although rT3 is not produced by the thyroid, it is produced by T4, via three deiodinase enzymes (D3). D3 is upregulated under stress. Reverse T3 is the inactive form of thyroid hormone. The T4 to rT3 conversion occurs when the body needs to lower its metabolic rate to conserve energy. Instead of producing active T3 to rev things up, the body produces rT3, to slow things down. This can happen during illness, fasting, severe stress, and starvation (extreme dieting) (4).

It should be noted that reverse T3 is not a bad thing, as it can work to protect you in times of stress. You don't want your body to have an increased metabolic rate when fuel is not available for a long time, as your body would have to use more of you (your organs, muscles, skin) as its fuel source. It's like trying to heat your entire house but using the house as the wood (fuel). It would be smarter to heat only one room (slow metabolism) so that you can limit the house breakdown.

At the same time, you must remember what rT3 is doing—it is slowing down energy production. When you are converting more T4 to rT3, you are producing less active thyroid hormone. Less T3, less energy production. In addition, rT3 can compete with T3 for binding sites to thyroid hormone receptors. Yet, unlike T3, rT3 does not activate the receptors (5). Which means that when rT3 occupies the receptor site, it blocks T3 from binding to receptors, reducing thyroid activity even more. This competition is particularly relevant in conditions where rT3 stays elevated like chronic stress or illness, which can lead to symptoms of hypothyroidism despite normal thyroid levels (more on this later).

This is another reason why measuring your T3 levels may not give you a complete picture as to what is going on in your cells. You can have completely normal T3 levels, but with excessive rT3, the T3 may be unable to get into the cell, as rT3 is bound to the receptor site. This may make you ask the question, "Are blood thyroid labs a good metric for thyroid levels?"

The Problem with Thyroid Blood Labs

The problem with testing blood levels of thyroid hormones is they only tell you what is in the blood, not the cell. And the cell is the only place that really matters as it is where all the action takes place. The blood is just the highway system thyroid hormone is traveling through—it is not the destination where thyroid hormone works.

Like I said above, for T3 to work, it must enter the cell directly or get produced inside the cell. Inactive reverse T3, which is produced under stress, can bind to the same receptor sites as T3. Thus, rT3 will block T3 from getting into the cell. This can lead to normal levels of free T3 and free T4 in the blood, but less activity in the cell.

In addition, most medical doctors only measure TSH to test for thyroid health. Oddly enough, TSH is a pituitary hormone, not a thyroid hormone. TSH tells the thyroid to release T3 and T4. High levels of TSH can mean your thyroid is unable to produce enough thyroid hormone, leading to hypothyroidism. While very low levels of TSH can mean you are producing too much thyroid hormone, leading to hyperthyroidism.

What most people are unaware of is chronically high cortisol can suppress TSH, giving the illusion that you are hyperthyroid, when you might just be hyper-cortisol. Meaning if you have been under a lot of stress, and get your TSH checked, you may come back with normal, high, or lower TSH levels. Yet, your thyroid production has slowed down, due to cortisol suppressing TSH. This occurs as an adaptive measure to deal with your stressed state. This is one reason why some people will experience higher levels of TSH once they start to heal and lower their cortisol levels, as cortisol is no longer suppressing TSH (6, 7, 8).

FUN FACT: Chronically high cortisol levels can suppress TSH, but acute (short term) stress can increase TSH. The initial response by the body can be to produce more thyroid hormone to keep up with the increased demands. Yet, if the stress continues, and resources are limited, the body will suppress TSH and thyroid production, to limit energy production, particularly in non-life-threatening areas (digestion, hormone production, energy levels, hair growth).

All this means is blood labs are not the end all when it comes to understanding your thyroid health. They can give you some insight, but they do not tell you everything. So, if your doctor tells you that your thyroid levels are normal, and you still feel like sh#t, just know you are not alone and you are not crazy. You can still have issues with thyroid activity (in the cell) with normal blood levels.

Thyroid Blood Labs 101

Here is a list of thyroid tests, what they represent, and why they can be deceiving.

Thyroid stimulating hormone (TSH) - TSH tells the thyroid to produce T3 and T4. Yet, it can be suppressed by cortisol, giving the illusion that thyroid levels are fine, when they are not.

Free T3 - Free T3 is a thyroid hormone that is not bound to a transport protein. Free T3 is considered active because it can enter the cell. Yet, you can have normal levels of free T3 in the blood, but it is unable to get into the cell due to excessive rT3.

Free T4 - Free T4 is T4 that is not bound to a transport protein. Free T4 is active, as it can enter the cell—yet still needs to be converted to T3 in the cell. Free T4 is only slightly active and still needs to convert to T3 in the liver and kidneys or in the cell.

Total T3 - Total T3 consists of free T3 and bound T3 in the blood. Most of the T3 in the blood is bound—only 0.3% is free. Bound T3 is inactive and needs to become unbound to enter the cell.

Total T4 - Total T4 consists of free T4 and bound T4 in the blood. Like T3, most of T4 is bound in the blood—only 0.3% is free. Bound T4 is inactive, and needs to become unbound to enter the cell.

Reverse T3 (rT3) - Reverse T3 is inactive T3 produced via the 3-deiodinase enzyme when the body is under stress.

Excessively high levels of rT3 can inhibit T3 from getting into the cell.

Thyroid peroxidase antibodies (TPOAb) - These antibodies are directed against the enzyme that is involved in thyroid hormone production. Remember TPO is needed to add iodine to the tyrosine backbone. It is very possible to have elevated antibodies without any thyroid dysfunction.

Thyroglobulin antibodies (TgAb) - These antibodies work against thyroglobulin, the protein (scaffolding) that helps produce thyroid hormones. TgAb can be elevated without any other signs of thyroid dysfunction.

Cholesterol - Although cholesterol is not a thyroid metric, checking cholesterol is a good marker to see if you are having thyroid issues. Most people with low T3 (either from low production or conversion) will have elevated cholesterol, since T3 is needed for cholesterol to convert into your steroidal hormones. If you are low in T3, less cholesterol will convert, and cholesterol (total and LDL) will be elevated.

What Nutrients are Needed for Thyroid Production?

If you remember from Chapter 3, nutrients are essential substances our bodies need to produce energy and maintain structure, including macronutrients (carbs, fats, protein) and micronutrients (vitamins and minerals). Some of these same nutrients (and a few others) are needed for thyroid production and conversion. The amino acid tyrosine, vitamin A, the minerals iodine, selenium, zinc, and iron, and glucose are all needed to produce or help convert inactive T4 into active T3. A lack of any of these nutrients could contribute to a low thyroid state.

Like I said above, the amino acid tyrosine makes up the backbone of all thyroid hormones. This means consuming enough quality protein is essential for thyroid production. Your best sources of tyrosine come from animal proteins, like eggs, milk, meat, fish, and organs. Tyrosine is also found in plant proteins like soy and tempeh. Your body can also produce its own tyrosine through the synthesis of phenylalanine in the liver.

When it comes to thyroid production, the mineral iodine is crucial for producing both T4 and T3. The thyroid gland, regulated by TSH, absorbs iodine from the bloodstream and incorporates it into thyroid hormone molecules. Inside the thyroid, iodine binds to tyrosine to form MIT (1 iodine) and DIT (2 iodine). The molecules then couple up to form T4 (4 iodine) and T3 (3 iodine).

Without enough iodine, you will have low thyroid production. This is the reason salt became iodized back in the early 20th century—as a health measure to combat widespread iodine deficiency. These deficiencies lead to significant health problems including goiters (enlarged thyroid due to low iodine) and hypothyroidism. Despite iodized salt being a source of iodine, it is not something I normally recommend—at least if you are consuming a healthy diet.

Why?

For every ¼ tsp of iodized salt you get about 85 mcg of iodine. You only need about 150 mcg a day. Thus, most people overconsume iodine if they consume a lot of this salt. And just like everything in nutrition—too little can produce a negative response, and too much can do the same. Too little iodine can create hypothyroidism and so can too much—yikes! Excessive iodine intake can inhibit the thyroid's ability to produce thyroid hormone by temporarily shutting it down to protect the body from an overproduction of hormones—this phenomenon is known as the Wolff-Chaikoff effect.

This is why I don't ever recommend iodine supplements either—as someone can easily overdo their iodine intake. My recommendation is to always get your nutrients from food. Good iodine sources include milk, seafood, eggs, and other dairy products. If you are looking for a plant alternative, you can get plenty of iodine from kelp and seaweed.

Another important mineral needed for active thyroid production is selenium. Remember the deiodinase enzymes from earlier? The deiodinase enzymes are needed to convert T4 into T3. The deiodinase enzymes are considered selenoproteins, as selenium is a key component of their structure. A deficiency in selenium can lead to reduced activity of the deiodinase enzymes, leading to lower levels of active T3 thyroid. Foods rich in selenium are seafood, organ meats, eggs, and Brazil nuts. A daily intake of 55-200 mcg is generally recommended (9).

The mineral zinc is also needed in thyroid hormone production and conversion. Zinc plays a crucial role in the activity of TPO (thyroid peroxidase), the enzyme that is essential for thyroid production. Zinc is also a cofactor for all the deiodinase enzymes, which are needed to convert inactive T4 into active T3. If this conversion is impaired, someone will experience low peripheral T3 levels, leading to hypothyroid-like symptoms. Essentially, zinc is needed for both thyroid hormone production and conversion (10, 11). As I have said before, a weekly serving of oysters (about a dozen each week) is your best food source of zinc, yet other shellfish, white fish, and dairy can also provide you with adequate zinc.

Iron is the fourth essential mineral that is needed for normal production and conversion of thyroid hormones. Iron is a cofactor for TPO. Without sufficient iron, TPO activity is impaired, reducing the thyroid gland's ability to produce adequate levels of T4 and T3. In addition, iron is also needed for T4 to T3 conversion, as iron is needed for proper function of the deiodinase enzymes (12, 13). Beef liver, red meat, and oysters are great iron sources.

What is also interesting about the connection between iron and thyroid is, when someone is hypothyroid, iron absorption decreases. Iron absorption is dependent on thyroid levels, and thyroid levels are dependent on iron availability. This viscous cycle can create an even deeper state of slow metabolism.

In addition, the deiodinase enzymes rely on proper gene expression to function effectively. Vitamin A, through its active form, retinoic acid, can modulate the expression of genes involved in encoding these enzymes. This helps ensure that the deiodinase enzymes are available and functioning properly to convert T4 into the more active T3. In other words, vitamin A acts like a coach, it helps "train" the deiodinase enzymes so that they can maximize thyroid conversion.

All this means is a deficiency of vitamin A can negatively impact thyroid levels (14). It also means that if thyroid levels are low due to low vitamin A, increasing your vitamin A consumption can improve thyroid levels. Foods high in vitamin A are beef liver (I know this recommendation is getting annoying, but you can see how powerful it is), egg yolks, whole milk and dairy, and salmon.

FUN FACT: Plant-based foods like carrots contain no vitamin A. Vitamin A is only found in animal foods. Plant-based foods contain beta-carotene, which is a provitamin (precursor to vitamin A). Your body cannot use beta carotene directly, it can only use Vitamin A—thus, your body must convert beta carotene into vitamin A. If someone is low thyroid, the conversion of beta carotene to vitamin A becomes inhibited (15). You can see these types of people from a million miles away as they will have orange skin (16). Instead of converting the beta carotene, you will store it in your tissue, making you look like an Oompa-Loompa from Charlie and the Chocolate Factory.

And finally, considering most T3 is produced in the liver, it is essential that the liver is well-fed. Glucose is the primary fuel source of the liver, thus making sure you are eating enough carbohydrates will support T3 production. It has been shown in numerous studies that those on a low-carb or keto diet produce lower levels of T3 (17,18,19). As I have talked about numerous times in this book, any time you restrict carbohydrates, you will be pushing your body into a stressed response. This stress response will hinder thyroid production and conversion.

How is Thyroid Hormone Transported to the Cells?

Thyroid hormones (T4 and T3) are transported to the cells via the blood. Most T4 and T3 are bound to transport proteins, consisting of thyroxine (thyroid)-binding globulin (TBG), transthyretin, and albumin. A small fraction (less than1%) of thyroid hormones is unbound or free. Thyroid hormone bound to transport proteins is believed to be inactive. Most research suggests that only the free unbound thyroid hormone is considered active, as it can cross cell membranes.

However, just to keep things interesting, there is evidence that protein-bound T4 and T3, specifically *within the mitochondria—* can play a metabolically active role. In his article, titled, "Thyroid: Therapies, Confusion, and Fraud," Dr. Raymond Peat points to numerous studies showing that mitochondrial thyroid hormone-binding proteins can directly affect mitochondrial function, disputing the belief that "only" free thyroid hormones are metabolically active (20, 21). To be clear, those bound to TBG, transthyretin, and albumin in the blood, are not metabolically active.

FUN FACT: Transthyretin also transports Vitamin A (retinol) indirectly by binding to retinol-binding protein (RBP), forming a complex that delivers vitamin A to various tissues. Consuming an excessive amount of vitamin A can limit the ability of transthyretin to carry thyroid hormone, which could contribute to a hypothyroid-like state. This means too little and too much vitamin A can contribute to hypothyroidism.

The fact that so many nutrients can have good and bad properties, depending on their dosage, is a huge reason why I suggest eating food for your nutrients. It is harder to overdose on nutrients with food alone as most excessive nutrient consumption comes from supplements.

Thyroxine-binding globulin (TBG) has the highest affinity for thyroid hormone; due to this, it transports most of the thyroid hormones throughout the bloodstream. Approximately 75% of circulating T4 and 70% of T3 is bound to TBG (22). Transthyretin and albumin can both carry other substances, thus limiting their ability to carry thyroid hormone.

How Does Thyroid Hormone Work in the Cell?

Alright, buckle up, because this is where the science of thyroid hormone goes from "What?" to "Whoa, that's pretty damn amazing!"

Once in the bloodstream, free (unbound) T3 and T4 are like the head managers of a sprawling factory (cell). They've got important work to do, but before they can make all their decisions, they need to get inside. Unfortunately, their chaperones—the transport proteins—are too large to enter the plant, so they drop off T3 and T4 at the cell membrane (think of it as the power plant's security gate).

Now, even though T3 and T4 are the big CEOs, they can't just stroll into the factory. They need to pass through the security guards, aka the membrane transporters. The two most important guards on duty are monocarboxylate transporter 8 (MCT8), which specializes in letting T3 through, and organic anion transporting polypeptide (OATP), which is flexible and can bring in both T3 and T4. Without these membrane transporters, T3 and T4 cannot enter the cell—so they are very important!

Once they get inside the factory (the cell), T4 must go through a little upgrade—this is when the Type 2 deiodinase (D2) enzyme comes in and converts T4 into T3. *Yes, this happens inside the cell!* The D2 enzyme is used inside the cell, allowing the cell to make its own T3 as needed. Just another reminder why blood levels of T3 can be misleading, as they do not measure the thyroid inside the cell!

At this point, T3 is ready to influence cellular metabolism. It has two main choices; head to the nucleus (the factory's control room) where it can adjust how the whole cell (factory) is run, or head directly to the mitochondria (the power plant), where it can boost ATP production.

Getting into the Nucleus—The Control Room

First let's look at T3 in the nucleus of the cell. Now that T3 is in the cell, what's next? Well, your cell is like a big energy-producing factory, and the nucleus is the control room where all the big decisions are made. Our newly arrived T3 is like a manager—ready to make things happen. When T3 enters the nucleus, it binds to thyroid hormone receptors (TRs) already sitting on specific spots of the DNA called thyroid response elements (TREs). TRs form with T3, forming a TR-T3 complex which affects gene expression in the cell. TREs act as binding sites for the TR-T3 complex. This binding activates or represses the transcription of specific genes.

Ummm—what?

Think of the TR-T3 complex as a specialized manager that comes with an instruction manual in hand, deciding which machines (genes) should be turned on or off in the factory (cell). These genes control all the critical processes that power the factory—like metabolism, protein synthesis, and energy production. The TR-T3 complex acts on the TREs (control panels) to either activate (crank up the energy) or repress (slow it down) depending on what's needed.

But Wait, What About Mitochondria?

If the nucleus is the control room, then remember that the mitochondria are the power plants inside the cell—the place where most of your energy is made. T3 can also head straight to the mitochondria to boost ATP production. This is where we see T3 bind to specific mitochondrial-specific proteins, rather than the typical thyroid hormone receptor (TR) found in the nucleus. This is the one place that "bound" T3 is metabolically active.

In the mitochondria, T3 increases the efficiency of the electron transport chain (ETC) and increases the rate of oxidative phosphorylation, thereby increasing oxygen consumption and ATP production. Essentially, this can give the cell an instant energy boost, whether it's building muscle, keeping your heart beating faster, keeping your bones, hair, and skin healthy, or producing heat to warm you up in cold environments.

Whether it is being used in the cell's mitochondria or nucleus, T3 is critical to nearly every cell in the body. Yet, depending on the cell's location, T3 can produce different metabolic effects.

Finally, here is the amazing part about T3—it has a role in almost everything!

Here is a list of how T3 acts on certain tissues and cells:

1. In the **liver** and **muscles**, T3 increases carbohydrate and fat metabolism to increase energy and heat production.

2. **Liver.** T3 promotes the conversion of cholesterol into bile acids and steroidal hormones, which can help reduce blood cholesterol levels (23, 24). T3 also supports liver enzymes that support detoxification of chemicals, hormones, drugs, etc.

3. **Muscles.** T3 promotes protein synthesis and breakdown. This helps maintain muscle mass and overall energy production.

4. **Heart.** T3 helps the heart pump stronger and faster, increasing heart rate, stroke volume, and cardiac output. Dr. Broda Barnes, a prominent physician, was well known for linking hypothyroidism to numerous chronic diseases including atherosclerosis (hardening of arteries) and heart disease. He discussed in his book, *Hypothyroidism: The Unsuspected Illness*, how he successfully treated his patients with thyroid hormones to "cure" chronic degenerative diseases, including heart disease (25).

5. **Brain.** T3 can regulate mood, memory, and cognitive function. This is why those with hypothyroidism can

have impaired cognitive function and memory problems.
These are people who are under stress, aging, or
anything that could be connected to being stressed—
like menopause. Yes, menopause can be a stress to
your system. Go to Chapters 6, 10, and 11 for more
information on this.

6. **Adipose tissue.** T3 stimulates thermogenesis (heat
    production). This is particularly important for
    maintaining body temperature in cold environments.
    This is also a big reason why measuring your body
    temperature can give you insight on your thyroid
    usage. When using thyroid hormone effectively, body
    temperature will elevate—ideally to 98.6 F or 37 C.
    When thyroid (or other factors lowering metabolism) is
    low, body temperature will drop—this is a sign you are
    conserving energy.

7. **Bone.** T3 influences both bone formation (via
    osteoblasts) and bone resorption (via osteoclasts),
    playing a key role in bone growth and bone density. Yes,
    bone health has a lot to do with thyroid function.

8. **Skin.** T3 promotes normal skin cell turnover, helping to
    maintain healthy skin.

9. **Hair.** T3 also regulates hair's growth cycle. Thus, those
    who are hypothyroid can experience hair thinning or loss.

10. **The gut.** T3 helps regulate enzyme production, gut
    motility, and stomach acid production. T3 also helps
    maintain the intestinal lining, helping maintain the gut's
    integrity and function. Those with hypothyroid can have
    decreased enzyme production, gut motility, and stomach
    acid production leading to constipation, SIBO, poor
    nutrient absorption, bloating, and other gut issues.

11. **The ovaries.** T3 enhances the survival, proliferation, and
    follicle development during a women's cycle (26).

The bottom line is, thyroid hormone, particularly T3, is damn amazing. This single hormone can influence almost every metabolic process in your body. T3 is your body's go-to manager for keeping every cell healthy and functioning properly. Whether it's turning up the energy production in the mitochondria, keeping the heart beating fast, helping to make more muscle, building strong bones, or making sure your brain stays sharp, T3 is a rock star!

Things that Interfere with Thyroid Production and Conversion

Alright, now that you know about how your thyroid hormone is made, how it moves through the body and acts in each individual cell, it is important to understand what can interfere with thyroid hormone production and conversion. Some people may not be able to produce enough thyroid hormone and are truly hypothyroid, while others do not have a thyroid issue, but rather an inability to convert T4 into T3—so they show signs of low thyroid hormone, even though their thyroid is working properly.

Just for a quick reminder, someone who has low thyroid production or conversion will end up creating less ATP, due to glucose or fat moving through the cell's mitochondria more slowly. Remember thyroid hormone is the dial that turns up energy production. Low thyroid levels will have similar symptoms to anything that inhibits energy production. This includes all the things we have already talked about like lack of fuel, nutrients, and oxygen. Each one of these, including thyroid, plays a role in how well (and fast) your fuel sources are converted into ATP.

This is why symptoms of low thyroid look very similar to the symptoms of other health issues including a deficiency in B vitamins, iron anemia, poor breathing, low fuel intake, etc. They all are working toward the same goal, to produce energy for your body. Each one is equally important when it comes to making ATP, as a lack of any of these can contribute to a low energy state, including fatigue, slow digestion, infertility, low libido, feeling cold, hair loss, painful periods, anxiety, depression, etc.

Ok, back to things that interfere with thyroid hormone production and conversion.

Let's talk about the inhibition of thyroid hormone production first, or what most people refer to as hypothyroidism.

Hypothyroidism -Hypothyroidism is when your thyroid gland does not produce enough thyroid hormone. This can occur for a variety of reasons including:

Hashimoto's - Hashimoto's is an autoimmune disease where the immune system mistakenly attacks the thyroid gland, reducing its ability to produce hormones. Doctors will check for Hashimoto's by testing TSH, Free T3, Free T4 and thyroid antibodies. A blood panel showing high TSH, low free T3, low free T4, and elevated antibodies can be a sign you have Hashimoto's.

It should be noted that the interpretation of high thyroid antibodies is controversial. Most medical and functional doctors suggest that high thyroid antibodies are harmful and attack your thyroid. Yet, there is emerging research that suggests elevated antibodies might not always be harmful but could play a protective or regulatory role in certain contexts (27, 28). Researcher Dr. Ray Peat often stated that thyroid antibodies are there to protect your thyroid—thus, their elevation is a protective response vs. a destructive response.

*It should be noted, Hashimoto's has been linked to digestive disorders—thus, sometimes healing your gut can fix your thyroid (more on that in the digestion Chapters 7 and 8).

Thyroiditis - Thyroid inflammation caused by infections, damaged thyroid cells, an autoimmune response (see above), certain medications and/or being postpartum.

Thyroid surgery - Removing all or part of the thyroid due to cancer, goiters, or nodules can reduce thyroid production.

Radiation therapy - Treatments for cancer in the thyroid, neck or head may affect thyroid hormone production, creating hypothyroidism. Those that have thyroid cancer normally have normal thyroid levels, it is not until after the treatments that they can suffer from hypothyroidism.

Nutrient deficiencies - The thyroid gland needs the amino acid tyrosine, iodine, iron, and zinc to produce thyroid hormones. Thus, a deficiency in any of these could inhibit thyroid hormone production. At the same time, excess iodine can also trigger hypothyroidism—one reason why iodine supplementation can make you worse.

Fluoride exposure - Fluoride (yes, the stuff in your water and toothpaste) can compete with iodine for absorption in the thyroid gland. Thus, fluoride exposure can suppress thyroid hormone production (29).

Medications - Certain drugs like lithium, amiodarone (treats heart arrhythmias), interferons (treat viral infections), Tyrosine kinase inhibitors (cancer treatment), glucocorticoids, anti-thyroid drugs like methimazole (used to treat hyperthyroidism), and excessive iodine containing agents.

Elevated cortisol - As I talked about earlier in this chapter, chronically elevated cortisol levels can suppress/lower TSH. If you suppress TSH, due to high stress, then your thyroid hormone production will slow, as an adaptive response to the increased cortisol. Thus, you may be truly hypothyroid (poor sleep, wired but tired, anxious, poor digestion, poor hormone function, hair loss, etc.), yet be told you are normal or possibly hyperthyroid due to the low TSH (30).

As you can see, there are numerous things that can negatively affect thyroid hormone production. To treat hypothyroidism, some people need to be on thyroid medication, as their thyroid is unable to produce enough thyroid hormone. Others may not need medication; they just need to correct a nutritional deficiency or reduce their stress levels (more on this later).

What about those that do not have a thyroid hormone production issue, but rather a thyroid conversion issue?

Impaired Thyroid Hormone Conversion Or Low T4 To T3 Conversion

If you have impaired thyroid hormone conversion, your body has difficulty in converting T4 (thyroxine), the inactive thyroid hormone, into T3 (triiodothyronine), the active thyroid hormone. Thus, you might experience hypothyroid symptoms, without having elevated TSH.

Here is a list of everything that can impair thyroid conversion:

Nutrient deficiencies - For optimal T4 to T3 conversion, you need optimal deiodinase enzyme production. The deiodinase enzymes need selenium, zinc, iron, and vitamin A for optimal deiodinase function and production.

Chronic stress and elevated cortisol - Yes, chronic stress can inhibit both thyroid production and conversion. High cortisol will inhibit the activity of the deiodinase 1 and 2, while increasing the deiodinase 3 enzyme. The deiodinase 3 enzyme will increase the production of rT3, which decreases the availability of active T3.

Estrogen. Yes, the hormone estrogen—whether produced in your body or taken externally through birth control or hormone therapy—can affect thyroid hormone availability and conversion. Estrogen increases levels of thyroxine-binding globulin (TBG), the protein that carries thyroid hormone in the bloodstream. Higher TBG means more thyroid hormone becomes "bound," leaving less free T4 and free T3 available for your cells (31). This may be one reason women experience hypothyroidism more frequently than men (32).

In addition, some research suggests that excess estrogen, particularly from exogenous estrogen use, may interfere with the deiodinase enzymes responsible for converting T4 into active T3 in the liver and other peripheral tissues (33). This can further reduce thyroid hormone activity, leading to hypothyroid-like symptoms in some women.

If you're experiencing thyroid symptoms and are taking estrogen-containing medications (birth control, HRT, or MHT), it's worth discussing with your healthcare provider. Dose, delivery method, and your personal physiology matter. There's much more to this estrogen–thyroid relationship, which is why I dive deeper into it in Chapters 9 and 10.

Inflammation and chronic illness - Chronic illness, infections, and inflammatory conditions can increase the production of cytokines, which can down regulate deiodinase enzyme activity, resulting in lower peripheral T3 production.

Liver and kidney dysfunction - The liver and kidneys are the primary sites for T4 to T3 conversion. Liver (including fatty liver) or kidney diseases can impair this process, leading to reduced T3 levels (34).

Poor gut function - Poor gut health will impact nutrient absorption, as well as increase bacterial toxins, both of which can negatively impact T4 to T3 conversion.

Medications - Certain medications can interfere with T4 to T3 conversion. These include beta-blockers (like propranolol), glucocorticoids (like prednisone), and amiodarone (used to treat arrhythmias).

Low-carb diets - Low-carb diets can hinder T4 to T3 conversion in the liver and other peripheral tissue, leading to hypothyroid-like symptoms. This primarily occurs because glucose is needed for optimal T4 to T3 conversion. Low-carb diets tend to increase rT3, while decreasing T3 (35, 36).

Low-calorie diets, fasting and starvation. Eating a lot less than your body needs will lower thyroid conversion, primarily due to the increase in stress hormones, from the lack of fuel and nutrients (37). So, yes, you can create hypothyroid-like symptoms by eating less.

As you can see there is some overlap when it comes to things that can hinder thyroid hormone production and conversion. Nutrient deficiencies and elevated stress (cortisol) play a role in both thyroid hormone production and conversion. This is why I place so much emphasis on eating foods that contain tons of bioavailable nutrients and finding ways to mitigate the stress response. Literally, these two things can be the answer to most of your thyroid issues.

The reason I wanted to write all the things out that can affect thyroid hormone production and conversion is so you can see how many things can affect your thyroid levels. Thus, the answer to fix your low-thyroid symptoms may have nothing to do with taking exogenous thyroid hormone, but rather with improving your overall nutrition, lowering stress and inflammation, or learning how to mitigate the stress response, reducing estrogen exposure, consuming more carbohydrates, and/or researching medication alternatives (if you are on one that is interfering with thyroid hormone production or conversion).

Which brings us to the next part in this chapter. How to improve your thyroid levels without taking thyroid medication. If you are looking to improve your thyroid hormone production and conversion, without taking exogenous thyroid, then listen up, this next part is for you.

Here are eight things you can do to support your thyroid hormone production and conversion— without taking thyroid medication.

1. **Make sure you are eating enough food.** If you are experiencing low-thyroid symptoms, then it could be due to not eating enough. Low fuel intake (carbs, fats, proteins) can increase the stress on the body, lowering thyroid hormone production and conversion. This is one reason why low-calorie diets stop working long term, as they are increasing rT3, while decreasing T3.

2. **Make sure you are eating enough carbohydrates.** Low-carbohydrate diets decrease T3, while increasing rt3. Glucose is needed for T4 to T3 conversion in liver and

kidneys. Low-carb diets tend to be more stressful on the body, increasing stress hormones. These same stress hormones will increase rT3.

3. **Consume nutrient-rich foods.** For you to produce and convert ample T4 into T3 you need numerous nutrients. Consuming a diet rich in dairy (tyrosine, iodine, zinc, vitamin A), shellfish (tyrosine, iodine, zinc, selenium, iron), beef liver (iron, zinc, vitamin A, tyrosine), eggs (Vitamin A, tyrosine), and fruits and roots (glucose, zinc, selenium) should help you meet your nutritional requirements for good thyroid health.

4. **Reduce stress.** Trying to find ways to reduce the stress on your body and life is helpful. Get to sleep on time, get outside, walk, practice breathing exercises, laugh, use therapy, reduce screen time, and spend time with people you love.

5. **Support liver and kidney health.** Your liver and kidneys need B vitamins, protein, and glucose to function optimally. Consuming foods like coffee (caffeine) can help liver function (38).

6. **Support gut health.** Remove processed foods. Reduce hard to digest foods like beans, grains, nuts, and seeds. See the next 2 chapters on fixing your gut.

7. **Reduce estrogen exposure.** Reducing estrogenic foods (soy, alcohol, PUFA), xenoestrogens (plastics, BPA, phthalates, parabens, PCBs, dioxins, herbicides, PBDE's, pesticides, alkylphenols), phytoestrogens, and exogenous estrogen (birth control, HRT, MHT).

8. **Check your medications.** As stated above, some medications can interfere with thyroid hormone production and conversion. If you are taking any of the above medications, talk with your health care provider to see if there are other options to support your medical condition. *Please do not stop any medication without talking with your healthcare provider.

Now, I am not suggesting that all thyroid issues can be fixed by doing the above list.

Many hypothyroid people may still need exogenous thyroid medication, even with a good diet, low stress, and low estrogen exposure. These people may have a true thyroid hormone production or conversion issue, and the only way this can be corrected is with thyroid medication.

However, there are some people, and you may be one, who have been placed on exogenous thyroid hormones and don't need the medication. Your functional medical doctor saw your free T3 and free T4 were low, so they gave you thyroid hormones to help support your thyroid levels. The problem with this is, if your free T3 and free T4 are low due to a nutritional deficiency, excess estrogen or cortisol exposure, then taking exogenous thyroid hormone is not really solving your problem—it is only overriding the problem.

Your body is decreasing thyroid hormone production, availability, and conversion for a reason, and if you try to override this just by taking thyroid hormones, your body might not respond the way you would like. For these people, they might see an initial improvement with the medication, but then the improvement fades, and they need to take more thyroid hormone. For others, they don't see any improvements at all and wonder why the thyroid is not working. Either way, the slow results can be tiresome and frustrating—as you can continue to be exhausted from not feeling any better.

This is why, if you know you have gone through a stressful time, or you know your diet has been less than great, I suggest working on your diet and lifestyle first, before jumping on the thyroid hormone bandwagon. Instead of taking an exogenous thyroid medication you might only need to improve nutrition, so the body has the resources to produce and convert its own thyroid hormone. For others, reducing cortisol and estrogen exposure will allow more free-T3 and free-T4 to become available. This can improve T3 activity in the cell, allowing for an improved metabolic rate, without exogenous thyroid hormone replacement.

With that said, if you have been working on your thyroid health, and are still experiencing low-thyroid symptoms, then an exogenous thyroid medication might be the thing you need.

What About Exogenous Thyroid Medications?

First, I want to be clear, I am not a medical doctor. The information in this section is based solely on my own research, the research of Dr. Ray Peat, Dr. Broda Barnes and numerous others, and conversations I have had with clients who have tried different thyroid medications. Ultimately, the thyroid medication that works best for you is the one you should take. This decision should be based on your thyroid labs, a conversation with your doctor, your own experimentation with different thyroid medications, and improvements with your symptoms. What I can say is, if the medication you have been prescribed is not helping you, and you have already worked on improving your diet and health, don't be afraid to ask your doctor for a different option—and if they refuse, find a different doctor.

The Four Main Types of Thyroid Medication

When it comes to thyroid medications, there are several types that include synthetic and natural "desiccated" thyroid hormone (normally from a pig's thyroid gland).

1. T4-only therapy or Levothyroxine. Levothyroxine is the synthetic form of T4. Common brand names are Synthroid, Levoxyl, and Tirosint. Most medical doctors prefer to prescribe T4-only medication as T4 has a longer half-life, which allows for more consistent blood levels and easier dosing. The hope is your body will be able to convert the T4 into the T3 as you need it.

2. T3-only therapy or Liothyronine. Liothyronine is the synthetic form of T3. The most common T3 prescribed in the US is Cytomel. Cytomel is often added to patients who are not fully responding to T4-only therapy, indicating they might have a thyroid hormone conversion

issue. T3 has a short half-life, so must be taken frequently throughout the day to keep levels stable. For this reason, T3-only therapy is normally added to T4 therapy and not taken alone.

3. Combination, synthetic T4 and T3 therapy. There are few synthetic thyroid hormone versions. The most popular and widely used is Cynoplus, made in Mexico. Cynoplus is made of 80% T4 and 20% T3. This combination is to resemble the thyroid hormone amounts produced by your own thyroid.

4. Desiccated, combination thyroid therapy. Desiccated thyroid is made from porcine (pig) thyroid gland, which is why it's often labeled "natural." Armour Thyroid, Nature-Throid, and NP Thyroid are the most common desiccated thyroid medications in the U.S. These medications are prescription drugs and are subject to FDA oversight in how they are manufactured and dispensed. However, they have never gone through the modern FDA approval process and are not officially FDA-approved medications.

    There are also desiccated thyroid products sold online without prescriptions. These are not regulated in the same way and may not contain consistent, or even real, thyroid hormone.

What Thyroid Medication is Best?

The best thyroid medication for you is the one that makes you feel the best. If you need additional thyroid hormone, then a good medication should make you feel more energized, warmer, happier, improve digestion, support hormone production, improve hair and nails, and improve your sleep.

Just like everything else I talk about, thyroid medication is very individualized. How well a thyroid medication works can depend on your current physiology, other medications, stress level, and diet. For many people, T4-only therapy works quite well, and their body can convert the T4 into active T3 as needed. However, for others who have a thyroid conversion issue (genetic issue, high stress, low-nutrient diet, excess estrogen, dieting, medications), a T4-only approach has either no effect, or can possibly make them feel worse.

You see, T4-only therapy will suppress your thyroid stimulating hormone (TSH). Remember, TSH is a pituitary hormone that elevates to tell your thyroid to produce both T4 and T3—if you take T4-only, suppressing TSH, your body will decrease its own production of not only T4, but also T3. And, if you are having a hard time converting the synthetic T4 into T3, you are at risk of having even less T3 (as your own production is suppressed by a suppressed TSH), than before you were taking the medication. This can be a frustrating situation, because your thyroid blood labs will return as "normal," while you don't feel any better.

This is why when you start taking any thyroid medication, you should monitor your symptoms and take your morning body temperature and pulse to make sure they are increasing. Thyroid hormone should increase energy production, which will increase both your body temperature and pulse. In addition, if thyroid hormone is working effectively, other symptoms should start to improve. You should feel warmer, have more energy, improved digestion, lower cholesterol, improved sleep, feel happier, and experience a possible adjustment in scale weight.

Thus, if you are someone who has been taking T4-only medication for at least a few months with no relief, or a few years and are starting to feel worse, it might make sense to add in some additional T3 or switch over to a combination T4/T3 therapy. As your life and health change, it is very possible that your thyroid needs will change. Please discuss with your doctor or hormone specialist as to which thyroid medication will work best for you.

Well, there you have it, you now have a much better understanding of how your thyroid gland and hormones work, how your thyroid hormones are produced, transported, and used in the cell. You should also have an understanding as to what nutrients are needed for production and conversion, and what things can interfere with optimal thyroid hormone production and conversion. All of this should help you understand if you really need to take exogenous thyroid hormone, or if maybe you just need to work on your diet and stress levels.

As you can see, your thyroid hormones are big players in the energy production equation. They are the CEOs of your cells, telling your cells, depending on what they need, to speed up energy production or slow it down. This is why there is such a big focus on thyroid health when discussing the bioenergetic guidelines—as without enough thyroid hormone, the entire process would come to a grinding halt.

With this said, we have now finished discussing the big four contributors to energy production, they include fuel, nutrients, oxygen and now thyroid hormones. Understanding and working on these four things should greatly increase your overall health and happiness. However, we are not done, there is still more to discuss, primarily all the things that can block energy production. Some of those I have already touched on in the previous chapters, but I want to go into far more detail in the chapters to come, so you can have a deeper understanding of all the energy blocks and what you can do to improve them!

CHAPTER 5

THE BOTTOM LINE

Your Thyroid—Your Cell's Energy Dial

1. Thyroid hormone sets your cellular ATP rate. T4 is mostly inactive, while T3 is the active thyroid hormone that revs mitochondria and gene expression. When thyroid drops, everything that depends on ATP (heat, digestion, hair/skin, mood, libido, sleep) slows.

2. The HPT axis (hypothalamus → pituitary → TSH → thyroid) makes T4/T3. Additional T4 to T3 conversion happens in peripheral tissues via deiodinases enzymes.

3. Tyrosine, iodine, selenium, zinc, iron, vitamin A, and glucose are required to make and convert thyroid hormone.

4. Chronic stress/cortisol, inflammation/illness, estrogen excess/ TBG rise (e.g., some HRT/BC), liver or kidney dysfunction, fluoride, certain meds (lithium, amiodarone, glucocorticoids, some beta-blockers), and classic nutrient deficits.

5. A full thyroid panel (TSH, Free T3, Free T4 and RT3), cholesterol, vitamin D, metabolic panel, as well as symptoms is the best method to understand if you are hypothyroid.

6. Support thyroid health by eating enough carbs, nutrient dense foods, reducing stress, estrogen exposure, increasing sleep, sunlight, breath work,and possible thyroid medications.

PART 2

ENERGY BLOCKS AND HOW THEY
CAN AFFECT ENERGY PRODUCTION

Since I've already covered all the wonderful things that support optimal energy production, it's only fair to get into the not-so-wonderful stuff, the little pests I like to call "energy blocks." Yep, just as there are things that make you feel like a well-oiled machine, there are also things that can make you feel like you're running on fumes.

Sure, you already know that energy production can tank without the right fuel (carbs, fats, proteins), essential nutrients, enough oxygen, or a well-functioning thyroid. Hopefully, after reading the last section, that is obvious, right? No fuel, no nutrients, no oxygen, no thyroid function, no metabolic fire. So yes, if any of these are out of whack, your energy production will feel like a car running on empty.

But what you *might not know* is that there are sneaky little energy drains lurking around that you may not even suspect. Chronic stress, poor digestion (hello, endotoxins!), excess estrogen, excess iron, and those nasty polyunsaturated fats can each mess with your ATP production. Yep, each one is like a clog in your personal fuel injection system (cell's mitochondria), preventing you from creating the energy you are looking for.

So, in the next section, I'm going to dive into all these sneaky energy blocks. This part is for those of you who have been trying to do everything right, eating well, breathing deeply, supporting thyroid health, but still feel like something's off. If you're asking, "Why am I still dealing with energy issues?" then this section is for you.

Turns out, one (or more) of these energy blocks might be the roadblock standing between you and vibrant health. Let's get into it, because without removing these blocks, you might just stay, well... stuck.

CHAPTER 6

STRESS—THE ENERGY
(METABOLISM) CRUSHER

In today's world, unless you live under a rock (though, let's face it, even a rock on top of you would be stressful), stress is as unavoidable as death, taxes, and spam emails. Stress can pop up from anywhere—your diet, your job, your environment, relationships, the news, that new workout program, social media, the lack of sunlight, EMFs, and, oh yes, even your own thoughts, which apparently, for most of us, are working overtime.

But here's the deal, it doesn't matter where the stress is coming from. To your body, stress is stress, and regardless of where it stems from, your body has the same physiological/biological reaction. You see, your body perceives all stress the same way, as a need to produce more energy to deal with the increased demands.

So yes, whether you're sprinting from a lion (rare, but hey, it could happen), fighting with your partner over the laundry, giving a speech, or eating a low-calorie, processed food diet, your body goes into action mode. The response? A need for more energy, which increases stress hormones, basically a biological alarm system to help you manage the drama.

When you experience stress, the body releases your primary stress hormones, including glucagon, adrenaline, and cortisol. These three hellions kick in for what is called the "stress response," a process designed to rev up your energy production and keep you from keeling over. And don't get me wrong; in the short term, this response is a lifesaver. If you're on the run (literally or metaphorically), it mobilizes fuel fast, keeping you ready to tackle whatever chaos comes your way.

Remember, all the cells in your body require a constant flow of fuel. This constant flow of fuel allows them to produce energy (ATP) to maintain their structure and function. Without enough energy, the cell's energy production will slow down, leading to a decrease in function and structure. In other words, when your energy production starts to dwindle, cells go on strike, and everything slows down: your heat production, digestion, sleep, energy levels, you name it. So, yes, this stress response is crucial because it's what keeps you alive when life's throwing punches. Without it, you'd be toast.

But what happens when these stressors don't take the hint and stick around indefinitely, keeping your stress response on permanent overdrive?

Well, as crucial as the initial stress response is to keep you going when the world becomes insane, running it nonstop is going to backfire. Chronic doses of stress hormones will tell your body to cut corners and redirect energy away from "non-essentials" (you know, digestion, balanced hormones, energy levels, and sleep) just to keep up with all those relentless external demands, be it workload, gym goals, or your own overthinking mind.

This energy diversion is your body's way of saying, "I am trying to protect you from breaking down while you are working on overdrive, but if you keep going, I am going on strike!"

Essentially, the stress response is like a fire alarm: it is there to save you in a crisis, but if it's blaring nonstop, you will soon go crazy or you might just throw yourself out the window. Which means, yes, excessive stress can be deadly.

In this chapter, we'll start by exploring what stress really is and the different forms it can take. From there, we'll take a deep dive into how your body responds physiologically to stress and how this impacts energy production, whether the stress is short-term or long-lasting. Finally, we'll look at practical strategies to help you reduce the impact of stress while building a stronger, more resilient body that's better equipped to handle whatever life throws your way.

First, What Is Stress?

Put simply, stress is the body's natural response to any demand, challenge, or threat that disrupts its balance, or what scientists call homeostasis. It's the body's way of adapting to change, activating a series of physical, emotional, and mental reactions designed to protect and prepare you for action.

Defined another way, stress occurs any time the demands placed on the body are more than the body has the available energy to keep up with. This is a more general term, so that you can understand that your body perceives all stressors the same way, a need for more energy.

This need for more energy can come from external or internal physical stressors, emotional or mental stressors, or anything that reduces the amount of incoming fuel—like dieting, starvation, or fasting to keep up with normal function.

Of course, so I am clear what all these stressors are, I created a short list of the four biggest stressors that can create a need for more energy.

Here are four types of stressors that will require more energy to keep your body in balance.

External Physical Stressors

External physical stressors are, you guessed it, external things that force your body's systems to work a little harder, demanding more energy and resources to maintain balance. These include the usual suspects: manual labor, extreme temperatures (too hot or too cold), lack of sun, lack of sleep, and even exercise. Don't get the wrong idea—physical stressors aren't "bad" by nature. They're simply anything that adds a bit of extra external pressure, nudging your body to produce more energy to keep up with the demand.

Of course, if your body can't keep pace with these increased energy demands, whether they're from "good" or "bad" stressors, it must make some tough choices. To keep up with the added demands, it will often reroute energy from internal systems—such as digestion or hormone production—to handle the strain from these external physical stressors.

Let's break it down with a classic example: exercise.

Exercise is an external physical stressor, which means it increases the body's energy requirements. When these needs are met with enough fuel and nutrients, exercise can lead to muscle growth, cardiovascular health, stability, coordination, improved brain function, and positive body composition changes. Fantastic, right?

But if you're under the weather or your body's running on fumes nutritionally, even a "good" stressor like exercise can turn to sh#t. Without adequate fuel or efficient energy conversion, exercise can start to break down tissue, wear you out, and increase your risk of injury. Which means it is important to be well fueled and rested before you start an intense exercise program, so that your body has the resources to do the workout and recover.

Internal Physical Stressors

Internal physical stressors are those delightful internal irritants that force your body to work overtime just to keep things running. These include all the fun stuff like injuries, pain, illness, post-surgery recovery, infections, fevers, burns, bone fractures—basically, if it's a hassle and happening inside you, it's an internal stressor.

Just like external stressors, these internal ones crank up your body's energy demands. And just like with external stressors, these demands aren't "bad." In fact, they're essential. Your body needs these stressors to kick into high gear to repair, recover, and handle the chaos. But they sure don't make it easy on you.

Let's look at some examples:

1. **Bone breaks**: Break a bone? Your body's energy needs (or metabolism) can jump up by 15–25% to repair and remodel the bone. Think of it as your body's construction crew clocking in extra hours just to patch things up (1, 2).

2. **Fever**: With a fever, every degree Celsius (that's about 1.8°F) above normal turns up the energy demand by a cozy 7–13%. Why? Because your immune system's going into overdrive to clear out the infection (3). It's like your body throws a huge party, and your white blood cells must come in and clean up after the party—and this cleanup requires a lot of energy.

3. **Critical injuries and weight loss (not just the bad hospital food)**: If you're critically injured, expect your metabolism to skyrocket—sometimes by over 30% above your resting rate (4). This energy surge is what your body needs to fuel healing and recovery.

FUN FACT: The weight loss people experience in the hospital? It's not just from dodging the Jell-O. It's because your body's burning through calories to put you back together.

So yes, internal physical stressors might be doing a number on you by increasing your energy needs, but it's all for a good cause. They're keeping you alive, repairing what's broken, and fighting what shouldn't be there. And, as it turns out, all that work requires some serious fuel to keep up with these increased demands.

Mental or Emotional Stressors

Mental and emotional stressors? Oh, those are the ones that sneak in, set up camp, and just *refuse* to leave. They're primarily driven by stressful situations, whether past or present, that keep circling around in your head like an annoying song you can't shake. Think; divorce, moving, loneliness, past trauma, death, financial stress, and, of course, the worst culprit—your own thoughts obsessing over what happened, what's happening, or what might happen. These stressors can sometimes be even tougher than physical ones because, unlike that workout that eventually ends, emotional stressors can run 24/7 in your mind without a moment's break.

And let's be honest, how many people do you know who went through something emotionally rough and then suddenly started dealing with digestive issues, low energy, poor sleep, or even a nonexistent sex drive? They're not just "being dramatic." Mental and emotional stressors drain your body's resources just like physical ones, stealing energy away from systems like digestion, hormone production, and sleep, and handing it over to your always-on, overactive nervous system. Because why should anything be easy?

If you're dealing with mental or emotional stressors, here's the best advice: give yourself some grace, time, and patience. When I was recovering from a neurological injury, the most helpful thing I did was to slow down (and stop trying to pretend I was fine). Sure, it's frustrating to feel like you're not yourself, but stressing about it only makes it worse. I learned to give myself a break, using stress-reducing practices to help calm my system and keep my mind from turning every minor issue into a national emergency. I'll share more on this later in the chapter, but for now you should know—it's okay to take a break and let yourself breathe.

Calorie Restriction

Yep, you heard right, whenever you cut calories below what your body needs to keep things running smoothly, you're setting off a stress response. When you're dieting (a.k.a., eating less than your body needs), your body turns up the stress hormones to start breaking *you* down for fuel. After all, you're a walking storage tank, using fat, glycogen, and yes, even muscle to produce energy when food is lacking. You should always remember, if you're not eating enough, your body's strategy is to tap into its reserves—it's survival 101.

Now, don't panic, calorie restriction isn't "bad" in and of itself. But you should know that doing it for extended periods can come with some not-so-great side effects. Like any stressful experience that goes on too long, restricting calories for months and years on end can hit your body's energy production in ways you might not enjoy.

Remember back in Chapter 1, when we talked about Ancel Keys and his (now infamous) Minnesota Starvation Experiment? In this study, Keys put a group of healthy young men on a severe diet, slashing their calories by 55%. They went from eating about 3,500 calories a day to under 1,600. After 24 weeks, these men lost 24% of their body weight and saw their metabolism crash by 39%. Their energy plummeted, they felt fatigued, depressed, had zero libido, dealt with constipation, headaches, insomnia, and felt like they'd been moved to Antarctica without a coat. The body was basically in "self-preservation mode," redirecting energy away from luxuries like sleep, digestion, and mood to keep up with the basics.

Here's where most people get it wrong; they think weight loss is purely about self-discipline, not realizing the toll it takes on your body's energy production. When you eat less than your body needs, it raises stress hormones to pull fuel from fat, muscle, and glycogen. Keep this up for too long, and your metabolism adapts by slowing down—aka, "survival mode."

Have you ever tried cutting calories to lose fat for months or years and noticed you suddenly feel cold all the time? Or your sleep goes downhill? Or your hair decides to stop growing? Libido drops, energy tanks…this is all thanks to long-term metabolic adaptations as your body adjusts to prolonged calorie restriction.

Does that mean that "fat burning (oxidation)" is stressful?

Well, my answer is *"yes and no."* It all depends on the context and the conditions under which fat burning occurs.

Like I discussed in Chapter 2, your body is constantly burning fat, whether it's the fat from your meals or the reserves in your fat tissue. When you're chilling (think lounging on the couch or sleeping), your body is in a low-stress state and naturally leans on fat as its primary fuel. Your muscles and heart, in particular, love using fat during these restful periods because it's efficient and doesn't require activating your stress response. So yes, in a calm state, fat burning is as smooth as homemade churned ice cream. (For more on this, check out the "Are You Ready for Fat Loss?" chapter.)

But things take a sharp turn when stress enters the conversation.

When you're stressed, your body activates its three main stress hormones: glucagon, cortisol, and adrenaline (more on these in a minute). Their mission? Mobilize fuel (glycogen, muscle, fat) for quick energy to deal with whatever chaos you're facing. If glycogen (your stored sugar) runs out, these hormones signal your body to ramp up lipolysis, the breakdown of fat into free fatty acids. Your cells then use the incoming fat to make energy, and you lose fat. Sounds great, right? Well, not so fast.

Here's the deal, stress-induced fat burning isn't ideal—at least long term. Unlike the chill, steady fat burning during rest, this version is turbocharged by stress hormones, which can wreak havoc if overused. Running on stress hormones creates numerous adaptive responses, responses which lower internal functions, lower thyroid hormone, lower CO_2 production, and can increase the breakdown of muscle and other connective tissues. In addition, excessive fat in the blood can inhibit your body's ability to use glucose (Randle cycle—more about this later), and anything that inhibits glucose oxidation, can increase the stress response.

Remember in your 20's when fat loss was relatively straightforward, you skip a meal, reduce calories, and your body would efficiently mobilize fat stores without much protest? It's as if your metabolism was on autopilot, readily adapting to these minor changes. Yet, over time and repeated low-calorie diets, and stressful experiences, your body's tolerance to these stressors diminishes significantly. The same calorie-cutting strategy that once worked seamlessly now triggers a cascade of physiological repercussions: energy levels plummet, sleep becomes fragmented and unrefreshing, anxiety or low mood may surface, and overall recovery slows. Your body's response shifts from adaptation to resistance, signaling that it can no longer handle the additional stress of extreme calorie restriction.

Does this mean you should avoid weight/fat loss because it stresses the body?

Absolutely not!

Most people carrying extra weight could benefit from shedding a few pounds. The trick is to do it the *right* way. The faster you lose weight, the more stress you're putting on your body. So, if you're aiming for sustainable, healthy weight loss, think "slow and steady." For more on how to lose fat without torching your metabolism, jump to Chapter 13.

In the end, how well your body handles any stress, whether from physical stressors like exercise, a bone break, or sickness, emotional stressors like the loss of a loved one, or some sort of calorie restriction, comes down to how efficiently you're producing energy and the resources you've got on hand.

If you're eating well, sleeping enough, and giving your thyroid and metabolism some love, congratulations! Your body is likely humming along and ready to handle most stressors like a champ. But if you're under-eating, skipping meals, cutting corners on rest, and living in a constant state of "just trying to keep up," your metabolism will slow down faster than you can say, "Why do I feel like crap?" Suddenly, even a short walk feels like you're scaling Mt. Everest without oxygen.

Which makes you ask the question, "What happens when you're unable to meet your body's increased demands?" Whether it's from too many external and internal stressors, or some sort of restrictive eating or fasting, here's the biology of what's happening when stress hits, and how it affects your energy production.

The Biology of the Stress Response

Stress starts with the amygdala, your brain's emotional alarm system. Think of it as your brain's overanxious friend who loves to scream, "OMG, WE'RE ALL GOING TO DIE!" at the first sign of trouble. This trouble can come from anything, your eyes spotting a lion (or just a nasty comment on your social media), your ears picking up a strange noise, your nerves signaling pain or heat, or even your own crazy thoughts. Yes, your thoughts can produce a stress response—in fact, it is you thinking about the stressful thing (not the actual event) that creates the stress. The amygdala immediately alerts the hypothalamus, which runs the show when it comes to coordinating your stress response.

The hypothalamus is like the CEO at stress headquarters, working overtime to keep your body balanced, or at least trying to. It is involved in detecting hormone levels in the blood from other endocrine organs and glands, and it responds accordingly by adjusting its own hormone output—either increasing or decreasing hormone levels depending on what the body needs. Essentially, the hypothalamus orchestrates the stress response through multiple connections with organ systems and glands, which communicate with each other via hormonal signaling pathways, commonly referred to as "axes."

Now, before we dive deeper into the hypothalamic axes, let's take a moment to meet the hypothalamus's right-hand partner: the pituitary gland. If the hypothalamus is the CEO, then the pituitary is the COO (Chief Operating Officer), responsible for turning all those brilliant plans into action. Often referred to as the "master gland," the pituitary has a big job: bossing around every other endocrine gland. Whether it's the thyroid, adrenals, or gonads, they all take their orders from the pituitary, who takes orders from the hypothalamus.

Despite being no bigger than a pea, the pituitary is a big player in the hormonal world. Nestled snugly in the sella turcica (a bony structure at the base of your brain), the pituitary gland is divided into two departments: the anterior pituitary and the posterior pituitary. These divisions don't just exist to sound impressive; they handle distinct jobs. The anterior pituitary is the real multitasker, producing and releasing a host of important hormones, including TSH (thyroid-stimulating hormone), ACTH (adrenocorticotropic hormone), GH (growth hormone), prolactin, and reproductive hormones like LH (luteinizing hormone) and FSH (follicle-stimulating hormone). Basically, if it involves metabolism, growth, or reproduction, the anterior pituitary is on the job.

The posterior pituitary, on the other hand, is more like the warehouse manager. It doesn't produce its own hormones but stores and ships out two hormones made by the hypothalamus: oxytocin (the connection hormone) and ADH (antidiuretic hormone, also known as vasopressin, your body's water conservation expert). So, while the anterior pituitary is busy manufacturing hormones in response to energy demands, reproduction, and stress, the posterior pituitary ensures its stored hormones are distributed precisely when needed.

Together, the hypothalamus and pituitary form a kick ass team. The hypothalamus sends out detailed instructions, and the pituitary ensures they're carried out with precision. It's the kind of teamwork that keeps your body running smoothly, or at least gives it a fighting chance when faced with stress, hunger, or a poorly timed deadline. Without the pituitary, the hypothalamus's big plans would never make it past the brainstorming stage, and without the hypothalamus, the pituitary would be like an overachiever with no clue what to do. Truly, a match made in endocrine heaven!

Now that we've met the hypothalamus-pituitary duo, let's dive into how they work together with other glands to keep you alive when life gets a little chaotic and stress rears its ugly head.

The Four Main Hypothalamic-Pituitary Stress Axes

Here's what each axis does when you're under stress, and how they (sometimes grudgingly) adapt to keep you alive.

The HPA Axis: The Major Player of Your Stress Response

First up is the Hypothalamic-Pituitary-Adrenal (HPA) axis, your body's primary stress-response system. The HPA axis upregulates in times of stress. Think of the HPA axis as the first responders on the stress management team, rushing in to handle any crisis. Its job is to make sure you have enough fuel to keep up with the increased demands. When stress strikes, the hypothalamus releases CRH (Corticotropin-Releasing Hormone), which signals the pituitary to release ACTH (Adrenocorticotropic Hormone). ACTH then tells the adrenal glands to release cortisol, one of your body's most powerful stress hormones.

Cortisol acts as your body's energy manager, first by stimulating the liver to break down glycogen into glucose via glycogenolysis, and then by driving gluconeogenesis—making new glucose from muscle, tissue, and other non-carbohydrate sources. It also mobilizes fat from adipose tissue (lipolysis), releasing fatty acids for fuel and glycerol for more glucose. These processes supply energy for whatever demand you're facing, whether you're escaping a lion (unlikely) or racing a deadline (more likely).

But there is a caveat, if stress sticks around for too long, the HPA axis becomes overworked, leaving you exhausted, burned out, and vulnerable to a host of physical and emotional issues. It's like forcing your CEO to work 80-plus hours a week with no breaks, eventually, they're going to crash. Although it might not seem like it at the time, this slowdown is an adaptive measure by your body to make sure it does not continue to keep breaking you (your tissue) down.

At the same time, the hypothalamus activates the sympathetic nervous system, the fast-acting branch of the autonomic nervous system. This system directly signals the adrenal medulla (the inner part of the adrenal glands) to release adrenaline and norepinephrine into the bloodstream. These hormones deliver the immediate "fight-or-flight" response, increasing heart rate, dilating airways, and boosting blood flow to your muscles. While this rapid response bypasses the pituitary gland entirely, it's often discussed alongside the HPA axis because it's such an integral part of the stress response.

The HPT Axis: The Energy Manager

Next, we have the Hypothalamic-Pituitary-Thyroid (HPT) axis, which oversees your metabolism and energy production. Under normal circumstances, the hypothalamus releases TRH (Thyrotropin-Releasing Hormone), which prompts the pituitary to produce TSH (Thyroid-Stimulating Hormone). TSH then activates the thyroid gland, which churns out T3 and T4, the hormones that keep your metabolism running smoothly.

During short-term (acute) stress, like I explained in the thyroid chapter, the HPT axis steps up to meet increased energy demands by increasing TRH, TSH, and thyroid hormone production. But if stress becomes more chronic, cortisol steps in like a micromanaging boss, slowing down TRH and TSH production to conserve energy. Your metabolism essentially shifts into "power saver" mode, leaving you tired, sluggish, and wondering why you can't function like you used to. Long-term, this slowdown will lower non-essential functions (like digestion, hormone production, hair growth), to conserve energy to survive (6).

Essentially, the HPT Axis can upregulate under acute stress and downregulate under chronic stress. The initial response is to help you make more energy, while the secondary response (the slow down) is there to make you conserve energy.

The HPG Axis: Reproduction Takes a Back Seat

The Hypothalamic-Pituitary-Gonadal (HPG) axis is next on the chopping block when stress comes into play. Yes, the HPG Axis downregulates under stress. This axis is responsible for regulating your reproductive hormones, but when survival is at stake, reproduction gets put on the backburner, because let's be honest, who is thinking of having a baby when you are running from a lion (or hiding from your boss)? When stress hits, the hypothalamus reduces GnRH (Gonadotropin-Releasing Hormone), which lowers LH (Luteinizing Hormone) and FSH (Follicle-Stimulating Hormone). As a result, estrogen, progesterone, and testosterone production drops significantly (7).

For women, this can mean irregular cycles, missed periods, a lower sex drive, and infertility, while men may notice a lower sex drive and sperm production, also contributing to lower fertility.

FUN FACT: Currently, 1 in 6 couples faces fertility issues. In the last year, using a bioenergetic diet and lifestyle, I helped five out of five women get pregnant and have a healthy baby. Supportive nutrition and stress reduction are the foundation of procreation.

Interestingly, during stress, ovarian estradiol production can be reduced, while peripheral estrogen production can increase. High cortisol and prolactin will suppress the HPG axis—reducing estrogen, progesterone, and testosterone production in the gonads. However, at the same time, elevated cortisol enhances the aromatase enzyme. Aromatase converts adrenal androgens (DHEA, testosterone) into estrogen, which can increase estrogen production in the peripheral tissues (8, 9, 10). Peripheral estrogen production can lead to hormonal imbalances, and a mess of other issues, but more on that later when I discuss estrogen in Chapters 9 and 10.

The HPP Axis: Prolactin Is a Stress Hormone?

Finally, we have the Hypothalamic-Pituitary-Prolactin (HPP) axis, which upregulates under stress by increasing prolactin levels. While prolactin is best known for its role in milk production, it takes on additional responsibilities during stress. Prolactin is activated by TRH and doesn't have downstream hormones to delegate to—it's the end hormone of this axis.

During stress, prolactin contributes to immune regulation, tissue repair, and even bone metabolism. It's like the overachieving intern who says "yes" to every task. However, when prolactin levels remain high for too long (like so many things), it can suppress reproductive hormones, increase aromatase and peripheral estrogen production, increase cortisol, and even contribute to bone breakdown. You know, like when that same overachieving intern works too late, for too long, and starts crashing and messing up all his work.

Elevated levels in both men and non-lactating women can be a sign of a prolactinoma (non-cancerous tumor), hypothyroidism, PCOS (only women), and/or an overstressed body.

What you should know is all these hypothalamic axes work together to keep your body running effectively. Yet, under chronic stress, these axes can get disrupted, leading to widespread physiological effects and stress-induced energy production.

Now, to round out your major endocrine glands that are involved in the stress response and energy production, we must discuss two additional glands and the hormones they produce. The first is a dynamic duo in charge of keeping you going, when your resources (food) are limited, let's hear it for your adrenal glands! I'll have more on Prolactin in Chapter 9.

The Adrenal Glands: Your Hyper Friend

The two adrenal glands, small but mighty, are your body's first responders to stress. These walnut-sized powerhouses sit atop your kidneys, forming part of the HPA Axis (Hypothalamic-Pituitary-Adrenal Axis) alongside the hypothalamus and pituitary gland. Together, they orchestrate your stress response and help maintain balance, particularly when your energy demands increase.

Each adrenal gland has two distinct parts, each with specialized roles:

- **The Adrenal Cortex:** Produces hormones like aldosterone (for salt and water balance), androgens (precursors to sex hormones), and most importantly, cortisol, your primary stress hormone that mobilizes energy for long-term adaptation.

- **The Adrenal Medulla:** Acts as your emergency responder, releasing catecholamines like adrenaline and noradrenaline to provide quick bursts of energy in moments of acute stress.

While all adrenal hormones play vital roles, adrenaline and cortisol are the stars when it comes to energy production under stress. These two hormones make sure you can keep going by mobilizing stored fuel when immediate energy sources, like food, are unavailable.

Adrenaline: The Quick Energy Liberator

Adrenaline, or epinephrine, is the adrenal medulla's star player during the fight-or-flight response. Derived from the amino acid tyrosine, adrenaline is a catecholamine that enables your body to react swiftly in emergencies. When released, adrenaline increases your heart rate and breathing, enhances blood flow to critical areas, and most importantly raises your blood sugar levels by breaking down glycogen in the liver (a process known as glycogenolysis) and creating glucose from non-carbohydrate sources (gluconeogenesis) (11).

In addition to mobilizing glucose, adrenaline will impair insulin secretion, which reduces glucose uptake by peripheral tissues. This ensures that critical systems like your brain and nervous system have priority access to fuel. All of this occurs so that your body has resources (glucose, fat, protein) to create enough energy to keep you going. Essentially, adrenaline helps keep you going when you are running on empty.

FUN FACT: Tyrosine is the backbone of both adrenaline and the thyroid hormones. Thus, when stress cranks up and your body is flooded with adrenaline, it is possible, adrenaline can hog tyrosine, leaving your thyroid a bit short of its needed building block. This is one possible reason why chronic stress can slow your thyroid function—your adrenal glands are stealing all the tyrosine.

However, chronic elevation of adrenaline due to prolonged stress can cause significant metabolic disruptions. Persistently high adrenaline levels mean persistently elevated glucose levels, which over time can lead to impaired glucose tolerance, insulin resistance, and an increased risk of diabetes (12, 13). In other words, when stress overstays its welcome, your blood sugar can go haywire—more on that in a moment.

Cortisol: The Energy Manager Under Long-Term Stress

Cortisol is your body's stress-time CEO, a steroidal hormone produced from cholesterol in the adrenal cortex. It belongs to a group of hormones called glucocorticoids, which means it plays a central role in regulating glucose. One of cortisol's primary functions is to increase blood sugar through gluconeogenesis—a fancy way of saying it converts whatever your body can spare (like muscle and connective tissue) into glucose when food isn't available. This ensures a steady fuel supply for critical organs, particularly the brain and nervous system, during times of scarcity.

Although cortisol is vital for survival, it's not your health's best friend when it overstays its welcome. Like adrenaline, cortisol impairs insulin secretion to ensure available glucose is reserved for vital systems and organs—especially your brain. Cortisol also blocks protein uptake, so forget about building sexy legs or big biceps if you're living in a chronic stress state. Instead, cortisol shifts into full-on catabolic mode, breaking down precious muscle, connective tissue, and even organs to churn out more glucose to keep you alive.

Cortisol is also a key player in lipolysis, the breakdown of triglycerides into glycerol and free fatty acids (FFAs). While this may sound great for fat burning, excessive fat oxidation driven by high cortisol can wreak havoc on your body. Chronic stress-related cortisol spikes can lead to metabolic adaptations such as high blood sugar, insulin resistance, and even diabetes. So, while cortisol might be trying to save the day, it often leaves behind a metabolic dumpster fire. (Don't worry—I cover blood sugar in more detail below.)

Finally, chronic cortisol elevation also dampens the immune system. In the short term, this reduces inflammation, but over time, it increases susceptibility to infections and chronic diseases. Interestingly, some individuals experience a temporary increase in aches and inflammation when they begin to heal, and cortisol levels drop. This reaction occurs because the immune system, no longer suppressed by cortisol, starts working again. Over time, however, balanced nutrition and reduced stress hormones can lead to improved inflammatory control.

Ok. So now that you know about the adrenal glands' main stress hormones, let's put it all together and talk about the adrenal glands' role in energy production.

The Adrenals and Energy Production Under Stress

When stress strikes and incoming fuel is limited, your adrenal glands spring into action. The adrenals release adrenaline and cortisol to mobilize stored energy. These hormones break down glycogen into glucose, convert fat into fuel, and even transform amino acids from muscle tissue into glucose through a process called gluconeogenesis. In essence, the adrenal glands ensure your body has the resources it needs to meet increased energy demands—whether you're running from a bear, running a race, or just trying to survive a tough day.

To be clear, this process isn't just about using up your stored resources; it's also about reallocating existing energy. Under stress, adrenal hormones prioritize critical systems—like your heart, lungs, and brain—giving them first dibs on fuel, even if it means borrowing energy from "non-essential" processes like digestion and reproduction. It's your body's way of saying, "Let's survive now and worry about everything else later."

Think of the adrenal glands as your backup energy production team. In an ideal world, your body produces energy efficiently by using carbohydrates and fats from your diet, along with nutrients, oxygen, and sufficient thyroid hormones. This is your primary energy system—the well-oiled machine that powers your cells under normal conditions. You know, everything we talked about in the first part of this book.

But when stress kicks in and immediate fuel isn't readily available (or your body perceives a threat), your HPA axis activates the adrenal glands to step in. They act like an emergency generator, keeping you running by mobilizing stored energy. It's not the most efficient system, and it's not meant to run for long periods, but it works beautifully in the short term to keep you alive and functioning.

While the adrenal glands are incredibly effective at providing energy during acute stress, problems arise when the stress response becomes chronic. If you're constantly dipping into your backup system—relying on cortisol and adrenaline to keep you going—your body starts to pay the price. Here's the deal: your body's number one job is to keep you alive. If it feels you're pushing too hard (overworking, overexercising, overstressing), it adapts by slowing down internal functions. It's the physiological equivalent of robbing Peter to pay Paul.

This reallocation of energy takes its toll. Thyroid function often slows, which in turn reduces energy production for your internal systems (reduces basal metabolic rate), leading to compromised digestion, hormonal imbalances (PMS, low libido, infertility), poor sleep, reduced heat production, and overall declining health. Some people might refer to this as "adrenal fatigue," but in truth, it's not—it's a metabolic adaptation designed to conserve energy. These adaptations are usually the result of low thyroid function, nutrient deficiencies, insufficient fuel, excessive stressors, or other energy blocks.

FUN FACT: Adrenal "fatigue" does not exist. There's no clinical diagnosis for adrenal fatigue, and research shows just as many people with supposed adrenal fatigue have low, high, or normal cortisol levels (14). What many call "adrenal fatigue" is often a systemic response to prolonged stress and energy depletion, not the adrenal glands "burning out."

The bottom line? Your adrenal glands are your body's stress warriors, stepping in to provide extra energy and resources when life gets tough. They're like your hyped-up caffeinated friend who makes sure you can rise to the occasion, whether it's a short-term crisis or a temporary increase in demands. But, just like that friend who drinks too much coffee, they can't run at full speed forever. Supporting your adrenals means giving your body the fuel it needs—carbs, fats, nutrients, and rest—so you can rely less on the backup system and more on the efficient, thyroid-supported system that keeps you thriving in the long term.

While the adrenal glands take the lead in mobilizing energy during stress, they don't act alone. Enter the pancreas, another key player in the endocrine system's stress response team. While the adrenals focus on activating stress hormones like cortisol and adrenaline, the pancreas works behind the scenes to regulate blood glucose levels, ensuring there's enough fuel to meet your body's heightened energy demands. Let's dive into how the pancreas steps up during stress to keep your blood sugar and energy production on track.

The Pancreas, Blood Sugar, and Energy Production

The pancreas is a critical player in regulating energy production, especially during stress, by managing blood glucose levels through two opposing hormones—insulin and glucagon. Let's be clear: you can't talk about stress and energy production without diving into blood glucose, the body's favorite quick-energy fuel. After all, the whole point of a stress response is to make more fuel (fat and glucose) available, so your body has the energy to fight a bear or meet a deadline. Because, let's face it, in today's wacky world, either one could be true.

Since stress is essentially your body screaming, "We need more energy!" It's no surprise that the gland and its hormones responsible for balancing blood sugar play a major role in this discussion.

Insulin: Your Blood Sugar Lowering Hormone

Let's start with insulin, the pancreas's better-known hormone. Produced by the beta cells, insulin is a peptide hormone released when blood sugar rises—like after you devour a bagel or accidentally finish the entire sleeve of Girl Scout Thin Mints. Its main job? Shuttle glucose out of the blood and into cells to be used for energy. If your cells are fully stocked, or the glucose gets "stuck" in the cells, insulin stores the extra glucose as glycogen in the liver or muscles. If those storage bins are full, the leftovers are packed away as fat. YAY! (Yes, that's sarcasm.)

But wait, there's more! Insulin also helps amino acids leave the blood so they can be used for protein synthesis, making it critical for maintaining muscle and tissue health (15, 16, 17). In short, insulin is the cleanup crew after a meal, ensuring everything is stored properly. Elevated insulin levels in response to rising glucose are normal and healthy, if the system works as intended. (Spoiler alert: for many, it doesn't. More on this later.)

Glucagon: Elevates Your Blood Sugar— and Increases Under Stress

Glucagon, the pancreas's lesser-known blood sugar hormone, is produced by the alpha cells and steps into the spotlight when blood sugar dips—like when you haven't eaten in hours, you're dieting, or you're under stress. Think of glucagon as your body's anti-hypoglycemic hormone, raising blood sugar through:

1. **Glycogenolysis**: Breaking down stored glycogen in the liver to release glucose.

2. **Gluconeogenesis**: Converting non-carbohydrate sources (like amino acids and fats) into glucose.

3. **Inhibiting glycolysis**: Slowing glucose breakdown to conserve it for essential functions (18).

Glucagon works as insulin's opposite. When insulin rises to lower blood sugar, glucagon decreases. Conversely, when glucagon elevates to raise blood sugar, insulin decreases.

In a healthy individual, glucagon does its job beautifully, stepping in to raise blood sugar when levels dip. It taps into your stored energy, including glycogen, amino acids, and fats, to meet your body's demands. Once you eat carbohydrates, glucagon levels naturally drop because your body no longer needs to produce its own glucose. This means carbs (yes, carbs!) lower glucagon, making them an anti-stress food.

Think about it, have you ever wondered why you crave carbs when you're stressed? It's simple, your body wants quick, usable energy to fuel the stress response. Eating the right carbs (fruits, root vegetables, honey, or juice) calms the stress response and helps you feel better. But if you rely on ultra-processed, low-nutrient foods (like those thin mints mentioned above), or worse, ignore those carb cravings entirely, the stress response continues. That's when other hormones in addition to glucagon, such as cortisol and adrenaline, step in to keep you going (19).

Elevated glucagon doesn't just fuel the stress response, it also impacts thyroid hormone metabolism in your peripheral tissues (20). High glucagon levels can reduce the active thyroid hormone, triiodothyronine (T3), while increasing the inactive form, reverse triiodothyronine (rT3). This shift lowers cellular energy production, as T3 is essential for driving metabolic processes.

These changes are part of your body's natural adaptation to stress, designed to conserve energy when resources are scarce. While helpful in the short term, prolonged glucagon elevation, especially when paired with cortisol and adrenaline, can slow down energy production, leading to a sluggish metabolism and decreased vitality.

Prolonged elevated glucagon levels are observed in people dealing with a wide variety of physiological stressors, including trauma, burns, surgery, heart attacks, hypoxia, blood sugar issues like diabetes, and anyone following a low-carb diet.

The bottom line is glucagon elevates when blood sugar drops, as its job is to raise blood sugar. The simplest way to lower glucagon naturally? Eat carbohydrates. If you're not eating enough carbs or your body struggles to convert them into energy (due to low fuel intake, nutrient deficiencies, low thyroid function, or other energy blocks), glucagon and other stress hormones will stay elevated, keeping your metabolism stuck in stress mode.

You might be wondering: what about people with blood sugar issues who don't respond well to carbs? If that sounds like you, let's dive into what's happening and what you can do to fix it.

What About People Who Have Elevated Blood Sugar Levels?

For individuals with chronically high blood sugar (like prediabetic, insulin resistance, and diabetics), the system doesn't work as well. Instead of carbohydrate intake lowering glucagon and other stress hormones, ingesting carbohydrates may increase glucagon levels, making blood sugar spike even higher. This happens because of poor cellular health and impaired glucagon regulation, creating a situation where both insulin and glucagon are elevated at the same time. It's like having two captains steering the same ship in opposite directions—chaos ensues.

Now, before I talk about what is going on with someone with high blood sugar, let me give you a little understanding of blood sugar and how it works.

What Is Blood Sugar?

Blood sugar, or glucose, is the sugar in your bloodstream that fuels your cells and powers your body. It originates from carbohydrates in your diet (think bread, fruits, milk, and vegetables), glycogen stored in your liver and muscles, and a process called gluconeogenesis, where your body converts non-carbohydrate sources like protein and fat into glucose. Normal blood sugar levels range from 70–100 mg/dl when fasting and up to 140 mg/dl after meals. Your body carefully regulates glucose levels using hormones, and maintaining this balance is crucial since extreme highs or lows can lead to serious health problems.

When you eat, especially carbohydrates, your body releases insulin to help transport glucose into your cells for energy. Conversely, during fasting or stress, hormones like cortisol, glucagon, and adrenaline signal your liver to release stored glycogen as glucose. If glycogen is depleted, your body starts producing glucose from other resources, like muscle tissue, to meet its energy demands.

What Is High Blood Sugar?

High blood sugar, or hyperglycemia, occurs when fasting levels exceed 125 mg/dl or post-meal levels rise above 180 mg/dl. Contrary to popular belief, sugar itself isn't the villain here. It's more like an innocent bystander caught in the crossfire when your cells can't process glucose efficiently.

Picture your body as a system of pipes. If a pipe gets clogged (poor cellular function), water (glucose) backs up, causing high blood sugar. Sure, you can temporarily shut off the water (cut carbs), but that won't fix the clog. The real solution? Clear the pipes (restore cellular function) so glucose can flow smoothly.

When cells aren't doing their job, they struggle to use glucose. Even if glucose makes it into the cell, it may struggle to get through the mitochondria (your cellular power plant), leaving energy production sputtering and glucose lingering in your blood. This dysfunction leads to a buildup of glucose in the blood and reduced energy production. And when you don't have enough energy being produced and your demands stay high, stress will occur—as it is a need for more energy. Thus, stress hormones signal to the body to release more glucose (even though you have enough in your blood), leaving you trapped in a vicious cycle.

Remember, the answer to fixing this is never about removing carbohydrates, but rather restoring proper glucose oxidation.

What About Low Blood Sugar?

Low blood sugar, or hypoglycemia, occurs when levels drop below 70 mg/dl. This can happen due to skipping meals, intense exercise, alcohol consumption, liver dysfunction, and all things stress. If glycogen stores are depleted, stress hormones raise blood sugar, which is why hypoglycemia can wake you up at night with a racing heart.

Since the liver stores glucose as glycogen, its health is critical for maintaining blood sugar levels, especially overnight. If your liver can't store enough glycogen, hormones like adrenaline and cortisol rise to produce more glucose, but this process can wake you up (22).

The fix? A little glucose-rich snack before bed can calm those stress hormones and help you sleep through the night without your body staging a glucose emergency.

How Do You Improve Glucose Oxidation?

Improving your body's ability to oxidize glucose is key. When glucose moves efficiently into and through cells, blood sugar levels decrease naturally, energy improves, and stress hormones stabilize

So, to improve glucose oxidation, reducing stress is a good place to start. Let's face it, your body can't regulate energy levels properly when it's in full panic mode. Stress can signal your body to keep making glucose, even when there's already plenty in the bloodstream. Reducing the stressor can decrease your need for more energy, shutting this process off. Numerous studies have shown that stress-reducing techniques like meditation, yoga, and mindfulness (being present with your body, thoughts, and feelings), have led to significant reductions in blood sugar levels in individuals with type 2 diabetes (23, 24).

(Check my top 9 healthy stress reducers at the end of this chapter.)

Another great way to improve glucose oxidation is to move your body. During exercise, muscles contract and stimulate glucose uptake independent of insulin. This means even people with insulin resistance can improve glucose metabolism if they use their muscles—this can work with aerobic exercise, strength training, or anything that uses muscular contraction. Even after exercise, muscles remain more insulin-sensitive for up to 48 hours, making glucose oxidation more efficient.

How well you produce energy is directly tied to how well you oxidize glucose. If your body has trouble producing energy, you'll be pushed into a stress response more easily, which negatively impacts glucose oxidation. (Remember, a stress response only occurs when your body needs more fuel to produce energy.)

Therefore, optimizing energy production is key to improving glucose oxidation. By focusing on strategies discussed earlier in this book, you can enhance energy production, which lowers the body's need for additional energy and reduces stress responses. Eating a nutrient-rich diet, supporting oxygen transportation and utilization, and ensuring proper thyroid hormone production and conversion all play vital roles in optimizing glucose oxidation.

In addition, as mentioned in Chapter 2, decreasing excessive fat oxidation can improve glucose oxidation. Excess free fatty acids (FFAs) in your bloodstream can interfere with glucose entering your cells, largely due to a biochemical tug-of-war called the Randle Cycle. It's named after P.J. Randle, who discovered in 1963 that excessive fat metabolism can inhibit glucose oxidation and vice versa (25).

Here's the deal, our cells can use either fat or glucose for energy, but they can't efficiently process both at the same time. When FFAs are elevated, whether from a high-fat diet or stress hormones prompting fat release, your cells prioritize fat metabolism. As a result, glucose isn't taken up as easily and is left circulating in the bloodstream instead of being used for energy. This contributes to elevated blood sugar, along with fatigue, increased thirst, hunger, and frequent urination.

The good news is that reducing dietary fat can significantly improve this dynamic. Lowering fat intake reduces FFAs in the bloodstream, which decreases the competition between fat and glucose for cellular energy production. This allows cells to become more sensitive to glucose (improved insulin sensitivity), helping glucose enter cells more freely and supporting both blood sugar regulation and optimal energy production.

Interestingly, research has shown that high-carbohydrate, very-low-fat diets (HCVLF) are particularly effective in improving glucose oxidation. These diets, usually around 10–15% fat, have even been shown in some cases to help reverse high blood sugar conditions, including diabetes. In essence, when excess FFAs step aside, glucose gets back to doing what it does best—fueling your body efficiently.

Still not convinced? Let's look at the research!

First on the list is Dr. Walter Kempner's Rice Diet. Developed in 1939, it consisted of white rice, fruit, sugar, and minimal protein and fat—a 95% carbohydrate diet. Originally designed to treat hypertension and kidney disease, it unexpectedly improved diabetes as well. After treating over 100 diabetics, Kempner found that most patients experienced lower fasting blood sugar and reduced insulin needs. Many even discontinued insulin all together (26, 27).

Many participants on the Rice Diet lost significant weight, which led some to wonder if it was the weight loss itself that improved glucose utilization.

To answer this, in 1977, researchers James Anderson and Kyleen Ward tested the Rice Diet on 20 long-term diabetics while ensuring calorie levels prevented weight loss. Within just 16 days, half of the participants stopped all diabetes medications, while the rest reduced insulin doses anywhere from 9% to 98%. This demonstrated that the diet—not just weight loss—was responsible for the improvements (28).

In the 1980s, Dr. John McDougall introduced a starch-based diet called The Starch Solution. It focused on rice, potatoes, corn, and other starchy foods. McDougall's starch-based diet consisted of 80% carbs, 10% fat, and 10% protein. It showed improvements in insulin sensitivity and glucose control. Many participants, who had type 2 diabetes, reduced or eliminated their diabetic medications (29).

In a 1982 study published in *Diabetes Care*, Dr. James Barnard, PhD, and colleagues found that combining a high-complex carbohydrate, low-fat diet with regular exercise reduced fasting glucose, on average, by 25%. Of the 23 patients who were taking blood sugar-lowering medications, all but two were off their medications by the end of the program. Of the 17 patients who were taking insulin, all but four discontinued insulin at discharge (30).

More recently, a study published in the *Endocrine Society's Journal of Clinical Endocrinology and Metabolism* found that consuming two or more servings of fruit a day lowered the risk of developing type 2 diabetes by 36%, compared to consuming less than half a serving. This suggests that fruit, which contains sucrose, glucose, and fructose, does not increase diabetes risk but may lower it (31).

Now, I want to pause for a moment because I can already hear the low-carb, high-fat enthusiasts saying, "But I fixed my high blood sugar by cutting out all carbs and eating mostly fat and protein." And yes, it's true, eliminating carbs can improve blood sugar levels. Think of it like turning off the water supply to stop a leak, it does work, at least for now, but as soon as you turn the water back on (eat carbs), the leak returns. Similarly, removing carbs may stabilize blood sugar in the short term, but the underlying issue of poor glucose oxidation often resurfaces when carbohydrates are reintroduced.

To be clear, I'm not dismissing the fact that some people feel better and see improvements on a low-carb diet. In many cases, these improvements come from eating less overall and, more importantly, losing weight, particularly visceral fat (the fat stored around your organs). This type of weight loss can enhance insulin sensitivity and improve glucose oxidation. So, it is not all bad, and if low-carb is working for you and you enjoy it, then do what works for you.

It's also worth noting that low-carb diets often eliminate highly processed foods, like breads, pastas, cookies, and cakes. These foods are loaded with refined flours, unhealthy fats, and sugar. Cutting these out can lead to weight loss and metabolic improvements, but this doesn't mean carbs themselves are the enemy. A low-carb lifestyle filled with animal fats and proteins and a sprinkle of vegetables can be a huge improvement over a diet filled with ultra-processed foods (often high fat and high carb) and excess calories.

If you opt to go low carb and feel better, the goal should not be to avoid carbs forever but to improve your body's ability to oxidize glucose efficiently. Better glucose oxidation means less reliance on stress hormones and better energy production.

In addition, I'm not suggesting that everyone with blood sugar issues should immediately abandon higher-fat foods and jump straight into a high-carb, low-fat diet. The purpose of this information is to highlight that sugars (carbs), the primary source of glucose, are not the evil villain causing high blood sugar problems. Instead, it's the cells' inability to efficiently utilize glucose that leads to elevated blood sugar. Increasing carbohydrates while reducing fat intake appears to help improve this issue by enhancing glucose oxidation.

That said, I'd recommend starting with the basics, which include reducing stress, supporting cellular function, and prioritizing nutrient-dense foods. If blood sugar levels remain stubbornly high, exploring a high-carb, low-fat diet (HCLFD) may be worth considering. Just be sure to keep a food log while experimenting, as lowering fat intake to 10–15% does take some planning. With the right approach, your body can become better equipped to handle glucose and maintain balanced blood sugar levels.

If you've made it this far, then pat yourself on the back! You're now armed with a deeper understanding of how stress, whether from physical, mental, or dietary sources, can wreak havoc on your energy production and overall health, particularly if it lingers too long. Chronic stress can overwhelm your body's systems, leading to metabolic slowdowns, hormonal imbalances, and impaired glucose oxidation.

So, what's next? How can you build resilience to stress and ensure you're better equipped to handle it when it strikes? And if stress has already knocked you down or worse yet, knocked you out, what can you do to recover and rebuild? Don't worry, in my 15 years of working with thousands of stressed-out people, I have never found anyone who can't get better. Let's dive into practical strategies to mitigate stress and strengthen your body for whatever challenges come your way.

How to Manage and Recover from Any Stressful Event

First, let me tell you; if life has recently decided to body-slam you into the pavement, kick you in the face, and then throw you into a very deep ditch—I feel you! Life has got a dark sense of humor sometimes, doesn't it? But hey, you've taken a step forward by reading this book, and that's a win. Your next mission is to understand what your body needs (vs. what it might want) to help you heal and recover.

Here are my top strategies to help you bounce back from any kind of stress:

1. Slow Down and Take a Break

One of the most important things you can do after hitting a wall at 100 mph is to simply slow down and take a break. It's simple advice, but often the hardest to follow. You might think, "But I have so much to DO!" Sure, I get it. But trust me, if you're sick in bed, or worse, hospitalized, none of it will matter. Wouldn't you rather operate at 100% with regular breaks than at 75% with no rest? A systematic review published in 2022, involving 2300 people, found that taking short breaks throughout the day dramatically improved vigor, while reducing fatigue and stress. Another study by the American Psychological Association found that taking as brief as 5–15-minute breaks early in the day helped restore energy and reduced afternoon health symptoms (fatigue, stress levels) (32, 33).

2. Get Outside

Rain, shine, snow, or frost, if it's weather permitting, get outside. Nature has a magical way of calming the nervous system and reducing stress. In fact, a 2019 study in *Frontiers in Psychology* found that just 20–30 minutes in nature significantly reduced cortisol levels (34). You don't need a mountaintop retreat, your backyard or a local park will do the trick.

Bonus points if you can soak up some sunlight. Sunlight supports your circadian rhythm (your body's internal clock), helps regulate cortisol (if you're not overexposed), and provides the immune and thyroid-supporting vitamin D your body needs (35, 36, 37).

3. Take a Walk

If you're physically able, take a walk—inside or outside. A study published in *Health Promotion Perspectives* found that a 10-minute walk significantly reduced anxiety, depression, and stress levels. Walking outdoors amplified these effects (38). If walking feels overwhelming right now, start with simply stepping outside. As you heal, you can gradually increase your walking time and intensity.

4. Fuel and Nourish Your Body

Healing starts with adequate fuel and nutrition. Your body needs energy to recover from stress, and that means eating. However, stress often hijacks appetite, either killing it or causing you to crave high-calorie, low-nutrient comfort foods. Neither is ideal.

Here's where I'll tell you not to "listen to your body" (at least not completely). When you feel stressed, I want you to eat, even if your body is saying you don't want anything. I also want you to eat nutrient-rich foods, even when your body wants salty, fatty, processed crap. Stress increases your energy and nutrient demands, so the only way to keep up with this stress is to eat foods that provide quality energy and nutrients. You can eat nutrient rich smoothies, soups, or solid meals, whatever works. One of the biggest drivers of chronic stress is continuing to undereat or overeating ultra-processed, fatty-sugary foods. Your system needs all nutrients, and when it's in overdrive, it needs even more!

For more guidance, revisit the first part of this book and my earlier book, *How to Heal Your Metabolism.*

5. Balance Your Meals

Balanced meals with ample carbohydrates (40–60%), proteins (20–30%), and fats (15–30%) help stabilize blood sugar and provide sustainable energy for recovery. Everyone's ideal macronutrient ratio is different, so don't get stuck on what worked for your friend. Experiment and find what fuels you.

Take into consideration the breakdown of your current diet before jumping into the above macronutrient ratios. If you are currently on a low-carb, higher-fat diet, you need to move slowly when adding carbs and lowering fat. Jumping quickly can have adverse effects on your health, weight, and overall well-being. I discuss this in more depth in my last book, *How to Heal Your Metabolism.*

6. Your Thoughts Matter

As I've mentioned before, the stress you feel often has more to do with your thoughts about the situation than the event itself. Stressful things are happening everywhere, all the time—but they're not stressful to you unless you focus on them.

When my nervous system was at its worst, I noticed that dwelling on how bad I felt only made me feel worse. Shifting my thoughts to focus on even the smallest positives made a world of difference. Training your mind to focus on what's good rather than what's going wrong can be transformative.

If you're feeling stuck, one option you might want to investigate is finding a "brain retraining" class. These types of classes help you get out of your stinking thinking, putting your nervous system at ease, and allowing your cells an opportunity to heal. The one I have used and often refer some of my clients to is Dynamic Neural Retraining System (DNRS). DNRS is a program designed to help rewire unhelpful thought patterns. I have no affiliation with this program, only that I have seen it work for not only myself, but numerous other people.

7. Get Enough Sleep and Rest

Sleep is where the magic happens—it's when your mitochondria (the energy powerhouses of your cells) regenerate. Increased energy production allows you to meet the demands of stress. Of course, sleeping well can be challenging when you're overwhelmed. If this is you, try to focus on the other strategies in this list: eating enough, proper nutrition, sunlight, movement, mindfulness, and being in nature, as each of these will help improve your sleep naturally.

In addition, you can also try supplements like magnesium, progesterone, added salt, taurine, and L-theanine to help with sleep—see below.

8. Control Your Controllables

While you don't want to avoid all stress, you should aim to reduce or reframe stressful situations whenever possible, especially while you're trying to recover. This means setting firm boundaries, limiting exposure to toxic people, chemicals, sensational news, avoiding doom-scrolling on social media, and anything else that might feel triggering. By lightening the overall stress load on your body, you'll create more bandwidth to handle the stressors you can't control with greater ease.

9. Stress-Reducing Supplements

As many of you know, I'm not the type to overhype supplements. I'd much rather you soak up some sunshine, take a walk, eat nourishing foods, and focus on positive thinking to recover from stress and boost energy. However, sometimes life throws more challenges our way, and a few well-researched supplements can provide valuable support during the stress reducing process.

Niacinamide (B3)

Niacinamide, also known as vitamin B3, is an essential nutrient that plays a vital role in energy production and stress reduction. As discussed in Chapter 3, niacinamide is crucial for forming NAD+, the coenzyme your cells need for energy metabolism.

When it comes to helping mitigate the stress response, B3 helps limit the excessive release of free fatty acids (FFAs) by slowing down lipolysis. This is important because high levels of FFAs can disrupt glucose metabolism, and your body performs better when it can utilize glucose easily. By keeping FFAs in check, niacinamide supports more efficient energy production, which will reduce the stress response. Better glucose oxidation means more efficient energy production, which will always limit the stress response.

Aspirin

Ah, aspirin. The MVP of the medicine cabinet and your grandma's favorite remedy for pretty much—everything. Believe it or not, it can also help with managing stress. Like niacinamide, it helps regulate FFAs, but it works differently. Aspirin inhibits the COX-1 and COX-2 enzymes, which are responsible for producing inflammatory prostaglandins. These prostaglandins contribute to pain, inflammation, menstrual cramps, and even lipolysis.

By reducing prostaglandin production, aspirin decreases FFA release from fat tissue. This allows your body to focus on glucose oxidation and energy production, ultimately helping to mitigate the stress response. It's a classic remedy with benefits that extend beyond pain relief.

Magnesium

Magnesium is a crucial mineral for managing the body's stress response. A deficiency in magnesium can lead to symptoms such as high blood pressure, elevated blood sugar, fatigue, and poor sleep—all of which can worsen stress. While magnesium-rich foods like cooked greens are excellent sources, supplementation can be particularly helpful during times of high stress.

Here are my preferred forms of magnesium:

- **Magnesium glycinate.** This highly absorbable form is known for its calming properties, thanks to glycine, an amino acid that promotes relaxation and better sleep (39, 40).

- **Magnesium taurate.** This combines magnesium with taurine, an amino acid that supports GABA, a neurotransmitter with calming effects. It's particularly useful for reducing stress-induced tension (41).

- **Combination of magnesium glycinate and taurate.** Personally, I find this blend most effective for promoting relaxation and improving sleep. (For those interested, you can find my recommended supplements on my website at katedeering.com).

Sodium Chloride (Salt)

Salt, a staple in the kitchen, can also support your body during stress. Adequate salt intake helps regulate cortisol and aldosterone, two hormones that rise under stress. When sodium levels are low, due to sweating or restrictive diets, the body triggers the stress response. Adding a pinch of salt to your meals can restore sodium balance, helping to lower stress hormones and support overall well-being.

However, moderation is important. If your diet is already high in processed foods, additional salt may not be beneficial. On the other hand, for those consuming a whole-foods diet rich in fruits and vegetables, a little extra salt can support your nervous system and enhance the flavor of your meals.

While supplements aren't a substitute for foundational practices like proper nutrition and mindfulness, they can be valuable tools to help manage stress and restore balance.

In summary, stress is an inevitable part of life, but it doesn't have to rob you of your energy and vitality. While your body's stress response is brilliantly designed to help you survive immediate challenges, chronic stress can leave your energy production systems sputtering on fumes. Understanding how stress impacts your energy, whether through disrupted glucose oxidation, hormonal imbalances, or metabolic slowdowns, puts you in the driver's seat, empowering you to restore balance and vitality.

Think of your energy production system as a finely tuned engine. When stress hits, your body shifts gears, redirecting resources to meet immediate demands. This works beautifully in the short term, but prolonged stress is like driving your car at full throttle without stopping for fuel or maintenance. Sooner or later, parts start to break down, leading to fatigue, poor digestion, hormonal chaos, and an inability to bounce back from even minor challenges.

Here's the good news, you can repair and optimize your body's energy systems by addressing stress head-on. Start by fueling your body with what it truly needs, nutrient-dense foods and balanced meals, to stabilize blood sugar and reduce reliance on stress hormones. Support your mitochondria with oxygen, glucose, and proper thyroid function. And by prioritizing rest, movement, and mindfulness, you can shift your body out of survival mode and back into efficient, thriving energy production.

The link between stress and energy production is undeniable. By reducing stress, you reduce your body's demand for emergency energy production, allowing your systems to return to their natural, steady state. When life inevitably throws stress your way, remember to slow down, breathe, and refuel, not with a shot of tequila and a

Big Mac, but with rest, sunlight, and a brisk walk. Stress will still knock on your door now and then, but with a well-fed body and a calm mind, you'll be ready to answer it, maybe even holding a glass of warm milk instead of waving the metaphorical white flag.

Alright, are you ready for the next energy block? The one so many people suffer from, but few understand how it affects energy production—you guessed it, it is your digestion.

CHAPTER 6

THE BOTTOM LINE

Stress—The Energy (Metabolism) Crusher

1. Stress occurs any time the demands placed on the body are more than the body has the available energy to keep up with. Stress occurs when there is a need for more energy.

2. All stress starts with the amygdala and then its connection to four different hypothalamus-pituitary axes. These axes communicate with the thyroid, adrenals, gonads and prolactin.

3. Glucagon, adrenaline, and cortisol are your primary stress hormones. Each elevates to mobilize fuel and raise your blood sugar.

4. The primary reason for chronically elevated blood sugar is stress.

5. The best methods to mitigate the stress response are slowing down, taking a walk, going outside, a nourishing diet, balancing your blood sugar, positive thoughts, controlling your controllables, and possible supplementation.

CHAPTER 7

WHAT YOUR GUT HEALTH SAYS ABOUT
YOUR ABILITY TO PRODUCE ENERGY

Good digestion is essential for optimal energy production. This intricate process involves breaking down macronutrients into their usable forms, absorbing sugars, fats, amino acids, vitamins, and minerals, and then eliminating the waste efficiently. It's your body's way of keeping the lights on and the engine running.

However, various health and digestive issues, like hypothyroidism, anemia, enzyme deficiencies, low stomach acid (HCl), poor bile production, malabsorption, endotoxins, or gut microbiome imbalances, can turn your digestive system into complete chaos. These disruptions don't just slow things down; they leave you feeling like you're running on fumes.

When your body can't access the nutrients and fuel it needs, cellular energy production takes a nosedive and stops you from performing at your best. This is why I have listed digestive and absorption issues as your second energy block.

Digestive issues have become so common that it's now more unusual to NOT have any chronic issues than to have one. Over 70 million Americans are affected by gastrointestinal (GI) diseases each year. And that's just the ones who report it, many people just grin (or grimace) and bear it. Let's face it, some of us have normalized bloating and stomach aches as if they were part of our personality.

The interesting (and annoying) thing is digestion doesn't stop at the gut. Those with digestive problems often report higher rates of depression, anxiety, skin issues, low energy, and sleep disturbances. Essentially, if your digestion is struggling, every system in your body can be affected. Without proper breakdown and absorption of food, your cells are left without the nutrients, proteins, and fuel they need to produce energy. Less energy for your cells means less energy to keep your entire body functioning optimally. It's a vicious cycle that leaves every system shorthanded.

I've been there. Over a decade ago, I dealt with daily bloating, gas, and the occasional roulette game of diarrhea or constipation. My diet back then? Raw veggies, plant milks, and sugar-free processed "health" foods. I thought these issues were just part of life, everyone around me seemed to be dealing with the same, uh, crap. In fact, my friends and I even made it a bonding activity. We'd discuss our bowel movements (or lack thereof) mid-workout or on a beach run. We called it "sh#t-talk," and we thought it was perfectly normal. Spoiler alert: it wasn't.

Had I known then what I know now, I would have realized that my gut issues were giant red flags waving frantically. The gas, bloating, constipation, and diarrhea were all signs of a digestive system under stress. Even though I "looked" healthy on the outside, my insides were struggling to keep up. It wasn't until the issues started showing up externally as weight gain, skin problems, and mood swings, that I finally started paying attention.

The good news? By understanding how digestion works, identifying obstacles, and adopting strategies to optimize digestive health, you can unlock your body's full energy-producing potential. And yes, that includes pooping like a rock star!

What Is Digestion?

Digestion is the process of breaking down food into its most basic components so your body can absorb it and send it off to your cells to be used as energy, structure, or backup reserves (glycogen or fat).

Your gastrointestinal (GI) system, often called your enteric nervous system (ENS) or "second brain," is a powerhouse that operates semi-independently of your central nervous system. With 400-600 million neurons, second only to your brain and spinal cord, the GI system is like your wise grandparent that tells everyone in the family what to do (1). It's constantly in touch with your other organs and glands to help them digest, absorb, and transport your nutrients while sending status updates to your brain about whether you're hungry, full, stressed, or under the weather. Basically, it's one of your body's communication centers.

The GI system is a long, muscular, multi-organ marvel that starts with your mouth and continues through your esophagus, stomach, small intestine, and colon. Key supporting players include the pancreas, liver, and gallbladder, which produce enzymes, bile, and hydrochloric acid to help keep the system running smoothly. Together, this amazing team handles breaking down food, absorbing nutrients and energy, removing waste, and protecting you from unwanted invaders like bacteria, fungi, and viruses.

> *FUN FACT: The GI system, along with your respiratory system, acts as the gatekeeper between the outside world and you. Your GI system contains 80% of your protective (immune) system. Every bite of food you take is scrutinized and processed to make sure only the good stuff gets in, it's like having a hyper-efficient bouncer at the door of Club You.*

The Digestion Time Frame

Complete digestion of food takes anywhere from 15 to 72 hours to move from your mouth to the toilet (2). Yes, it's a journey, not a sprint. Here's how the timeline typically breaks down:

- **Chewing:** 10-30 seconds per bite. (Unless you're a speed eater, in which case, slow down and let your teeth do their job.)
- **Esophagus:** Peristalsis (the muscle movement that pushes food) takes about 10 seconds to deliver your food to your stomach.
- **Stomach:** Emptying takes around 2-5 hours, depending on what you ate. Fat, fiber, and proteins like to linger, while carbs make a quicker exit.
- **Small intestine:** Food spends about 2-6 hours here, getting broken down into its nutrient building blocks.
- **Colon:** The final leg can take anywhere from 10 to 59 hours, depending on your metabolism, hydration, and fiber intake.

So, from first bite to the big finale, digestion spans about 15 to 72 hours, with the state of your metabolism, overall health, and food type influencing the journey. A slower metabolism can slow gut transit time, hello constipation. While an irritated or inflamed bowel can quicken transit time. In addition, meals filled with fat, protein, and fiber will take longer to digest than a liquid meal.

Digestion Starts Before the First Bite

Believe it or not, digestion kicks off before food even enters your mouth. Just the sight or smell of your favorite food (hi there, french fries!) can send signals along your vagus nerve (3), communicating to your stomach, triggering saliva production and prepping gastric juices for action. It's your body's way of saying, "Let's get ready to rumble...digestively."

The Vagus Nerve

Your vagus nerve is like the unsung hero of your nervous system. It's the longest cranial nerve, stretching from your brain to almost all your organs (except your adrenal glands and bladder) (4). It plays a key role in your parasympathetic nervous system (PNS), often called the "rest and digest" system.

When your vagus nerve is activated, your body feels relaxed and calm, creating the perfect environment for digestion (4). On the flip side, the sympathetic nervous system (SNS), your "fight or flight" mode, slows or halts digestion entirely. If your body thinks you're running from a lion, it doesn't care about breaking down your lunch, it cares about not becoming the lion's lunch.

Here's the deal:

- The PNS (via your vagus nerve) upregulates digestion and gets everything moving efficiently.

- The SNS (via stress hormones) downregulates digestion, inhibiting stomach and intestinal activity.

When your body is under chronic stress, digestion slows or even stops. This means that if stress has been your constant companion, your digestive system is probably struggling to keep up.

The takeaway? Your gut thrives on calm, not chaos. Later in this chapter, I'll explain how to activate your vagus nerve and get your PNS back in charge. But for now, remember stress is the digestive system's kryptonite. Relaxation, on the other hand, is its superpower.

Chew Your Food!

Digestion officially begins in the mouth, where your saliva, a true multitasking hero, gets to work. Saliva contains enzymes such as amylase, which starts breaking down starches, and lingual lipase, which kicks off fat digestion. Your mouth is essentially the opening act for your digestive system, and a good performance here sets the stage for the rest of the show.

To make the most of this first step, experts recommend chewing each bite of food 20-40 times. It might sound excessive, but the logic is solid: softer, well-chewed food is easier for your stomach and intestines to process. Of course, chewing a piece of watermelon will take far fewer chomps than a steak, but you get the idea, the tougher the food, the more effort required.

Now, let's be real. Most people chew each bite about 10 times before gulping food down, which means they're starting the digestive process at half-speed. If this sounds like you, it's time to slow down and let your teeth do their job. Research (while not conclusive) suggests that chewing thoroughly can increase nutrient absorption, decrease stomach upset, and even help with weight management (5). So, if you're looking for an easy way to upgrade your digestion, start by simply chewing more, your gut will thank you.

Pro Tips for Better Chewing

1. **Eat distraction-free:** Step away from your computer or TV.

2. **Sit down while eating:** Your stomach likes it when you're relaxed.

3. **Put your fork down between bites:** It's not a race.

4. **Count your chews:** Aim for at least 30 per bite.

5. **Swallow each bite before adding more to your mouth:** Again, it's not a race.

The Beginning of Peristalsis

Peristalsis is your digestive tract's version of a moving walkway, a series of muscle contractions and relaxations that propel food along its journey. Once you swallow, peristalsis kicks in, sending the broken-down food, now called a bolus, down the digestive tract. These muscles work in a single direction, pushing the bolus through your upper esophageal sphincter (UES) and into the esophagus. The UES is the bouncer, keeping air out of your esophagus and food out of your windpipe (6).

When the bolus reaches the end of the esophagus, the lower esophageal sphincter (LES) steps in. This clever valve relaxes to let food into the stomach, then closes to keep it there. When it works well, you don't even notice it. But when it malfunctions, you get this lovely burning feeling most of us know as heartburn! If the LES doesn't close properly, food and stomach acid can sneak back into the esophagus, causing gastroesophageal reflux disease (GERD). Symptoms of GERD include a burning sensation in the chest (classic heartburn), belching, regurgitation, and even nausea (7), more on GERD below.

Most of us know what happens next. You're probably prescribed an antacid to reduce stomach acid, which provides temporary relief. But here's the problem, this approach doesn't fix the underlying issue, at least, not long term. Yes, it will further decrease your stomach acid (so it doesn't splash up into the esophagus), allowing your esophagus to heal, but it is not fixing the reasons you have GERD, which means, over time the situation is bound to happen again. It's like using a bucket to pour water out of your leaking boat, without plugging the hole. It works, at least until you stop using it, but eventually the boat will fill up again (GERD will come back).

How Does a Weak LES Affect Energy Production?

A weak LES can lead to chronic inflammation of the esophagus (esophagitis) due to your stomach acid repeatedly damaging the tissues. This inflammation will lead to inflammatory cytokines (signaling proteins that regulate immunity and inflammation) being released, which can trigger mitochondrial stress and dysfunction.

These damaged mitochondria produce less ATP, while generating excessive reactive oxygen species (ROS). Remember ROS is naturally produced in cellular respiration, yet excessive ROS can lead to oxidative stress and damage to the cells. The truth is any inflammatory condition can lead to a decrease in ATP production because the increase of pro-inflammatory cytokines disrupts mitochondrial function—which is the primary site of ATP synthesis.

In addition, due to the discomfort of GERD many people tend to eat less, further disrupting overall energy production, increasing the stress on the body, and further hindering healing. Later, I'll dive into how to address GERD at its source instead of just masking the symptoms.

Now I know the anatomy and physiology of the stomach, small intestine, and colon might not sound like thrilling bedtime reading. But stick with me—understanding their roles can reveal why you might be experiencing bloating, constipation, diarrhea, dull skin, low energy, mood swings, or other signs that something isn't quite right. When you know how these organs work, you can better troubleshoot what's going on in your own body.

So, without further ado, let's keep going...

Your Amazing Stomach

Your stomach is the next stop on the digestive journey, overseeing the continued breakdown of food while protecting you from external bacteria and pathogens. Your entire gut, starting with your stomach, plays a huge role in your immune system!

Once the food bolus enters your stomach, it mixes with powerful gastric juices—hydrochloric acid (HCl), lipase, and pepsin. These juices, produced by the stomach lining, are so essential that some experts consider the stomach a gland as well as an organ. After all, glands release crucial substances like hormones, sweat, and, in this case, digestive juices.

These gastric juices, particularly HCl, lower your stomach's pH to a range of 1-3, creating an incredibly acidic environment that can break down just about anything. HCl is required for directly breaking down proteins, activating digestive enzymes (like pepsin to help digest protein), signaling the release of bile and pancreatic enzymes (to help digest fats and carbs), killing harmful bacteria and pathogens, and triggering the LES to prevent acid reflux.

A Quick pH Lesson

The pH scale runs from 0 to 14:

- Anything below 7 is acidic.
- Anything above 7 is alkaline.
- A pH of 7 is neutral.

So, a stomach pH of 1? That's very acidic!

FUN FACT: Your stomach acid is slightly more acidic than battery acid. Humans share stomach acidity levels with scavengers like eagles and vultures, as well as carnivores like cats. By comparison, herbivores (vegetarians) have a stomach acid pH of around 4-5. What does this tell you? Hint: You weren't designed to be a vegetarian (8).

Moving On: Let's Talk Stomach Anatomy

Your stomach lining is an impressive multitasker, composed of three layers of muscle and a variety of specialized cells that work together to keep digestion running smoothly. These include:

- Mucous cells: Produce mucin, a protective mucus layer.

- Parietal cells: Produce hydrochloric acid (HCl) and intrinsic factor (needed for vitamin B12 absorption).

- Chief cells: Produce pepsinogen (precursor to pepsin) and lipase for protein and fat digestion.

- Epithelium cells: The inner lining of your stomach.

- G cells: Produce gastrin, a hormone that stimulates acid production.

- Enterochromaffin-like (ECL) cells: Produce histamine, which promotes acid secretion.

- Delta cells (D-cells): Produce somatostatin, which inhibits acid production.

To save your brain from exploding, let's focus on the first three cell types, as they are directly involved in breaking down food and protecting your stomach lining.

Parietal cells are particularly crucial because they produce hydrochloric acid, which breaks down proteins into absorbable nutrients, and acts as a first line of defense against harmful bacteria and pathogens. They also produce a protein critical for vitamin B12 absorption that's called intrinsic factor. Without enough intrinsic factor, a B12 deficiency can develop, potentially leading to pernicious anemia. A lower amount of stomach acid will result in poor protein digestion, reduced nutrient absorption (especially B12, iron, zinc, and calcium), and increased susceptibility to infections (10).

Chief cells play a key role in protein digestion by producing pepsinogen, which is converted into the active enzyme pepsin with the help of HCl. Pepsin breaks proteins down into amino acids, while lipase, also produced by chief cells, assists in fat digestion. When chief cell function is reduced, protein digestion may be compromised, potentially leading to deficiencies and further digestive issues.

Meanwhile, mucous cells work tirelessly to protect your stomach lining from its own acidic environment by producing mucin. This protective barrier is essential, as decreased mucin production can leave your stomach vulnerable to gastritis, peptic ulcers, or even stomach cancer.

Although your stomach is primarily involved in the breaking down of food, it can play a role in how nutrients and other substances are absorbed. As stated above, your parietal cells produce intrinsic factor, which is critical for B12 absorption. In addition, stomach acid converts dietary iron (Fe^{3+}) into ferrous iron (Fe^{2+}), the form that can be absorbed in the small intestine. Small amounts of water, sodium, and potassium can be absorbed through the stomach—this happens primarily when someone is dehydrated. In addition, alcohol, aspirin, and caffeine can be absorbed through the stomach lining. This is the main reason why you feel their effects so fast.

Beyond digestion, your stomach also acts as a storage tank for the food and gastric juice mixture known as chyme. The pyloric sphincter, located between the stomach and small intestine, controls the release of chyme into the small intestine at a manageable pace. Most stomachs hold about a liter of food before signaling fullness, but if needed, they can expand to accommodate up to four liters—useful fact if you're ever tempted to compete in a hotdog eating contest.

Common Stomach Issues that Affect Energy Production

When it comes to stomach issues, there are quite a few that can throw a wrench in your body's energy production—low stomach acid, GERD, gastritis, ulcers, and an *H. pylori* infection, to name a few. As you'll start to see, most of these problems have one thing in common: they stem from an energy production issue. When your body struggles to generate enough energy, stomach function takes a hit. And when function slows down, digestion, nutrient absorption, and immunity can suffer.

A quick reminder: your stomach, like the rest of your digestive system, thrives in a parasympathetic (rest-and-digest) state. Chronic stress shifts your nervous system into fight-or-flight mode, diverting energy away from digestion. This is where problems start—functions slow, acid levels drop, and stomach disorders set in. In other words, your stomach is just as stressed out as you are.

Low Stomach Acid (Hypochlorhydria) & GERD

Low stomach acid occurs when the stomach doesn't produce enough hydrochloric acid (HCl), a crucial player in breaking down food, absorbing nutrients, and keeping harmful bacteria at bay. Low acid levels lead to poor digestion, bloating, nutrient deficiencies, and acid reflux. Essentially, your stomach turns into a useless food storage unit instead of an efficient digestive machine.

The main culprits behind low stomach acid include chronic stress, nutrient deficiencies, low calorie intake, and low thyroid function, all factors that tie back to low energy production. Additionally, a processed food diet, *H. pylori* infection, alcohol, smoking, and eating too quickly or too much can further weaken stomach acid levels. In short, if your diet consists mostly of alcohol, ultra-processed snacks, and stress, your stomach probably isn't doing too great.

When stomach acid is insufficient, food isn't broken down efficiently, leading to poor nutrient extraction, especially B12, iron, zinc, and amino acids, all of which are essential for ATP (energy) production. Less fuel for your cells means a slower metabolism, increased fatigue, and sluggish digestion.

According to cardiologist Dr. Broda Barnes, MD, *"In hypothyroidism, digestion in the stomach and intestines is delayed. The concentration of acid and enzymes involved in digestion may be diminished. Motility of the gut is reduced, and food is propelled more slowly along the tract. Absorption through the intestinal wall is slower."*

Simply put, if your metabolism is sluggish and stress levels are high, your stomach produces less HCl, making it harder to extract energy from food. At the same time, poor digestion means your body struggles to get the raw materials it needs to generate more energy, yes, a vicious cycle. Symptoms like heartburn, nausea, bloating, gas, and fatigue become all too familiar. And here's the kicker: low stomach acid often contributes to GERD. Yes—GERD again.

The real cause of GERD often comes down to a weakened lower esophageal sphincter (LES) and poor stomach acid function. Low stomach acid and weak digestion increase intra-abdominal pressure (IAP), which can push stomach contents up into the esophagus. Chronically elevated IAP, often due to bloating, overeating, and low stomach acid, makes reflux more likely.

Don't worry, I'll get into how to fix this naturally by restoring stomach acid levels and improving digestion at the root. The goal isn't just to mask symptoms but to fix the actual dysfunction causing them. Because let's be honest, covering up symptoms with antacids is like slapping duct tape on a leaking pipe.

H. pylori, Gastritis, and Ulcers: Energy Saboteurs

H. pylori, gastritis, and ulcers are major disruptors of gut function and energy production. These conditions can lead to fatigue, poor digestion, and systemic inflammation, all of which make you feel like you're running on empty.

H. pylori: An Unwanted Visitor

Helicobacter pylori (*H. pylori*) is a spiral-shaped bacterium that burrows into the stomach lining, causing chronic inflammation and lowering stomach acid production. As stomach acid levels drop, digestion weakens, leading to poor nutrient absorption, increased inflammation, and a weakened immune system, all of which can drain energy and slow metabolism.

As of 2023, approximately two-thirds of the world's population is infected with *H. pylori* (11). Surprisingly, most people carry it without symptoms, while others develop gastritis, ulcers, or even stomach cancer. Some research even suggests that *H. pylori* may play a beneficial role in the gut microbiome, potentially offering protective effects in certain individuals.

Most people only require treatment if *H. pylori* is detected AND they have symptoms, such as ulcers, gastritis, stomach cancer, anemia, or chronic reflux. The bacteria spreads through contaminated food, water, or utensils, and symptoms can be triggered by stress, poor diet, and weakened immunity. So, if your gut feels like it's constantly in turmoil, these little bacteria might be the hidden culprit.

The standard treatment for *H. pylori* involves a combination of two antibiotics, typically clarithromycin and amoxicillin, along with a proton pump inhibitor (PPI) to reduce stomach acid and aid healing. Some research suggests that famotidine (Pepcid AC) may be a safer and highly effective alternative to PPIs for *H. pylori* treatment (12).

Of course, if you're looking for a more natural approach to eliminating this unwelcome guest, there are alternative methods that may help. Keep reading to explore ways to address *H. pylori* naturally.

Gastritis: Stomach Inflammation

Gastritis is inflammation of the stomach lining, often triggered by *H. pylori*, excessive NSAID use, alcohol, low thyroid function, smoking, and stress. This inflammation weakens the protective mucus barrier, leaving the stomach vulnerable to damage. Basically, it's like removing the spyware on your computer and then downloading sketchy files, things go downhill fast.

When gastritis is present, ATP (energy) production takes a hit. The inflamed stomach lining struggles to digest food properly, reducing the absorption of key nutrients needed for mitochondrial function. A sluggish digestive process leads to fewer nutrients being absorbed, a weaker metabolism, and an increased risk of infections, making energy production even less efficient.

Peptic Ulcers: When Stomach Acid is No Longer Your Friend

A peptic ulcer is an open sore in the stomach lining or upper small intestine, caused by excessive acid exposure, often due to *H. pylori*, chronic stress, or nutrient deficiencies. When the stomach's protective mucus barrier is compromised, acid can eat away at the lining, leading to pain, burning sensations, and even bleeding.

Ulcers disrupt energy production in several ways. Chronic pain leads to increased cortisol, which places a higher demand on energy stores. Poor digestion further reduces nutrient absorption, meaning fewer raw materials are available to fuel mitochondria. If an ulcer bleeds, anemia may develop, reducing oxygen delivery to cells and leading to extreme fatigue. Because nothing says "low energy" like having a hole in your stomach lining.

As you can see, your stomach isn't just responsible for digesting food—how it functions is a key player in energy production. When digestion slows down due to low stomach acid, infections, inflammation, or GERD, your body struggles to extract fuel and nutrients from food, leading to low energy, slower metabolism, and systemic dysfunction.

The good news? You can fix this. In the next section, I'll show you how to restore stomach acid, improve digestion, and address these gut issues at the root. Because let's be real, treating symptoms without fixing the system is like trying to drive a car with no gas and hoping the check engine light just goes away.

Fixing Your Stomach for Better Digestion and Energy

Your stomach isn't just a food processing machine, it's a key player in energy production, nutrient absorption, and overall health. When stomach function is compromised due to low stomach acid, infections, inflammation, or GERD, your body struggles to extract fuel and nutrients efficiently, leading to a sluggish metabolism, and lower energy production. Luckily, your stomach can heal remarkably well once you know what it needs.

Healing your stomach isn't about masking symptoms with quick fixes; it's about restoring proper function, so digestion works smoothly and efficiently, without bloating, reflux, or discomfort. Let's explore the steps to repair and optimize your stomach for better digestion and energy.

Step 1: Manage Stress to Support Stomach Function

Digestion is controlled by the nervous system, and chronic stress can slow stomach acid production and weaken digestion. When you're stressed, your body diverts energy away from digestion to prioritize essential survival functions like the nervous (brain) and circulatory systems (heart). This means digestion slows down, making it harder for your stomach to function properly.

Managing stress doesn't mean you have to quit your job and move to a beach (although, tempting). It can be as simple as:

1. Slowing down and taking things off your plate (your life plate not your food plate) when possible.

2. Going to bed earlier to improve recovery.

3. Cutting back on social media & news—constant stimulation isn't helping.

4. Getting outside and taking breaks on weekends.

5. Enjoying your life more—stress reduction is often about balance.

One of the easiest yet most effective ways to improve digestion is by stimulating the vagus nerve. This can be done through deep breathing, gargling, and even humming before meals. These simple actions help shift your body into "rest and digest" mode, allowing digestion to function optimally.

Finally, eat in a calm, distraction-free environment. Scrolling on your phone, rushing through meals, or eating on the go can disrupt digestion and lead to bloating and discomfort. Taking time to relax and enjoy your meals can make a big difference in how well your stomach processes food.

Step 2: Strengthen the Lower Esophageal Sphincter (LES) to Prevent Reflux

If you experience GERD or frequent heartburn, the issue isn't too much stomach acid—it's that acid is escaping where it shouldn't be due to a weakened LES, and too little stomach acid. Strengthening the LES keeps stomach contents where they belong and helps prevent reflux.

1. Eat smaller, balanced meals – Overeating puts pressure on your stomach, increasing the likelihood of acid reflux. Keep portions moderate to ease digestion.

2. Stay upright after eating – Lying down too soon can allow acid to creep into the esophagus. Wait at least 2-3 hours before lying down.

3. Sleep on your left side – This position has been shown to reduce reflux symptoms by keeping stomach acid lower.

4. Avoid things that weaken or relax the LES – Alcohol, smoking, caffeine, and high-fat meals can relax the LES, making reflux more likely.

Step 3: Repair & Soothe the Stomach Lining

If you have gastritis, ulcers, or stomach irritation, focus on healing the stomach lining before working on increasing stomach acid.

1. Soothe with aloe vera juice and bone broth – These help to reduce inflammation and support stomach lining repair.

2. Protect with DGL (deglycyrrhizinated licorice) – Take before meals to coat and shield the stomach lining.

3. Use slippery elm & marshmallow root – These herbs create a barrier that protects the stomach from further irritation.

4. Support with collagen & bone broth – These provide building blocks to help heal the gut lining.

5. Manuka honey – This honey has antibacterial properties that can help reduce *H. pylori* overgrowth and heal ulcers

from the stomach lining. Take a teaspoon on an empty stomach for added gut support. (Check my website for my favorite brand.)

Step 4: Restore Stomach Acid Naturally

If you deal with GERD, bloating, slow digestion, or poor nutrient absorption, you may have low stomach acid (hypochlorhydria). Instead of suppressing acid with antacids, focus on supporting natural acid production so your stomach functions optimally.

1. Increase zinc intake – Zinc is essential for HCl production. Eat foods like oysters, beef, and low-fat dairy to boost levels.

2. Get enough B vitamins (B1, B6, B12) – These are critical for stomach acid production. Best sources include beef liver, eggs, and grass-fed meats.

3. Taurine supplements. Taurine has been shown to induce acid secretion due to an increase in intracellular calcium (13).

4. Increase coffee. Of course, if you have reflux, you will want to wait on this since coffee can relax your LES. But coffee is known to increase stomach acidity.

5. Consume foods high in glycine (gelatin and bone broth)—glycine enhances gastric secretion in the stomach, while helping to restore the intestinal barriers (14). Glycine is also helpful in helping to treat *H. pylori*, in combination with other antibacterial drugs (15).

6. Consume adequate protein. Protein will increase HCl.

By focusing on strengthening digestion and supporting stomach acid, you can improve gut health at the root level instead of just masking symptoms.

Step 5: Sun Exposure and Vitamin D

Vitamin D plays a vital role in stomach health by protecting the gastric lining, supporting digestion, and potentially alleviating symptoms of digestive disorders. Research suggests that vitamin D3 helps protect gastric epithelial cells from acid-induced injury and oxidative stress, reinforcing the integrity of the stomach lining (16).

Additionally, studies have found a link between low vitamin D levels and worsened gastroparesis symptoms, such as nausea and vomiting, indicating that adequate vitamin D may contribute to better gastric motility and function (17). Since vitamin D also supports immune regulation and gut microbiome balance, ensuring sufficient sun exposure or dietary intake may be essential for overall digestive well-being.

How to maintain healthy vitamin D levels:

1. Aim for at least 10-15 minutes of full-body sun exposure daily.

    - If you have fair skin, start with 5 minutes and gradually increase.

    - Avoid sunburn—gradually build tolerance over time.

2. Supplement with Vitamin D3 when necessary.

    - In winter or areas with minimal UVB exposure, supplementation can help maintain optimal levels.

    - Safe daily intake ranges from 500 to 4,000 IU (18).

Some studies suggest that doses up to 10,000 IU/day may be safe for short-term use in individuals with very low vitamin D levels (19, 20).

It's best to check your vitamin D levels and consult a healthcare provider before supplementing with high doses.

Step 6: Improve Energy Production

Once your stomach is in better shape, you can gradually increase your fuel intake. To fully heal, your body needs to produce more energy, as energy is essential for cellular repair. Everything covered so far is about creating a stomach environment where your body can handle food better.

If you've ever dealt with GERD, gastritis, *H. pylori*, or ulcers, you know that eating can be a challenge. That's why supporting the stomach first is crucial. Once it improves, you can gradually increase food intake, allowing the energy from food to contribute to further healing.

I will dive deeper into this at the end of this chapter, as improving energy production is a recurring theme in all gut healing protocols, regardless of where your digestive issues originate.

Ultimately, by restoring stomach acid, strengthening digestion, repairing the stomach lining, managing stress, and improving energy production, you address the root cause rather than just masking symptoms. The goal is to help your stomach function as it was meant to.

In summary, your stomach is a multitasking marvel that produces gastric juices to lower stomach pH for efficient protein breakdown, protects you from harmful pathogens, and produces intrinsic factor to ensure proper vitamin B12 absorption. Keeping your stomach functioning optimally is crucial for maintaining a healthy digestive system and optimal energy production.

Up next, your digestion and absorption powerhouse—your small intestine.

The Small Intestine—Your Primary Digestive and Absorption Organ

Located just below your stomach, the small intestine is where most of the magic happens in digestion and absorption. Though it's only about 20 feet long, its surface area—thanks to countless folds, villi, and microvilli—spans over 250 square feet (roughly the size of a tennis court).

As Dr. Ray Peat explained, *"The upper part of the small intestine is sterile in healthy people. In the last 40 years, there has been increasing interest in the 'contaminated small-bowel syndrome,' or the 'small intestine bacterial overgrowth syndrome.' When peristalsis is reduced, for example by hypothyroidism, along with reduced secretion of digestive fluids, bacteria can thrive in the upper part of the intestine. Generally, the healthier a person is, the more sterile their small intestine."*

In other words, the cleaner your small intestine, the better it works. Think of your small intestine as the gatekeeper, carefully regulating what enters your bloodstream and lymph—absorbing vital nutrients, proteins, and fats—while keeping unwanted invaders out. It's the real MVP of digestion, transforming your food into fuel for your body.

The small intestine is divided into three sections: the duodenum, jejunum, and ileum, each with distinct roles in digestion and absorption (21).

The Duodenum: The King When It Comes to Digestion

After chyme passes through the stomach's pyloric sphincter, it enters the duodenum, the first and shortest section of the small intestine. Though only about 10 inches long, this region is where most of your digestion occurs. The duodenum neutralizes acidic chyme with bicarbonate from the pancreas, raising the pH of the small intestine to around 8.5—a stark contrast to the stomach's highly acidic environment (pH 1-3).

Key Digestive Enzymes in the Duodenum

The brush border enzymes, located on the microvilli, play a major role in breaking down food particles for absorption (22):

- Lactase – Breaks down lactose (milk sugar).
- Sucrase – Breaks down sucrose (table sugar).
- Maltase – Breaks down maltose (malt sugar).
- Lipase – Breaks down fats.
- Peptidase – Breaks down proteins.

Bile and Pancreatic Enzymes: Essential for Digestion

The duodenum is also where bile from the liver and gallbladder emulsifies fats (23). Bile acids are synthesized from cholesterol in the liver and stored in the gallbladder, then released when dietary fats are present. Once in the small intestine, bile acids help break down fats, allowing for better digestion and absorption. About 95% of bile acids are reabsorbed in the ileum (the final portion of the small intestine) and transported back to the liver via the portal vein, a process known as bile recycling or enterohepatic circulation. The remaining 5% of bile acids reach the colon, where they can influence the gut microbiome and metabolic health (more on this in the next chapter).

As chyme moves into the duodenum, the pancreas releases essential digestive enzymes:

- Amylase – Breaks down carbohydrates.

- Lipase – Breaks down fats.

- Proteases (Trypsin, Chymotrypsin, Carboxypeptidase) – Break down proteins.

Without bile acids and pancreatic enzymes, digestion would be incomplete, leading to malabsorption, bloating, and nutrient deficiencies.

FUN FACT: Pancreatic enzymes are inactive until they reach the duodenum—a protective mechanism that prevents the pancreas from digesting itself.

Micronutrients Absorption and Serotonin

The duodenum is the first site of micronutrient absorption, including iron, calcium, magnesium, phosphorus, copper, selenium, thiamin, riboflavin, niacin, biotin, folate, and fat-soluble vitamins A, D, E, and K (24). In addition to being the location of most digestion and some absorption, the duodenum (along with the jejunum) is responsible for 80-90% of serotonin production in the body. The colon produces an additional 10-15%, while only about 5% is produced in the brain. While serotonin is commonly referred to as the "happy hormone," it is more accurately a gut hormone, influencing gut motility, peristalsis, bile release, and enzymatic secretion rather than mood alone.

Serotonin—Not the "Happy Hormone," but a Gut Hormone

Serotonin is widely known as the "happy hormone," but this description is misleading. While serotonin does act as a neurotransmitter in the brain, 95% of it is produced in the gut, where its primary role has little to do with mood and everything to do with digestion, inflammation, and metabolism.

The enterochromaffin (EC) cells in the small intestine and colon produce serotonin in response to food and mechanical stimulation. Once released, serotonin increases gut motility— accelerating peristalsis and transit time. This explains why excess serotonin is linked to diarrhea and why SSRIs (Selective Serotonin Reuptake Inhibitors), which increase serotonin, list diarrhea as a common side effect. Conversely, serotonin antagonists like Zofran (ondansetron) and activated charcoal are effective in reducing diarrhea by blocking serotonin's effects in the gut. I'll discuss these more in the next Chapter.

Despite its reputation, serotonin is more of a stress-adaptive hormone than a happiness-inducing chemical. In times of stress, serotonin slows metabolic rate, promotes learned helplessness—a state in which individuals feel powerless over their circumstances, while increasing histamine, estrogen, and endotoxin activity, all of which can elevate under stress and contribute to inflammation, digestive disorders, and metabolic dysfunction.

This misconception about serotonin extends beyond gut health. A 2022 systematic review in Molecular Psychiatry found "no consistent evidence of there being an association between serotonin and depression" and no support for the hypothesis that depression is caused by low serotonin levels (25).

This metabolic slowdown isn't unique to humans, hibernating animals rely on high serotonin levels to suppress energy production (ATP), lower thyroid function, and conserve resources. While beneficial for survival during months without food, this same mechanism can leave humans feeling fatigued, inflamed, and metabolically sluggish.

Excess serotonin can contribute to gut disorders such as SIBO and leaky gut. It increases gut permeability and overstimulates motility, leading to rapid transit (diarrhea) and poor nutrient absorption. Paradoxically, chronic serotonin exposure can also desensitize serotonin receptors, slow motility and lead to constipation (26).

Rather than viewing serotonin as the hormone of happiness, it's more accurate to see it as a regulator of stress, digestion, and survival, one that must be kept in balance for optimal health.

The Jejunum: The Home to Nutrient Absorption

The jejunum, about 8 feet long, is where most nutrient absorption occurs. Its villi and microvilli provide an expansive surface area for absorbing broken-down proteins (amino acids), carbohydrates (glucose, fructose, galactose), and fats. Unlike proteins and carbs, fats (now in the form of chylomicrons) bypass the blood and liver (at least at first) and enter the lymphatic system through structures called lacteals. After traveling through the lymphatic system, the fat gets dumped into the blood, where it is sent directly to the cells to be used as energy.

This section is also where most of your fluid/water is absorbed along with micronutrients, including calcium, magnesium, phosphorus, iron, zinc, and B vitamins (except B12), chromium, manganese, molybdenum, and vitamin A, C, D, E and K, continue to be absorbed (27).

The Ileum

The ileum, the final 12 feet of the small intestine, continues absorbing nutrients, albeit at a lower rate. Key absorption tasks of the ileum include magnesium, folate, vitamin C, vitamin D, vitamin K, and it is the primary spot for reabsorption of bile acids and vitamin B12 (28).

The Ileum also contains Peyer's patches, a key part of the gut-associated lymphoid tissue (GALT), a critical part of your immune system. These patches identify and respond to bacteria, pathogens, and dietary antigens. The ileum also produces large amounts of secretary IgA, a protective barrier on the gut lining that neutralizes harmful microbes.

FUN FACT: Acute and chronic inflammation in the small intestine can reduce brush border enzyme production, leading to lactose intolerance. Which means if you fix your intestinal inflammation, you may no longer be lactose intolerant.

Common Small Intestine Issues that Interfere with Energy Production

When your small intestine can't absorb nutrients efficiently, your metabolism and energy production suffer. A vicious cycle begins; less absorption of energy and nutrients leads to fewer resources for energy production, which further compromises your ability to heal and digest properly. In this next section, I am going to talk about the top three issues caused by a compromised small intestine, including Celiac disease and gluten sensitivity, leaky gut, and SIBO, and how they affect energy production. In the conclusion, I will provide guidance from a bioenergetic perspective on how you can address these issues.

Celiac Disease and Gluten Sensitivity

Celiac disease is what happens when your immune system mistakes gluten for an invading army and decides to burn down the entire village (your small intestine) in response. Found in wheat, barley, rye, spelt, farro, kamut, and bulgur, gluten triggers an immune attack on the villi—the tiny, nutrient-absorbing fingers lining your intestines. Over time, this leaves your gut inflamed, your nutrients unabsorbed, and your energy levels stuck in "I just ran into a wall" mode.

Gluten sensitivity, on the other hand, doesn't warrant a full-blown autoimmune war, but it's still an annoying mofo. It can irritate the gut lining, disrupt digestion, and sabotage metabolism—all without causing the outright destruction seen in celiac disease. This is why some people test negative for celiac but still feel like an inflated balloon after eating a slice of bread.

Both conditions primarily target the duodenum, the first part of the small intestine, where most nutrient absorption happens. This is where your body soaks up essential nutrients like iron, calcium, copper, selenium, B vitamins, and vitamins A, D, E, and K. If this area is inflamed and absorption is compromised, you're basically running on nutritional fumes. In more severe cases, damage spreads to the jejunum and ileum, meaning even fewer nutrients get absorbed, and suddenly, every meal feels like you've been hit by a truck.

In the short term, an inflamed small intestine can lead to bloating, gas, diarrhea, brain fog, nausea, joint pain, brittle hair, and the kind of fatigue that even ten cups of coffee can't fix. You might also mysteriously gain or lose weight, depending on whether your body is dealing with full-body inflammation or complete malabsorption.

In the long term, it's a nutritional disaster, causing anemia, osteoporosis, thyroid dysfunction, blood sugar imbalances, muscle wasting, nerve damage, and infertility. If your small intestine isn't functioning properly, energy production, bone health, muscle growth, nerve protection, and reproductive function all take a hit.

Can You Heal from Celiac or Gluten Sensitivity?

The most important treatment for celiac disease is strict gluten avoidance, including cross-contamination risks. Those with celiac can heal their intestinal lining by removing gluten, but their immune response is permanent. Even if symptoms disappear, the body never forgets how to overreact to gluten, meaning reintroducing it is not an option.

For those with gluten sensitivity, avoiding gluten can relieve symptoms and improve gut health. However, unlike celiac disease, gluten intolerance isn't necessarily permanent. By optimizing small intestine function, increasing nutrient intake, and reducing overall stress, some people may be able to tolerate gluten again in moderation without adverse effects.

I've worked with numerous gluten-sensitive clients who, after improving gut function, energy production, and overall metabolic health, found that their gut no longer reacted negatively to gluten. At the end of this chapter, I'll dive deeper into how to strengthen your small intestine, so that gluten may no longer be the villain it currently is.

Leaky Gut (Intestinal Permeability)

Leaky gut syndrome, or intestinal permeability, is what happens when your gut lining starts acting like an over-tipped bouncer at a nightclub, letting in toxins, undigested food particles, and bacteria that have no business being in your bloodstream. This overlooked entry of the wrong guests triggers system-wide inflammation, immune overreactions, and sluggish energy production, essentially turning your body's internal engine into a complete mess.

Beyond letting harmful substances in, leaky gut also disrupts nutrient absorption, preventing your body from getting the essential vitamins and minerals it needs. In a well-functioning gut, nutrients enter the bloodstream through intestinal cells in an orderly fashion. But when the gut barrier weakens, nutrients escape through gaps between cells instead of being properly absorbed, leaving you malnourished, tired, and inflamed.

Worse yet, larger, partially digested food particles slip through these weak junctions and enter the bloodstream, where they trigger immune responses, causing further inflammation and food sensitivities. Instead of fueling your body with essential vitamins and minerals, these rogue nutrients end up triggering immune responses in the gut-associated lymphoid tissue (GALT), creating more chaos (29).

Symptoms of Leaky Gut

Wondering if you have a leaky gut? The symptoms can be annoyingly vague at first, bloating after meals, gas, stomach discomfort, diarrhea, constipation, and food sensitivities (think dairy, gluten, soy, eggs). But if this gut rebellion continues unchecked, things get worse. Fatigue, brain fog, anemia, hair loss, skin issues, low body temperature, frequent colds, anxiety, depression, poor sleep, and unexplained weight changes can all be part of the mix, resembling the mess seen in Celiac disease.

And here's the unfortunate news, the leakier your gut, the worse your nutrient absorption gets. More toxins flood your bloodstream, inflammation skyrockets, and energy production nosedives, trapping you in a vicious cycle of gut damage, inflammation, and exhaustion.

What Causes Leaky Gut?

One of the biggest culprits behind leaky gut? Stress, and not just the kind you feel when your computer shuts down right before you hit save after your 8 hours of work (yes, this happened to me). Chronic stress from over-exercising, working too much, skipping meals, and poor sleep (30, 31, 32) diverts blood flow away from digestion, slowly chipping away at your gut lining's integrity. Ever notice that sometimes you can handle certain foods, like dairy or starches just fine, but other times they wreck you? Well, if the food does not change, then the only change is your current state, or the stress your body is under.

But external stress isn't acting alone. Your gut lining is under constant attack from modern food and lifestyle choices. Alcohol (33), processed foods laced with gut-wrecking additives like polysorbate 80, carrageenan, and artificial sweeteners (34, 35), gluten and lectins from soy, corn, legumes, nuts, and seeds (36), polyunsaturated fats (vegetable, seed and fish oils), and high-fructose corn syrup (37) all contribute to gut permeability issues. And let's not forget dairy from grain-fed animals (38), glyphosates (39), and heavy metals (40) can further damage the gut barrier.

Adding insult to injury, medications like proton pump inhibitors (PPIs) (39), NSAIDs (40), and excessive antibiotic use (42) strip the gut of beneficial bacteria and damage the intestinal lining. Estrogen exposure, whether through your own production or exogenous sources, can also impact your gut lining (more on this in chapter 9). Other offenders include sauna-induced hyperthermia (44), H. pylori infections (45), parasites, and autoimmune conditions like Celiac disease, Crohn's, and Hashimoto's thyroiditis (46).

What You Can Do to Fix Leaky Gut (Besides Pray)

If you've read this far and realized you check most of the boxes for leaky gut, don't panic—there are plenty of things you can do to turn this leaky mess around.

1. **Eliminate gut irritants.** Any food that pokes holes in your gut lining (literally or figuratively) should be off your plate. This means avoiding ultra-processed foods, alcohol, high-fructose corn syrup, artificial sweeteners, and food additives. Hard-to-digest foods like gluten, soy,

corn, legumes, nuts, and seeds should also be shelved for now while your gut repairs itself.

2. **Rethink your fiber intake.** Yes, fiber is often labeled as "healthy," but for some people with leaky gut, too much can be a real irritant. This includes raw leafy greens, raw cruciferous vegetables, and high-starch foods. Some people need to limit even "safe" starches like rice, potatoes, sourdough, and masa harina—at least until the gut is strong enough to handle them. If you do eat them, proper preparation is key; soaking and boiling potatoes and rice, fermenting grains (hello, sourdough), and nixtamalized corn (aka masa harina) make them easier to digest.

3. **Support stomach acid production** (see the stomach section for details). If your stomach acid is too low, you won't break down food properly, which increases gut irritation and undigested particles slipping through the cracks.

4. **Eat foods that don't make your gut work overtime.** Stick to well-cooked vegetables, fruit juices, cooked fruits, honey, and properly prepared starches (if tolerated). These foods provide energy without adding stress to an already struggling gut.

5. **Load up on nutrient-dense, gut-healing foods.** Beef liver, dairy (if tolerated), shellfish (especially zinc-rich oysters), beef, and eggs are powerhouses for gut repair. Without these nutrients, your body simply won't have the tools to rebuild the gut barrier.

6. **Consume gut-cleansing foods.** The daily raw carrot salad (shredded carrot + vinegar + coconut oil + salt) helps bind bacterial toxins and disinfect the intestines. If carrots aren't your thing, boiled white button mushrooms or bamboo shoots can serve as effective alternatives. For more details on how these foods support gut health,

including the benefits of Ray Peat's carrot salad, white button mushrooms, and bamboo shoots, see Appendix A.

7. **Increase glycine-rich foods** like gelatin, collagen, and bone broth. Glycine is one of the best amino acids for gut repair, and these foods provide it in an easy-to-absorb form.

8. **Consider milk—if you can tolerate it.** Milk is low in fiber, high in bioavailable nutrients, and easy to digest if your body produces enough lactase. But if you're lactose intolerant, it will wreck your gut even more. If you have a lactose issue, raw cow's and goat's milk tend to be tolerated better, as they both contain the lactase enzyme. The key is to test and adjust accordingly.

9. **Reduce stress.** Stress will always pull blood flow and nutrients away from your digestion, making it more challenging to do its job and heal. Refer back to Chapter 6, so you can review what to do.

Leaky gut isn't just a digestive issue; it's the beginning of a failure to produce energy effectively. If you are unable to absorb and digest your nutrients, then your energy production will tank, and all the systems of your body can become compromised.

The good news is you can reverse the damage by cutting out gut irritants, improving digestion, eating nutrient-dense foods, and incorporating gut-healing compounds like collagen, glycine, and antimicrobial fibers. Managing stress is equally critical, because all the gut-healing protocols in the world won't help you like they should if your body is constantly in fight-or-flight mode.

Small Intestinal Bacterial Overgrowth (SIBO)

SIBO is what happens when bacteria decide to throw a party in the wrong neighborhood—the small intestine. Normally, gut bacteria should set up shop primarily in the large intestine (colon), but in SIBO, excess bacteria migrate to the small intestine, where they don't belong. This unwanted overgrowth disrupts digestion, messes with nutrient absorption, and throws gut function into chaos. The result? A delightful mix of bloating, diarrhea, constipation, malabsorption, and inflammation.

Like leaky gut, SIBO most commonly sets up camp in the duodenum (first part) and jejunum (second part), and only in severe cases does it sneak into the ileum (last part). This bacterial invasion usually happens due to a breakdown in the body's defense systems, low stomach acid, sluggish bile flow, inadequate digestive enzymes, or poor gut motility.

Structural issues of the small intestine, like diverticula, scars, tumors, and adhesions, can also invite SIBO to stick around. Another sneaky culprit? A weak ileocecal valve (the gatekeeper between the small and large intestines) that lets bacteria from the colon backflow into the small intestine.

How Does SIBO Interfere with Energy Production?

SIBO doesn't just mess with digestion, it actively drains your energy in several ways:

1. **Gut barrier breakdown** – SIBO can contribute to leaky gut, damaging the intestinal lining and leading to poor nutrient absorption.

2. **Excessive fermentation** – These bacteria ferment carbohydrates before your body can absorb them, leaving you running on empty. We want to feed you, not your bacteria!

3. **Mitochondrial suppression** – SIBO bacteria produce endotoxins (LPS), hydrogen sulfide, and D-lactate, which can impair your mitochondria, the powerhouses of your cells.

4. **Chronic inflammation** – The overgrowth triggers low-grade inflammation, releasing cytokines that shift your body into a stressed, energy-draining state.

5. **Hormone chaos** – SIBO can increase serotonin, estrogen, histamine, and cortisol, which throws off your stress response and further inhibits energy production.

Do You Have SIBO?

Do you experience bloating that worsens after meals, especially after fibrous or starchy carbs? Do you feel better on a low-carb diet? Do you feel tired, bloated, constipated, burp frequently, get gassy, or struggle with brain fog? Have you had food poisoning, H. pylori, leaky gut, low stomach acid, low thyroid, or anemia? Are you under a lot of stress? If you answered yes to multiple questions, there's a strong chance SIBO is in the mix.

How to Prevent and Treat SIBO

1. **Cut off the food supply** – Reduce fermentable carbs, resistant starches, and certain fibers. A low-FODMAP diet for 4-8 weeks can help starve the bacteria while supporting digestion and energy production (see Appendix B for a detailed food list).

2. **Eat a gut-cleansing food daily** – Yep, it's time for the legendary Ray Peat carrot salad again. This simple shredded carrot + vinegar + coconut oil + salt mix helps bind bacterial toxins and disinfect the gut. (See Appendix A for details.)

3. **Try herbal antimicrobials** – Natural compounds like berberine, oregano oil, and garlic can help kill off the overgrowth. If these don't work, don't fear antibiotics, sometimes, a targeted round of antibiotics can be necessary.

4. **Boost gut motility** – Support movement in the intestines by optimizing thyroid function, getting enough vitamin D, and eating nutrient-dense foods. Also, walking for 10-30 minutes after meals can help stimulate motility. Coffee, Cascara Sagrada, and magnesium can all help

with gut motility. See the next chapter to help stimulate colon motility.

5. **Increase stomach acid** – Low stomach acid allows bacteria to thrive. Support HCl production by consuming zinc, B6, B12, and salt.

6. **Improve bile flow** – Bile has antimicrobial properties that help keep bacteria in check. Support bile flow by eating adequate fat, ox bile, taurine, and digestive bitters.

7. **Use a soil-based probiotic** – Unlike traditional probiotics, soil-based probiotics, such as bacillus subtilis, bacillus coagulans, and saccharomyces boulardii are better tolerated in SIBO cases since they don't overpopulate the small intestine like lactobacillus or bifidobacterium can.

8. **Improve energy production** - Ultimately, this is what is going to heal your system and keep the bacteria away. If you don't work on energy production, your symptoms will eventually return. Refer to the first section of this book.

SIBO is like an unwanted houseguest that eats all your food, trashes your place, and leaves you exhausted. It hijacks digestion, drains energy, and throws off metabolism. But by clearing the bacteria, improving gut motility, balancing stomach acid and bile flow, and using targeted antimicrobials, you can reclaim your energy and gut health. With the right strategy, you can show those unwelcome bacteria the door, for good.

Candida, It's Not a Sugar Issue, but an Energy Issue

Most people think of Candida as a rogue invader that must be starved, killed, or purged with an intense, sugar-free diet and a long list of antifungal supplements. But what if that common view misses the point entirely?

Candida is not just an external pathogen, it's a naturally occurring yeast that lives in and on the body, particularly in the mouth, skin, vagina, colon, and most critically, the small intestine. In a healthy body, Candida is kept in check by good gut motility, healthy immune function, adequate bile flow, and a robust metabolism. It's when the body becomes stressed and under-energized that Candida becomes problematic.

What is Candida?

Candida albicans is the most common species of yeast found in the human body. It's part of the normal microbiota, and in small amounts, it doesn't cause harm. However, under the right (or rather, wrong) conditions, like antibiotic use, chronic stress, low stomach acid, excessive processed foods, or hormonal imbalance, it can grow out of control. This overgrowth is often referred to as Candidiasis.

Where Candida Overgrows

- Small Intestine: This is where it often does the most damage. Overgrowth here can lead to bloating, gas, sugar cravings, fatigue, food sensitivities, and nutrient malabsorption.

- Colon: Though less common, overgrowth here may contribute to inflammatory bowel symptoms, especially if there's constipation or sluggish motility.

- Mouth and Esophagus: Often seen as oral thrush, white coating on the tongue and inner cheeks.

- Vagina (in women): Vaginal yeast infections are a common symptom of local Candida imbalance, often after antibiotics or hormonal shifts.

- Skin and Nail Beds: Candida can live on the skin, especially in moist areas, causing rashes or fungal infections.

Why Cutting Sugar Isn't the Solution

Contrary to popular belief, cutting sugar to "starve" Candida can backfire. This idea stems from the logic that Candida feeds on sugar, so remove the sugar, and you'll kill the yeast. But as many of you have now realized, the body isn't that simple.

As Dr. Ray Peat often emphasized, Candida doesn't overgrow just because sugar is available, it overgrows when the host's energy metabolism is suppressed. Restricting carbohydrates slows down glucose oxidation, lowers CO_2 production, raises stress hormones like cortisol, and makes the body more reliant on fat metabolism and lactic acid production. This low-energy, low-oxygen environment supports fungal overgrowth.

As Dr. Peat put it, "The body's defenses against Candida include not just immune cells, but metabolic energy and carbon dioxide. A shift away from glucose metabolism supports fungal growth."

When someone restricts sugar or carbohydrates for too long, the result is often a colder body, an elevation of stress hormones, increased food cravings, dysregulated blood sugar, and a weaker digestive system, which can be the exact conditions that allow Candida to thrive.

Of course, I am not saying that removing all sugar/carbs will not temporarily improve your symptoms—because it will. What I am saying is this is only a temporary solution, and if you don't fix the system, the candida overgrowth will eventually come back.

Candida produces a toxic byproduct called acetaldehyde, which interferes with mitochondrial function and creates a hangover-like effect. It also promotes histamine release, damages the gut lining, worsens permeability, and can increase endotoxin absorption.

In the small intestine, Candida interferes with enzyme activity, nutrient absorption and immune regulation. This leads to a vicious cycle: weakened digestion > more fermentation > more fungal growth > more toxins > less energy.

How to Fix Candida Without Giving Up Sugar

Instead of going to war with Candida, the goal should be to support your energy production. When your body is metabolically strong, well-fed, and resilient, Candida doesn't have the environment it needs to grow. Addressing Candida from an energy-based perspective means focusing on restoring the body's core systems, blood sugar regulation, gut motility, thyroid function, and stress response.

Here's my five-step approach:

1. **Support glucose metabolism** - Include easy-to-digest carbs like orange juice, ripe fruits, honey, and well-cooked root vegetables. Avoid prolonged fasting or ketogenic diets that suppress metabolic function. Keep blood sugar stable by eating frequent, balanced meals that include protein, carbs, and fat.

2. **Improve gut motility and bile flow** - Use raw carrots or cooked bamboo shoots daily to bind endotoxins and reduce microbial burden. Support gut movement with magnesium glycinate or small amounts of cascara sagrada. Ensure optimal thyroid function, refer back to the thyroid chapter, to promote healthy peristalsis and bile flow.

3. **Reduce the stress load** - Prioritize deep, consistent sleep and daily sunlight exposure to regulate circadian rhythm. Choose restorative movement like walking or stretching over high-intensity exercise. Avoid carb-restrictive diets or under-eating, both of which signal a starvation response and suppress metabolism.

4. **Rebuild gut integrity** - Eat collagen-rich foods like bone broth and gelatin to support the gut lining. Prioritize saturated fats (from dairy, coconut oil, butter) over PUFA, which can damage intestinal cells. Ensure adequate intake of fat-soluble vitamins, especially A, D, and K2, for mucosal repair and immune regulation.

5. **Use antifungals strategically (if needed)** - If symptoms
    are severe or persistent, short-term use of gentle
    antifungals like flowers-of-sulfur (100-200mg once daily
    for 2-3 days) or even oregano oil (1-2 drops daily for
    3-4 days) may be helpful, but only after foundational
    metabolic support is in place.

From an energy production lens, Candida is a symptom, not a
root cause. It thrives in a body that is under-fueled, stressed, and
metabolically suppressed. The long-term solution isn't to eliminate
sugar, but to restore cellular energy production. When your cells
are well-nourished and producing energy efficiently, Candida has
nowhere to grow.

Histamine Intolerance—Allergy or Gut Issue?

For many, histamine intolerance is lumped into the same category
as seasonal allergies or food sensitivities. The symptoms, which can
include hives, flushing, congestion, and stomach cramps, can look
and feel a lot like an allergic response. But the truth is, histamine
intolerance isn't a true allergy. It's a sign that your body is struggling
to regulate and clear histamine, often due to a lower metabolic rate
and deeper issues in the gut. Rather than an overactive immune
response to an outside threat, histamine intolerance is more often
a breakdown in energy production, enzyme activity, and digestive
health.

When histamine builds up, either because it's being produced in
excess or not being broken down efficiently, it can affect nearly every
system in the body. And while it may look like a classic allergy on the
surface, its root cause is far more metabolic and microbial than most
people realize.

What is Histamine?

Histamine is a naturally occurring compound that plays several
important roles in the body. It functions as a neurotransmitter in the
brain, a regulator of stomach acid for digestion, and a key player in

immune responses, especially in allergic reactions. It also modulates vascular permeability and inflammation. In the right amounts, histamine is essential. It helps your immune system respond to threats, signals your stomach to release acid for digestion, and plays a role in alertness and sleep cycles. But like many things in the body, too much of a good thing often becomes bad.

Where is Histamine Produced?

Histamine is stored and released by mast cells and basophils, which are found throughout the body, but are especially concentrated in the small intestine (particularly the duodenum and jejunum), the skin, lungs and respiratory tract, the brain and central nervous system, and the uterus and reproductive organs. Histamine is also produced by certain types of gut bacteria, especially during dysbiosis or when Candida or SIBO are present. These microbes ferment amino acids like histidine into histamine, which can overwhelm your natural clearance systems.

Additionally, histamine is produced by enterochromaffin-like (ECL) cells, which are in the lining of the stomach. These cells release histamine in response to gastrin, stimulating parietal cells to secrete hydrochloric acid. While this is a normal and necessary function for digestion, excess histamine from ECL cells, especially in the context of chronic inflammation or stress, can contribute to acid reflux, gastritis, or histamine-related sensitivity in the upper GI tract.

What is Histamine Intolerance?

Histamine intolerance occurs when histamine builds up in the body faster than it can be broken down or when too much histamine is being produced internally. This isn't an allergy to histamine itself, but rather a disruption in the balance between histamine production and histamine clearance. The two main enzymes responsible for histamine breakdown are DAO (Diamine Oxidase), which is found in the lining of the small intestine and breaks down histamine from food and gut microbes, and HNMT (Histamine-N-methyltransferase), which is found mainly in the liver and central nervous system and breaks down histamine within cells.

On the other side of the equation, certain conditions can promote excess histamine production. Gut dysfunction, Candida, SIBO, and chronic stress can all stimulate overproduction of histamine, especially through microbial fermentation or mast cell activation. Excessive estrogen to progesterone can also increase histamine release. When both overproduction and impaired breakdown are at play, histamine intolerance becomes much more symptomatic and difficult to manage. This can be due to gut inflammation, poor gut lining health, or nutrient deficiencies. Ultimately, histamine builds up and leads to a wide range of symptoms.

Symptoms of Histamine Intolerance

Histamine affects multiple systems, which is why symptoms can seem unrelated or random. People with histamine intolerance may experience bloating, gas, and cramping after meals, as well as skin issues like rashes, hives, itching, or flushing. Headaches or migraines, nasal congestion, and sinus pressure are also common. Some may feel anxiety, irritability, or even panic attacks, while others notice heart palpitations, menstrual cramps, worsened PMS, or overall fatigue and brain fog. These symptoms are often worse after eating fermented foods, wine, aged cheeses, smoked meats, or chocolate, all of which are high in histamine or histamine-releasing.

What Causes Histamine Intolerance?

Histamine intolerance can stem from several factors. Gut inflammation, infections, dysbiosis, or food sensitivities, can impair the gut lining and reduce DAO production. Overgrowths like Candida or SIBO can increase histamine production in the small intestine. Estrogen excess is another factor, as estrogen stimulates histamine release and lowers DAO activity (more on this in Chapter 9). Chronic stress weakens gut lining and alters immune function, while nutrient deficiencies, especially in vitamin B6, copper, and magnesium can impair the enzymes responsible for breaking histamine down. Certain medications, like NSAIDs, antibiotics, or antidepressants, can also block DAO and worsen histamine overload.

How to Fix Histamine Intolerance

Addressing histamine intolerance requires a multi-layered strategy. Here are several targeted approaches based on supporting metabolic energy and restoring gut integrity:

1. Support DAO enzyme activity by rebuilding the gut lining with collagen, bone broth, and gelatin, all rich in glycine. Ensure adequate intake of copper, zinc, B6, and magnesium, all needed for DAO production.

2. Consume a daily gut cleaner. The raw carrot salad, well-cooked mushrooms, and/or bamboo shoots. See Appendix A.

3. Utilize sugar and salt to lower stress hormones and stabilize mast cells. Lower stress reduces the production of histamine.

4. Progesterone to oppose the pro-inflammatory effects of estrogen and histamine. *Please consult with your health practitioner.*

5. Cyproheptadine (an antihistamine and serotonin antagonist). Temporarily using an antihistamine can reduce symptoms while you work on improving metabolic health.

6. Coffee (caffeine) to improve metabolism and modulate histamine sensitivity when tolerated.

7. Limit ultra-processed foods that can disrupt gut integrity (foods high in PUFA oils, and contain carrageenan, gums, additives, and preservatives).

8. Improve metabolic health by eating balanced meals that include carbohydrates, protein, and saturated fats. Avoid restrictive or ketogenic diets that suppress metabolic rate and thyroid function.

9. Reduce stress. Practice restorative movement, get daily sunlight, and prioritize high-quality sleep.

10. If needed, temporarily reduce histamine load by avoiding high-histamine foods such as fermented (soy sauce, sauerkraut, kefir, kombucha), smoked or canned fish (tuna, sardines, anchovies), processed meats (salami, pepperoni, bacon, sausage) or leftover meats or fish, vinegar, certain fruits and vegetables (tomatoes, eggplant, spinach, citrus). Focus on freshly prepared, simple meals.

These strategies work best when used as part of a larger plan focused on energy restoration, gut healing, and nervous system regulation.

Histamine intolerance isn't about your body turning on you, it's about your system being underpowered. When your gut is inflamed, your metabolism is suppressed, your nutrients are depleted, and histamine builds up and starts misfiring. Instead of seeing histamine as the enemy, the real goal is to strengthen the systems that keep it in balance. By restoring energy, supporting gut function, and nourishing enzyme activity, histamine can go back to doing what it's meant to do, without wreaking havoc.

In summary, a compromised small intestine is more than just a digestive nuisance, it's a metabolic nightmare. Without proper absorption of nutrients, your body struggles to generate energy, leading to fatigue, brain fog, and a cascade of systemic health issues. Whether the culprit is celiac disease, leaky gut, SIBO, candida, or histamine intolerance, the good news is that healing is possible. By addressing gut irritants, supporting digestion, and replenishing key nutrients, you can restore energy production and metabolic function.

Now that we've tackled the small intestine, let's move to the colon, the final stop of digestion, where waste is processed, gut bacteria thrive, and metabolic health is fine-tuned. The next chapter will dive into how your colon impacts digestion, energy, and your overall well-being.

CHAPTER 7

THE BOTTOM LINE

What Your Gut Health Says About Your Ability to Produce Energy

1. Digestion fuels your body—it's the process of breaking down and absorbing macro and micronutrients. Poor digestion can lead to fatigue, skin and hair issues, depression, muscle loss, anemia, diabetes, and even cancer due to inadequate energy production.

2. Your digestive system is known as the enteric nervous system (your "second brain"). It functions best in a parasympathetic state (rest and digest) and shuts down in a sympathetic state (fight or flight). Chronic stress is the #1 factor that negatively impacts digestion.

3. Digestion starts before you eat. The smell and sight of food triggers digestive enzymes. Chewing is the first physical step of digestion, so eat slowly, without distractions, and avoid eating while driving, working, or multitasking.

4. Peristalsis is the rhythmic muscle movement that pushes food through your digestive tract, starting at the esophagus and ending at the colon. Healthy peristalsis ensures proper nutrient absorption and waste elimination.

5. The stomach breaks down food using gastric juices (HCl, lipase, pepsin) to digest protein, kill harmful bacteria, and signal the release of bile and pancreatic enzymes. Common stomach issues that disrupt digestion and energy production include low stomach acid, GERD, H. pylori, gastritis, and ulcers.

6. The small intestine is your main digestive organ, where most nutrient absorption occurs. Conditions like celiac disease, leaky gut, and SIBO impair nutrient absorption, leading to energy depletion and systemic inflammation.

CHAPTER 8

THE COLON AND ENDOTOXINS—
THE HIDDEN ENERGY BLOCK

Now that you've journeyed through the nutrient-absorbing maze of your small intestine, dodging leaky gut, malabsorption, and bacterial overgrowth, you might think you're in the clear. Nutrients have been absorbed, enzymes have done their job, and the body has gotten what it needs. Time to remove the waste, right?

Not so fast.

Just because the small intestine handles most of the digestion and absorption doesn't mean the rest is "waste." In fact, what happens next is just as important, maybe even more so when it comes to energy production and hidden energy blocks. Because now, everything heads to the colon, the place where balance is maintained or chaos is unleashed, and where your metabolism can either stay steady...or hit a wall.

As the final stage of digestion, the colon is responsible for water balance, mineral absorption, vitamin production, supporting gut bacteria, regulating endotoxins, and eliminating toxins, all of which directly impact how your body produces and uses energy.

When your colon is working optimally, it helps maintain steady energy levels, hydration, hormone balance, and metabolic flow. But when it becomes sluggish, inflamed, or out of sync, it can slow down metabolism, increase endotoxin load, and contribute to fatigue, inflammation, and systemic dysfunction.

In this chapter, I'll guide you through the winding pathways of your large intestine—helping you understand how it works, why it matters, and how these bacterial toxins, known as endotoxins, make up your third hidden energy block. We'll explore the microbiome, the most common colon-related issues, and, most importantly, what you can do with nutrition and lifestyle to support your colon, reduce endotoxin production, and unlock better energy and metabolic health.

Colon Physiology and Function

I know, I know—not more physiology?! I promise, the colon will be quick and simple—well, sort of (I did my best). The colon is a muscular tube stretching about 5 feet (150 cm) and framing the small intestine (1). The colon begins at the cecum, where it connects to the small intestine via the ileocecal valve. From there, undigested fibers, cholesterol, fats, and water travel through five main sections:

1. The Ascending colon (right side). Receives semi-liquid chyme from the small intestine. Its main job is water and electrolyte absorption. This is where bacterial fermentation begins, and where gut bacteria are most active. This is also the primary site of endotoxin production—but more on this later.

2. The Transverse colon (top-across upper abdominal). As the chyme moves horizontally from right to left, more water and electrolytes are absorbed, thickening the stool. Bacterial fermentation also continues in the transverse colon. Most of your gut microbiome is in your ascending and transverse colon.

3. Descending colon (left side). Once at the descending colon chyme is now semi-solid waste, at this point the stool is often referred to as feces. Less fermentation

occurs, but the remaining water is absorbed to firm up stool. Gut motility will slow down here, getting waste ready for the final transit toward elimination.

4. Sigmoid colon (left to center). Your stool is now fully formed and is temporarily stored. Once the stool (feces) builds up, signals are sent from the rectum to the brain to prepare for elimination. This communication happens through the ENS (the second brain) and your autonomic nervous system.

5. Rectum (final storage before elimination). Your rectum holds stool until it's ready to be expelled. The anal sphincter controls the release of waste, and once you are relaxed, can open to release your stool. If stool hangs out too long here, more water can be absorbed from it, leading to constipation.

As stool moves through the colon, water is reabsorbed to solidify it. If transit is too fast, diarrhea occurs; if too slow, constipation follows. By the time feces exits, it is composed of dead bacteria, undigested fibers, fats, water, bacterial toxins, and other waste (2).

Colon Functions—More than Just Waste Removal

The colon may not be the flashiest part of your digestive system, but it's one of the most underappreciated when it comes to your energy production, immunity, and overall metabolic health. Beyond simply removing waste, the colon fine-tunes your hydration levels, recycles key minerals, supports immune function, regulates bacterial populations, produces its own vitamins, impacts hormone levels, and handles elimination like a rock star, or at least it should.

Water and Electrolyte Absorption

One of the colon's most important jobs is regulating fluid and mineral balance. It reabsorbs roughly 90% of the remaining water from your intestinal contents, about 1 to 1.5 liters per day, to prevent dehydration and support the formation of well-shaped stool. In the process, it also pulls back critical electrolytes like sodium, potassium, and chloride, which your body uses for nerve signaling, muscle contractions, heartbeat regulation, and cellular energy production.

Too little reabsorption = diarrhea, electrolyte depletion, and fatigue. Too much reabsorption = constipation, sluggish digestion, and increased endotoxin absorption. Like most things in the body, balance is the goal, and the colon plays a large role in making sure your poop is well, pretty—don't try to pretend you do not know what I mean!

Later in this chapter I will discuss all the possible issues with your colon, including diarrhea and constipation.

Immune Function

The colon is a critical component of the body's immune defense system, serving as both a physical barrier against pathogens and a hub for immune cell activity. The colon also contains important immune structures that help regulate inflammatory responses, prevent infections, and maintain overall immune balance. Think of it as your own security team, scanning, screening, identifying and neutralizing threats before they cause harm to the body.

One of the primary immune functions of the colon is to maintain a strong mucosal barrier that prevents harmful substances from entering the bloodstream. The colonic lining is protected by a thick mucus layer, which acts as a first line of defense by trapping potential pathogens. Embedded within this mucus are antimicrobial peptides (AMPs) and secretory IgA (sIgA) antibodies, both of which help neutralize harmful bacteria and prevent infections.

Another key immune feature of the colon is the gut-associated lymphoid tissue (GALT). While the small intestine houses the highest concentration of gut-associated lymphoid tissue (GALT), the colon is responsible for distinguishing between harmful invaders and harmless dietary antigens, ensuring that the immune system does not overreact to normal food particles. This function is particularly important in preventing conditions such as food allergies, chronic gut inflammation, and autoimmune reactions.

Beyond just security, your colon also serves as a regulatory control center for inflammation. When inflammatory signals (pro-inflammatory cytokines) start rising, immune cells in the colon act like air traffic controllers, managing the response so that inflammation doesn't get out of hand. If this system fails, inflammation can spread throughout the body, contributing to arthritis, cardiovascular disease, and metabolic disorders.

So, if you've been wondering why your joints ache, your cholesterol is high, or your blood sugar is out of balance, your colon's "security system" may not be functioning at full capacity. A healthy gut means a well-regulated immune system, better inflammation control, and overall metabolic health. Keep your colon's security team well-equipped, and it will keep your whole body safe.

Nutrient Production

The colon, particularly the ascending and transverse sections, plays a role in nutrient production, specifically B vitamins and vitamin K2. Certain bacteria in the colon can produce B1 (thiamine), B2 (riboflavin), B3 (niacin), B7 (biotin), and B12 (cobalamin). However, due to the thicker walls of the colon, these vitamins are not efficiently absorbed into the bloodstream and are instead excreted in stool. While this may seem wasteful, research suggests that B vitamins serve a local function, helping to support bacterial growth, gut balance, and energy production for colon cells (3).

In addition to B vitamins, the colon can also produce vitamin K2 (menaquinones), which plays a critical role in calcium metabolism, cardiovascular health, and inflammation regulation. Unlike water-soluble B vitamins, which require active transport for absorption (a mechanism lacking in the colon), fat-soluble vitamins like K2 can be absorbed more efficiently (3,4).

However, it's important to note that gut bacteria produce less than 10% of the body's required K2 (approximately 10 mcg per day), and only a small portion of this is absorbed. While the K2 produced in the colon may contribute locally to gut health, particularly in regulating inflammation, supporting gut barrier integrity, and reducing endotoxin damage, it is insufficient to meet whole-body requirements (5).

For optimal vitamin K2 levels, dietary sources are far more reliable. K2 is abundant in animal-based foods, including eggs, butter, and liver, as well as fermented foods like natto, cheese, and sauerkraut. The body uses K2 to regulate calcium metabolism, ensuring that calcium is directed into bones rather than accumulating in arteries, thereby reducing the risk of arterial calcification and cardiovascular disease.

Understanding Vitamin K2

Vitamin K2, also known as menaquinone (MK), exists in multiple forms, classified by side-chain length. These forms are labeled MK-4 through MK-14, with at least 11 known variations. While the colon produces MK-7 through MK-12, this is not sufficient to meet daily needs. The two most essential forms for human health are MK-4 and MK-7, both of which must come primarily from dietary sources.

It is estimated that humans require 100-200 mcg of K2 daily. The most bioavailable form, MK-4, is found in animal-based foods such as butter, egg yolks, liver, and meats. It is absorbed in the small intestine and stored in the brain, pancreas, and arteries. Goose liver (foie gras) contains the highest amount of MK-4, providing 100 mcg per ounce, while two large egg yolks provide approximately 20-30 mcg, and a tablespoon of butter contains 10-15 mcg.

MK-4 plays a crucial role in bone health by activating osteocalcin, a protein responsible for binding calcium into bones, thereby increasing bone density (6). It also works synergistically with Vitamin D to improve calcium metabolism and activates matrix Gla-protein (MGP), which prevents arterial calcification, reducing the risk of heart disease and stroke (7). Additionally, MK-4 is believed to have neuroprotective (8) and anti-cancer (9) benefits.

MK-7, on the other hand, is primarily found in fermented foods, particularly natto, cheese (especially Gouda, Brie, and Jarlsberg), and sauerkraut. One ounce of Gouda cheese provides 60 mcg of MK-7, while one ounce of Jarlsberg cheese offers 75 mcg. Although gut bacteria can produce small amounts of MK-7, most of it is used locally in the gut, with minimal absorption into circulation.

Like MK-4, MK-7 supports cardiovascular health by preventing calcium buildup in arteries (10). It has also been shown to enhance bone mineral density, activate osteocalcin (11), and improve lipid profiles by lowering LDL cholesterol, increasing HDL cholesterol, and improving insulin sensitivity (12).

Although the colon produces some K2, this is not enough for overall health. To ensure optimal K2 levels, it is best to consume a variety of K2-rich foods, incorporating both MK-4 and MK-7 sources into the diet.

While the colon contributes to B-vitamin and K2 production, absorption limitations prevent these nutrients from meeting the body's full needs. Instead, these vitamins appear to play a more localized role in gut health rather than systemic nutrition.

For whole-body health, dietary sources remain the best way to obtain sufficient levels of vitamin K2. A diet rich in animal products and cheeses supports bone density, cardiovascular function, and overall metabolic health, ensuring that calcium is properly utilized, and inflammation is kept in check.

Your Microbiome: An Ecosystem like No Other

The colon is home to a vast and diverse ecosystem made up of thousands of microbial species, including bacteria, fungi, parasites, viruses, and phages, all of which coexist and interact within the digestive system (13). In fact, your microbiome contains about 10 times more microorganisms than your own human cells, considering that your body has approximately 37 trillion cells, that's an astonishing number of microbial residents! (14)

The human microbiome is often described as a delicate ecosystem, where beneficial and potentially harmful microbes exist in balance. When this balance is maintained, "good" bacteria support digestion, immune function, and metabolic health. However, when this balance is disrupted, due to stress, diet, infections, or medications, harmful bacteria can overgrow, leading to gut inflammation, immune dysregulation, and metabolic dysfunction.

Dr. Ray Peat offered an insightful perspective on the complexity of the microbiome:

"The interaction of the intestinal bacteria is far too complicated to neatly divide them up into beneficial and harmful bacteria. Even the so-called 'beneficial' bacteria have been shown to create injury in a germ-free animal. (15)"

This highlights just how intricate and dynamic the gut microbiome truly is, what is helpful in one situation may be harmful in another, depending on the environment and individual factors.

This concept also applies to the fermentation of dietary fiber into short-chain fatty acids (SCFAs), such as butyrate, acetate, and propionate. Under the right conditions, SCFAs can benefit the gut by providing fuel for colon cells, reducing inflammation, and strengthening the gut barrier. However, under certain conditions, such as chronic stress, gut dysbiosis, low thyroid function, or poor energy production, excess SCFAs can contribute to inflammation, intestinal permeability, endotoxin production, sleep disturbances, obesity, and imbalances in lipid and glucose metabolism (16,17, 18).

It is suggested that the body produces SCFAs as an alternative energy source to fuel your cells when glucose oxidation is insufficient. Basically, your colon produces fuel for your body to use. While this mechanism can compensate in times of need, it is not an ideal long-term strategy. Relying too much on gut fermentation for energy production can create a cascade of negative health effects.

Think of your metabolism like a fireplace. Glucose oxidation, your preferred energy source, is like burning clean, dry wood, producing steady, efficient heat with minimal waste.

SCFAs, on the other hand, are like using backup fuel, such as damp wood. In small amounts, it can still provide warmth and be beneficial, especially for gut cells. However, if your fireplace starts depending too much on damp wood, because dry wood (glucose oxidation) isn't available, it burns inefficiently, produces excess smoke (inflammation), and may clog the chimney (metabolic dysfunction and gut issues).

In a healthy system, SCFAs play a beneficial role in gut barrier function and immune support. But when gut dysbiosis, chronic stress, or low thyroid function disrupt metabolism, the body may produce or absorb SCFAs in excess, leading to systemic inflammation, endotoxin production, metabolic slowdown, and poor gut health. In essence, a healthy metabolism should primarily rely on glucose oxidation rather than excessive fermentation in the gut.

Hormonal Health – When Estrogen Fights Back

Your colon plays a significant role in hormone regulation, particularly estrogen metabolism. The connection lies in beta-glucuronidase, an enzyme produced by certain gut bacteria that can determine whether estrogen leaves the body or gets recycled.

Here's how it works: your liver metabolizes estrogen, breaking it down and binding it to a molecule called glucuronic acid. This process, called glucuronidation, makes estrogen water-soluble, allowing it to be excreted through bile into the intestines. Ideally, the estrogen continues its journey out of the body via stool, preventing excessive buildup in the bloodstream.

However, if your gut bacteria are producing too much beta-glucuronidase, the story changes. Instead of estrogen being eliminated, this enzyme deconjugates (reactivates) the estrogen, allowing it to be reabsorbed into circulation. This increases estrogen levels, leading to a hormonal imbalance, often tipping the scales in favor of estrogen excess disrupting the balance between estrogen and progesterone.

Diets high in excessive fat and protein, and lower in fiber, stress, and/or excessive antibiotic use are shown to produce more beta-glucuronidase in the gut. Symptoms can include PMS, weight gain, bloating, breast tenderness, mood swings, and an increased risk of estrogen-related conditions like fibroids or endometriosis (19, 20). More on this in Chapters 9 and 10.

Bile Recycling (Enterohepatic Circulation) & Endotoxins

Bile acids play a crucial role in digestion, helping to break down fats and absorb fat-soluble vitamins. Most of these bile acids are reabsorbed in the ileum of the small intestine, but about 5 percent escape into the colon. Ideally, very little bile should reach the colon, but some always does, and in small amounts, it serves a useful function. However, when excess bile acids accumulate in the colon, they can cause problems, kind of like when over-served guests stay too long at your dinner party, getting rowdy and disrupting the peace.

One of the biggest issues with excess bile acids in the colon is their interaction with endotoxins (lipopolysaccharides, LPS). Bile acids can bind to endotoxins, increasing their chances of being reabsorbed rather than eliminated. This allows harmful endotoxins to re-enter circulation instead of being properly excreted.

Once absorbed, these endotoxins travel back to the liver via the portal vein. If the liver is already overburdened, whether due to stress, poor detoxification, or a high endotoxin load, it may struggle to clear them efficiently. Instead of breaking them down and eliminating them, the liver packages them back into bile, which is then secreted into the duodenum (the first section of the small intestine) to restart the cycle (21).

If the small intestine is compromised, due to leaky gut, inflammation, or slow motility, these endotoxins can escape into circulation, triggering systemic inflammation. Once in the bloodstream, they disrupt mitochondrial function, increase oxidative stress, and interfere with energy production, essentially waging metabolic warfare on your cells. This endotoxin-driven inflammation has been linked to insulin resistance, liver dysfunction, obesity, cardiovascular disease, and neurodegeneration.

Now, before diving deeper into the damage endotoxins cause, let's look at the colon's final and most celebrated role: elimination.

Elimination: The Final Job of the Colon

The colon's most iconic and celebrated role is elimination, in other words, it is taking out your trash. This is where all the leftovers from digestion, detoxification, and microbial turnover are sent to be expelled from the body. When everything's working smoothly, your colon helps clear out a wide variety of waste products: endotoxins and other toxins, broken down hormones like estrogen, bile-bound toxins, dead microbes, undigested food fibers, and excess cholesterol.

But when motility slows down or the gut lining becomes compromised, things start to back up. Instead of exiting the body, many of these waste products can be reabsorbed into circulation, forcing the liver to detoxify them all over again. This creates a vicious cycle of overwork and inflammation, putting stress on your entire system, disrupting hormone balance, and ultimately compromising your body's ability to produce energy effectively.

When elimination is impaired, the body retains far more than it should. And as you'll see in the next section, when toxins like endotoxins aren't properly removed, they don't just sit quietly, they sneak back in and stir up chaos at the cellular level.

FUN FACT: Most of your stool is not undigested food, it's dead bacteria! Roughly 55-60% is made of microbial remnants. These cellular leftovers are part of your body's natural turnover process and play a key role in clearing out both waste and microbial debris. Here's the kicker: your colon turns over trillions of bacteria every single day–like a microscopic Roomba–and your poop is your final exit strategy. At this point, it is less about what you ate, and more about what lived (and died) in your gut ecosystem.

Endotoxins: The Hidden Energy Block

One of the primary functions of the colon is to act as a containment and elimination site for endotoxins (LPS). Endotoxins are toxic fragments released when Gram-negative bacteria die. While these bacteria are a natural part of the gut microbiome, excess endotoxin levels can become problematic when they leak into circulation.

A healthy colon should eliminate endotoxins through stool. However, when gut integrity is compromised, due to inflammation, increased permeability, bacterial overgrowth, or bile dysfunction, endotoxins can enter the bloodstream and cause systemic dysfunction.

Although endotoxins are primarily produced in the colon, they are not significantly absorbed there due to the protective mucus layer and tight junctions that prevent large molecules from entering circulation. Instead, most endotoxin absorption happens in the small intestine, where the gut lining is more permeable, particularly in the duodenum and jejunum.

This paradox is largely due to enterohepatic circulation, the process where the liver filters out endotoxins from the bloodstream and excretes them into bile as part of detoxification. However, since bile is released into the small intestine to aid in fat digestion, endotoxins hitch a ride along with the bile salts. Under normal conditions, bile salts are reabsorbed in the ileum, while endotoxins stay behind for excretion. But if gut integrity is compromised, some endotoxins sneak into the colon and get reabsorbed, slipping back into circulation instead of being eliminated.

It's like kicking out a rowdy drunk guy from a nightclub, only to have him sneak around to the back entrance and get right back in (oh, the good ole days). No matter how many times security throws him out, he keeps finding a way back in, causing even more problems each time he returns. This constant recycling of endotoxins creates a vicious cycle of inflammation, metabolic dysfunction, and liver overload, until you stop serving the pesky drunk (reduce endotoxin production) and improve the club's security (improve gut health).

Once endotoxins reach the bloodstream, they travel inside your cells, inhibiting cellular production in the mitochondria. Endotoxins interfere with the electron transport chain (ETC), at complex I and complex IV (refer to Chapter 1 for a refresh on complexes). This reduces ATP production, leading to less energy production, fatigue, blood sugar issues, and metabolic slow down (22).

In addition, endotoxins stimulate the release of Nitric Oxide, which binds to cytochrome C oxidase in Complex IV. This prevents oxygen from being used efficiently (remember oxygen is the final electron acceptor keeping your energy production working efficiently), forcing the cell to switch from aerobic respiration (with O_2) to anaerobic (without O_2) respiration (23).

And finally, endotoxins trigger excessive production of reactive oxygen species (ROS—oxidative stress) in the mitochondria, leading to excessive lipid metabolism, protein damage, and an increased susceptibility to chronic disease.

This endotoxin-driven inflammation can present as brain fog, fatigue, weight gain, high blood sugar, insulin resistance, anxiety, depression, and hormone imbalances. In addition, it has been implicated in obesity, diabetes, liver dysfunction, heart disease, neurodegeneration, and immune dysregulation (24, 26, 26, 27, 28, 29). Many chronic diseases thought to be caused by genetics or lifestyle choices may be driven by excessive endotoxin absorption and its inflammatory burden on the body.

In other words: If you're feeling tired, foggy, inflamed, gaining weight, or just feel "off," don't underestimate the power of your gut's unwanted party guests. Endotoxins may be microscopic, but they sure know how to trash the place—and your body. So, if your energy production feels like it's on the fritz, it might be time to tighten up the club's security, bouncing out the rowdy drunks for good (translation: improve gut health).

Other Toxins in the Colon – And Why Endotoxins Matter Most

While endotoxins are the main villains when it comes to gut-driven inflammation and metabolic slowdown, they're not alone. I know a few of you may be asking, *"What about all the other toxins the colon produces?"* And it's a fair question. The colon, especially when it's sluggish, inflamed, or overtaken by the wrong microbes, can churn out a cocktail of toxic byproducts that quietly wreak havoc on your health.

Here are a few of the key offenders:

Ammonia - Does your urine smell like window cleaner? That might be ammonia buildup. Produced when bacteria break down protein and urea, ammonia can irritate the gut lining, impair liver detox, and contribute to brain fog, poor focus, and even anxiety when levels rise.

Phenols and Indoles - Chemical sensitivities? Skin flare-ups? Brain fog or mood swings? Could be excess phenols and indoles. These compounds form when gut bacteria ferment amino acids like tyrosine and tryptophan. Once absorbed, they place extra strain on the liver and may contribute to mental sluggishness, skin issues, and even a sharp or chemical body odor.

Hydrogen Sulfide (H_2S) - Rotten egg gas, bloating, or fatigue after sulfur-rich foods? Excess H_2S could be the culprit. Produced by sulfur-reducing bacteria, H_2S can support gut lining repair in small amounts, but in excess, it impairs mitochondrial function and increases inflammation and gut discomfort.

Secondary Bile Acids - Heartburn, bile reflux, or fatty, watery stools?

When gut bacteria convert bile salts into secondary bile acids like deoxycholic acid (DCA), they can become irritating to the gut lining and serve as vehicles for endotoxins to sneak back into circulation.

Putrescine & Cadaverine - Smelly gas or body odor that won't quit, even after showering? These nasty protein-fermentation byproducts are created from undigested proteins, especially in low-acid or slow-moving guts. They can lead to bloating, halitosis, and a noticeable "funk" that seems to come from nowhere.

All these compounds can fuel inflammation, disrupt detoxification, and impact your mood, skin, digestion, and energy. But there's one reason I'm zooming in on endotoxins: their direct and measurable impact on your ability to produce energy at the cellular level.

Endotoxins don't just cause surface-level inflammation, they infiltrate your cells, damage your mitochondria, and interfere with your body's ability to generate ATP, your energy currency.

So, while these other toxins deserve respect, and certainly contribute to chronic symptoms, endotoxins are the ultimate energy thief. That's why they've earned the spotlight in this chapter.

What Increases Endotoxin Production and Absorption?

While small amounts of endotoxins (LPS) are normal, and even expected in a healthy gut, too much production or absorption becomes a major metabolic roadblock, especially when it comes to energy. So, what triggers the increase?

Here are the eleven most common culprits:

1. **Low stomach acid** - Less acid = less ability to kill off incoming pathogens → more bacteria reaching the colon alive (30, 31).

2. **Liver dysfunction** - A sluggish liver can't detox endotoxins efficiently, allowing endotoxins to make their way back into the blood.

3. **Slow motility or constipation** - Waste that lingers in the colon becomes a breeding ground for endotoxin-producing microbes (32, 33).

4. **Infections** - *(viral, bacterial, fungal, or parasitic)*

5. Infections shift the microbial balance, often increasing gram-negative bacteria, which release endotoxins as they die (34).

6. **Chronic stress & low thyroid function** - Both stress and low thyroid contribute to slow gut motility, weaken immune defenses, and increase intestinal permeability—allowing more LPS into circulation (35, 36, 37).

7. **Progesterone deficiency** - Progesterone helps stabilize mast cells and maintain tight junctions in the gut. Loss of progesterone, such as after menopause, anovulatory cycles, or with certain hormone contraceptives, may reduce this protective effect, potentially increasing intestinal permeability (38).

8. **Estrogen excess** – Estrogen can alter gut barrier function, bile flow, motility, and the microbiome in ways that may increase endotoxin (LPS) absorption. It also amplifies the body's inflammatory response to endotoxin, potentially worsening systemic inflammation. This is noted in mechanistic and experimental studies, as large human trials are limited (39, 40, 41).

9. **Alcohol consumption** - Alcohol can increase both LPS production and absorption, damaging the gut lining and weakening liver detox pathways (42). Alcohol can also increase estrogen production, which increases endotoxins.

10. **Excessive fiber intake** - Excess fermentable fibers can feed bacteria; this includes fiber from legumes, grains, raw leafy green and cruciferous vegetables (43). This occurs primarily in someone with existing gut issues— SIBO, constipation, dysbiosis.

11. **High-fat diets, especially those high in unstable polyunsaturated fats (PUFAs)** - Many seed oils, nut oils, and vegetable oils don't necessarily create more endotoxin, but they can increase how much of it gets into your bloodstream. PUFAs are highly prone to oxidation,

and their breakdown products can stress and weaken the intestinal barrier. When the tight junctions in the gut lining become compromised, more endotoxins can slip through into circulation, triggering inflammation and slowing metabolic function (44, 45).

12. **Medications** - Excessive use of antibiotics (46), PPIs (47), opioids (48, 49), NSAIDs (ibuprofen, naproxen, high-dose aspirin) (50), corticosteroids (51), chemotherapy (52), and radiation (53) can all increase endotoxins.

What is most interesting about endotoxins is they're rarely discussed in conventional medicine, at least, in the context of energy metabolism. However, once you understand their far-reaching, damaging effects, it becomes clear how they could be the reason for some of your health issues, as anything from fatigue, blood sugar issues, weight gain, hormonal issues and/or liver issues, could be linked to these sneaky little toxins.

Naturally, your next question might be:

"So how do I reduce them?"

Great question, and I will get to that by the end of this chapter. But first, let's take a closer look at the most common colon-related health conditions, many of which are deeply rooted in gut dysfunction, impaired motility, and an increased endotoxin burden.

Common Conditions of the Colon

Understanding colon health also means recognizing the common conditions that impair its function, many of which are tied to inflammation, motility issues, or an imbalance in the microbiome.

IBS (Irritable Bowel Syndrome)

IBS is a functional bowel disorder, meaning there is no visible damage on scans or labs. Rather, it is diagnosed based on symptoms, not biomarkers. IBS affects 10-15% of people globally, which means upwards of one billion people suffer with IBS.

Interesting enough, IBS is more common in women, and it often shows up between 20-40 years of age. Estrogen (the primary female sex hormone) tends to slow down gut motility, impact gut permeability, and reduce bile flow, which may explain why women experience IBS at double the rate over men. More on estrogen in Chapters 9 and 10.

IBS is characterized by abdominal pain, gas and gurgling, mucous in stool, bloating, altered bowel habits (diarrhea, constipation, or both). It can come with a feeling of urgency or a sense of incomplete evacuation. Symptoms normally get worse after eating, during stress, and during hormonal shifts (menstruation).

Although primarily a colon issue, IBS can be triggered by SIBO, poor enzyme secretion, and low stomach acid. So, it can be the result of a complete gut breakdown. Like other gut issues, IBS is connected to a dysregulated nervous system, since it can become much worse under stress.

What often goes overlooked in conventional conversations around IBS is the role of endotoxins. Whether IBS leans more toward constipation (IBS-C) or diarrhea (IBS-D), both situations can lead to an increase in endotoxin production or absorption. In constipation, stool sits too long and ferments; in diarrhea, contents move too quickly, impairing proper digestion and allowing bacterial overgrowth to thrive in the small intestine.

Once endotoxins leak through the gut barrier and enter circulation, they don't just irritate your GI tract, they disrupt your entire system. In many ways, IBS isn't just a gut problem—it's an energy problem, driven in part by these microscopic toxins overwhelming your system from the inside out.

Inflammatory Bowel Disease (or IBD)—Isn't just "Irritable"

It's inflammatory, meaning the immune system is actively attacking parts of the digestive tract, causing pain, damage, and dysfunction. Unlike IBS (which is more functional and symptom-based), IBD involves visible tissue damage, bleeding, and ulcers, which is normally diagnosed with a colonoscopy or biopsy. It can also be diagnosed with stool tests, testing for fecal calprotectin and lactoferrin, in addition to certain blood markers like C-Reactive Protein (CRP), Erythrocyte Sedimentation Ratio (ESR), Complete Blood Count (CBC) to check for possible anemia, low albumin, and nutrient deficiencies.

IBD includes two main conditions:

- **Crohn's disease** – Can affect any part of the GI tract from mouth to anus but often impacts the small intestine and colon. Inflammation is deeper and patchy.

- **Ulcerative colitis (UC)** – Primarily affects the colon and rectum. Inflammation is more superficial but continuous.

Inflammatory Bowel Disease (IBD) can affect anyone, but certain patterns emerge when we look more closely at age, gender, and environment. Most people are diagnosed with IBD between the ages of 15 and 35, with a second, smaller spike in incidence occurring after age 50. While ulcerative colitis appears to be slightly more common in men, Crohn's disease tends to affect women more often, suggesting a potential role for sex hormones like estrogen and progesterone. In fact, many people report symptom changes during hormonal transitions such as puberty, pregnancy, or menopause, which supports the idea that estrogen, cortisol, and serotonin may influence IBD expression and severity.

Genetics also play a role. If you have a first-degree relative, such as a parent or sibling with IBD, your risk increases significantly. However, like most health issues, genes alone don't explain everything, lifestyle factors seem to predominately "flip the switch."

Chronic stress, frequent use of antibiotics or NSAIDs, high intake of PUFA fats, low bile flow, sluggish digestion, and excessive endotoxin production and absorption can all increase your chances of IBD. In many cases, IBD seems to arise in people whose gut lining is already compromised, whose immune system is overstimulated, and whose metabolism is already suppressed.

When someone has IBD, their immune system is essentially in overdrive, mistaking food particles, gut bacteria, or even the lining of the intestine as a threat. This immune misfire creates a vicious cycle of chronic inflammation, mucosal injury, increased gut permeability, and elevated endotoxin absorption, resulting in systemic stress.

Over time, this leads to abdominal pain, diarrhea (sometimes bloody), weight loss, fatigue, anemia, and a range of nutrient deficiencies.

Like IBS, there is a strong link between endotoxins and IBD. In a 2009 study in *Molecular Immunology*, researchers found that lipopolysaccharides (LPS) directly trigger pro-inflammatory cytokine production in intestinal epithelial cells through the TLR4 and MyD88 signaling pathways. These cytokines, including TNF-α and IL-6, are well-established in IBD pathogenesis, suggesting that endotoxins are not just present, but may be actively fueling the inflammatory loop in both Crohn's disease and ulcerative colitis (54).

Additional studies have shown that individuals with Crohn's disease exhibit heightened sensitivity to LPS and increased expression of toll-like receptors, which may amplify immune reactivity to even small amounts of endotoxins. Elevated plasma LPS levels have also been correlated with disease severity in IBD, supporting the idea that compromised gut integrity allows for bacterial translocation and systemic immune activation (55).

Taken together, these findings suggest that addressing endotoxin load and strengthening gut barrier integrity aren't just complementary strategies, they may be central to long-term IBD healing and remission. Yes, we will get to this in a minute...

Diverticulosis / Diverticulitis

Diverticulosis is a condition where small pouches, called diverticula, form in the lining of the colon, most often in the descending colon (the left side). These pouches develop when the inner layer of the intestine pushes through weak spots in the muscular wall, kind of like small hernias in the colon wall.

On its own, diverticulosis doesn't always cause symptoms, and many people don't even know they have it. But when those pouches become inflamed or infected, it turns into diverticulitis, a more serious condition that can cause pain, fever, cramping, and even perforation in severe cases.

Diverticulosis becomes more common with age, especially after 50. It's estimated that over 60% of people over 70 have it to some degree. But it's not just an "old person" issue anymore, it's increasingly being seen in younger adults as well.

Diverticulosis can be caused by chronic constipation or straining during bowel movements, slow motility, sedentary lifestyle, low thyroid, excess estrogen exposure, stress, poor diet, nutrient deficiencies, alcohol, drugs, and you guessed it—high endotoxin load.

A 2021 study published in the *United European Gastroenterology Journal* found that individuals with diverticular disease often show signs of gut microbiome imbalance, increased mucosal permeability, and heightened immune activity, all of which can be triggered by endotoxins (lipopolysaccharides or LPS). These bacterial toxins activate inflammatory pathways in the gut, creating a state of chronic low-grade inflammation that weakens the integrity of the colon wall over time (56). In short, endotoxins not only drive systemic inflammation, but they can also compromise the local environment of the colon, making it more vulnerable to structural changes and flare-ups.

Are you starting to see a pattern yet? Let's keep going.

Constipation – When Nothing is Moving

Constipation is one of the most common digestive complaints, characterized by infrequent, difficult, or incomplete bowel movements. In the medical world, it is typically defined as having fewer than three bowel movements per week, which I feel is way too few. If you are not having at least one, even two bowel movements a day, I'd say you are somewhat constipated.

Most people will complain of hard, dry stools, straining, and that frustrating sense of "not quite done." While anyone can experience constipation occasionally, it's more common in those who are not eating enough, low nutrient diet, low thyroid, and or have an increase in stress. Remember high stress is going to shut down digestive function.

From a metabolic perspective, constipation is more than just annoying, it sets the stage for bigger problems. When stool sits too long in the colon, it allows more water to be reabsorbed, making stool harder to pass. Even more concerning, it allows for greater absorption of endotoxins (LPS) and other microbial byproducts that should've been excreted. This is a key reason constipation is considered an endotoxin amplifier, one that burdens the liver, slows metabolism, and raises systemic inflammation. Constipation also impairs hormone clearance, particularly estrogen, contributing to excess estrogen and further slowing motility. Yes, it is a vicious loop.

Diarrhea – When Things Are Moving Too Fast

On the other end of the spectrum, diarrhea is the result of hyperactive intestinal motility, when food and waste move too quickly through the colon for proper water reabsorption to occur. This leads to loose, watery, and often urgent bowel movements. While short-term diarrhea is usually tied to infections, food poisoning, or something you ate that might have irritated the gut lining, chronic diarrhea is often a symptom of deeper dysfunction, seen in IBS, IBD, SIBO, bile acid imbalance, high histamine or serotonin states.

Diarrhea can affect anyone, but it tends to occur more frequently in people with gut inflammation, poor gut lining integrity, or disrupted microbiome composition. It's also common during times of stress, due to elevated serotonin, adrenaline, and cortisol, all of which stimulate excessive motility and secretions. Like I said in the last chapter, serotonin is more of a gut hormone than a brain hormone, and when it increases, it speeds up digestion at the expense of absorption.

Matt's Story

Matt came to me with a classic case of chronic diarrhea and IBS. At 45, he was a busy dad of two, with a loving wife and a high-stress job in tech startups. His days were packed with deadlines, meetings, and pressure, and his body reflected it.

He lived on energy drinks, coffee, antacids, and fast, convenient meals. While his wife tried to cook healthy dinners, during the day, Matt was on his own. His "healthy" lunch choices included Chipotle bowls, pre-packaged salads, and the occasional pizza, all quick, but gut-irritating choices.

Working from home made his digestive urgency manageable, until he had to travel or attend in-person meetings. On those days, the stress skyrocketed. In business settings, Matt often drank 2–4 alcoholic beverages in the evening, as part of the social routine. To offset the aftereffects, he'd rely on Imodium and Pepto-Bismol the next day. He knew these were only masking the symptoms, not solving the issue, so he was ready for a real solution.

The first thing we addressed was nervous system regulation. I asked Matt to carve out short breaks throughout the day to breathe, reset, and not answer emails. He also began setting clearer boundaries around work hours, this included no more late-night messages. This alone began to reduce his stress load and give his gut some breathing room.

Next, we looked at food. I asked Matt to move away from fast food and salad-heavy meals. While some were seemingly "healthy," they were high in PUFAs, raw roughage, and processed grains that irritated his gut. Instead, we focused on easy-to-digest, gut-soothing meals:

- *Well-cooked starches like white rice, white potatoes, and sourdough*
- *Fruit juices and ripe fruit*
- *Soft-cooked vegetables*
- *A daily raw carrot salad for antimicrobial support*
- *Adequate protein with each meal*
- *Three structured meals a day, with rest in between to support proper motility*

We also talked about travel. Instead of defaulting to alcohol in social settings, Matt started ordering soda water with orange juice, a simple drink that looked like a cocktail but didn't wreck his gut or sleep.

For targeted gut support, I added:

Activated charcoal *every other day to reduce endotoxin load and slow gut transit.*

Saccharomyces boulardii*, a probiotic yeast, taken daily for 60 days to help regulate motility and strengthen his gut lining.*

Almost immediately, things began to shift. His stools became more formed, his urgency decreased, and his digestion noticeably improved. As his stress dropped, his gut calmed. And with more nourishing, less irritating meals, his entire system got a break.

After three months, Matt was completely off Imodium, antacids, and Pepto-Bismol. He was sleeping better, pooping better, and had far more energy. This all translated into stronger performance at work and more presence at home. As his confidence grew, he became more selective about his habits while traveling. He realized just how much social drinking had been affecting his digestion and sleep, so he let it go.

The biggest lesson? When you give your gut what it needs, less stress, more nourishment, and fewer irritants, it doesn't just positively affect your digestion. It also impacts your clarity, energy, mood, and the way you show up for your life.

While it may feel like the body is "getting rid of toxins," diarrhea often means that something is irritating the gut lining, or the gut barrier is compromised. Both can increase gut permeability and absorption of endotoxins into the bloodstream, and diarrhea can make the absorption of toxins worse, not better. In addition, the rapid transit doesn't allow for proper nutrient uptake, resulting in mineral deficiencies, dehydration, and increased inflammatory burden. Excess bile acids in the colon (due to not being reabsorbed in the small intestine) can also act as irritants, further contributing to endotoxin reabsorption and urgency,

IBS, IBD, diverticulosis, constipation, and diarrhea are not just annoying digestive issues—they are signs and symptoms of energy production issues. Whether your colon is inflamed, sluggish, racing, or has a microbial imbalance, they are linked to a common villain—endotoxins. Which all makes sense, once you understand that endotoxins are the third energy block. Now, the million-dollar question is, what do you do to fix the negative effects of endotoxins?

How to Reduce Endotoxins (And Why This Can Improve Most Colon Issues)

No matter which colon issue you're dealing with, IBS, IBD, constipation, diarrhea, or diverticulitis, endotoxins always seem to be in the mix. And in my experience, if you can work on decreasing these little buggers, every one of these colon issues can start to improve.

Instead of chasing every symptom at the surface level, the biggest game-changer is to focus on lowering your exposure to endotoxins. When you do that, you can increase energy production, decrease gut permeability and inflammation, and help your colon get back to its natural rhythm.

Here Is My Eight Step Process on How to Reduce Endotoxins:

Step 1: Remove the Things that Increase Endotoxin Exposure - This includes ultra-processed foods, fermentable fibers, seeds and nuts, polyunsaturated fats (seed, nut, and vegetable oils), alcohol, and medications like PPIs and opioids. *Please make sure to consult with your doctor before stopping any medications.* This helps with: IBS, IBD, diverticulitis, diarrhea, and constipation.

Step 2: Support Gut Motility - If you're experiencing an increase in endotoxin absorption, then you've got to make sure you're moving waste out of your body at a reasonable pace. When you're in a low-energy state, constipation can sneak in and increase bacterial toxins. So, until your energy improves, you might need a little help getting things moving.

- **Coffee** - Coffee is the most natural gut-stimulating, bile-releasing powerhouse out there. It's not just a morning ritual; it's a gut mover and shaker. It often triggers a bowel movement within 15–30 minutes and stimulates bile flow, which helps carry out endotoxins, estrogen, and other toxins. Pro tip: drink it with or after a meal to minimize stress and maximize the good stuff. Blend it with milk, cream, sugar, or collagen for a metabolically supportive version your gut and hormones will thank you for. If coffee is too stimulating, start small or skip it for now.

- **Cascara sagrada** - Cascara sagrada is a gentle herbal laxative that can help restore natural motility and bowel tone. A low-dose tincture, tea, or 1/16 tsp in water can reset a sluggish gut. Some people are sensitive, so start low, too much can lead to diarrhea.

- **Magnesium** - Magnesium is a calming and moving mineral. Citrate or glycinate forms help keep things flowing by pulling water into the colon and softening stools. Start slow, as too much can lead to diarrhea.

- **Take a walk** - Yep, walking helps motility. Gravity and gentle movement go a long way in assisting digestion. Try a 10-40-minute walk after meals.

This helps with: IBS, IBD, diverticulitis, and constipation.

Step 3: Boost Bile Flow to Remove Endotoxins - Endotoxins are detoxed by the liver and eliminated through bile. But if bile isn't flowing, those toxins can hang around and recirculate.

Support bile with:

- **Saturated fats** - Coconut oil, butter, ghee, and tallow tell the gallbladder to release bile, helping to remove endotoxins and reduce reabsorption.

- **Bitter foods** - Digestive bitters like artichoke, burdock, wormwood, and milk thistle stimulate bile flow from the liver and gallbladder. Be cautious with bitters if you have active ulcers, gastritis, or severe bile blockage, they might make you nauseous. Start slow.

- **Taurine** - This amino acid is conjugated (bound) to cholesterol to make bile. That process enhances bile flow and can increase bile acid excretion. Studies suggest 500–1500 mg/day of taurine can support bile production and liver function.

This helps with: IBS, IBD, diverticulitis, diarrhea, and constipation.

Step 4: Clean the Gut - Yes, the carrot salad again! Shredded raw carrot (with coconut oil, vinegar, and salt) acts like a street sweeper for your colon. It's antibacterial, antifungal, and antimicrobial. It binds endotoxins and helps escort them out. It's simple, cheap, and surprisingly powerful. Eat it once a day, ideally between meals.

If raw carrots aren't your thing or you get tired of them, cooked white button mushrooms or bamboo shoots can work just as well. See Appendix A.

Need something a bit stronger?

- **Activated charcoal (AC)** - Activated charcoal is a much stronger binder than carrot salad. It can be effective when symptoms flare up. AC is also a serotonin antagonist, so it can be used to treat nausea and diarrhea. Just be sure to take it away from meals and supplements so it doesn't bind nutrients. I recommend 1 heaping tsp of AC in 10 oz of water, away from meals. But not every day, it can cause constipation and reduce nutrient absorption.

- **Soil-based probiotics** - These are spore-forming bacteria naturally found in dirt, including Bacillus subtilis, Bacillus coagulans, Bacillus clausii, and Bacillus indicus. They tend to survive stomach acid better and are more shelf-stable than other probiotics. SBOs have been shown to suppress harmful bacteria, improve gut motility, and strengthen the gut lining (57).

- **Saccharomyces boulardii (SB)** - This probiotic yeast inhibits gram-negative bacteria, the big endotoxin producers. SB can bind endotoxins directly and keep them from entering your bloodstream. It also improves gut regularity and strengthens the barrier.

This helps with: IBS, IBD, diverticulitis, diarrhea, and constipation (58).

Step 5: Consider Additional Serotonin Antagonists - Excess serotonin is linked to gut inflammation, diarrhea, and low energy metabolism. Blocking serotonin (under guidance) with things like low dose cyproheptadine, Zofran (prescription needed) or progesterone can help regulate motility and reduce inflammation. This helps with: IBS, IBD, diverticulitis, and diarrhea.

Step 6: Eat Healthy Carbs to Support Energy - You don't want to avoid ALL carbs when healing your colon, your digestive cells still need fuel. Eat easy-to-digest carbs that don't leave a lot of waste behind. Think ripe fruits, fruit juice, honey, milk, and yes, even white sugar in moderation. This helps with: IBS, IBD, diverticulitis, diarrhea, and constipation.

Step 7: Reduce Stress - I know, I know, you hear this all the time. But seriously, if you're pushing your body when it's begging for rest, healing is going to be an uphill battle. Stress decreases motility, increases gut permeability, and raises hormones like estrogen, cortisol, histamine, and serotonin, all of which increase endotoxins.

Step 8: Consider Antibiotics - Excessive or repeated antibiotic use can weaken the gut microbiome, impair barrier integrity, increase permeability, and potentially raise endotoxin exposure. However, in the right context and dose, antibiotics can do the opposite by reducing the bacteria that produce endotoxin in the first place. By lowering bacterial overgrowth, antibiotics may help individuals whose endotoxin burden is driven by conditions such as SIBO, IBS flares, IBD, or liver-related endotoxemia.

It's important to note that as bacteria die, they can temporarily release more endotoxin, which may worsen symptoms before improvement occurs. If symptoms are severe or persistent, a short, targeted antibiotic course may be an appropriate therapeutic tool. Always work with a qualified healthcare practitioner before starting any antibiotic treatment.

So, slow down. Sleep. Take breaks. Get outside. Stay off social media. Whatever reduces your stress, do more of that. This helps with: IBS, IBD, diverticulitis, diarrhea, and constipation.

When it comes to healing your colon, it's not about doing one, or seven things perfectly (I see you, Type A people). It's about removing the blocks and supporting your colon where it's struggling. Lowering endotoxins isn't a quick fix, but it's a powerful and often overlooked strategy that can change everything.

These eight steps aren't here to overwhelm you, they're here to guide you and remind you that you're not stuck (literally or figuratively). These are simple, doable, at-home ways to lower inflammation, restore rhythm, and support your gut microbiome. Your colon was designed to work *for* you, not against you, it just needs the right environment to thrive. Start where you are. Pick one or two steps.

Layer as you go. This is how you begin to move an important energy block that might be keeping you stuck.

As you've seen in the last few chapters, the digestive system is nothing short of extraordinary. From the moment food enters your mouth to its final farewell through the colon, your body is orchestrating a beautifully complex process—extracting nutrients, neutralizing invaders, and maintaining inner balance. But as we've uncovered, digestion isn't passive. It's a high-energy, highly coordinated effort that only performs its best under calm, parasympathetic, well-fueled conditions—yes, the so-called "rest and digest" state. Just because digestion works best when you're resting doesn't mean your digestion is "resting." Quite the opposite, it's working hard.

The trouble starts when we hit obstacles; low stomach acid, thyroid dysfunction, malabsorption, SIBO, leaky gut, and bacterial toxins, all of which interfere with digestion and energy production. And when energy drops, digestion suffers even more. It's a vicious cycle, but now you've got real tools to help break it.

You've made it through the core of digestive healing, and now, it's time to shift gears. In the next chapter, we'll dive into your fourth energy block, one I've already hinted at many times throughout this section. It's powerful, complex, and often misunderstood. Yep, we're going there: the world of estrogen.

CHAPTER 8

THE BOTTOM LINE

The Colon and Endotoxins—The Hidden Energy Block

1. The colon is made up of five main sections (ascending, transverse, descending, sigmoid colon, and rectum), is about five feet long, and frames the small intestine.

2. The functions of the colon include water and electrolyte absorption, immune function, nutrient production (B and K vitamins), housing your microbiome, supporting hormone health, including estrogen detox, recycling bile acids, and removing waste.

3. The colon is the primary location of endotoxin production. Endotoxins are toxic fragments released when your bacteria die. In a healthy gut these are eliminated in the stool, in a gut that is compromised, these toxins can enter the blood creating systemic dysfunction.

4. Endotoxins can inhibit cellular energy production in several ways. They inhibit cellular production in the mitochondria, they stimulate nitric oxide—preventing oxygen from being used properly, slowing down energy production, and they trigger excessive oxidative stress.

5. To improve colon function, it is important to lower endotoxin production and absorption. This can include lowering PUFA, reducing alcohol consumption, supporting stomach acid production, supporting gut motility, supporting thyroid function, improve estrogen to progesterone balance, reducing excessive fermentable fibers, reducing medications that can increase endotoxins, using supportive supplements like activated charcoal and soil-based antibiotics, reducing stress, and supporting overall energy production. In other words, everything I talk about in the beginning of this book.

CHAPTER 9

ESTROGEN UNMASKED:
FROM FEMININE TO FRAZZLED

Estrogen is often described as *the* female hormone, the one that makes a woman, a woman. It's linked to curves, fertility, menstrual cycles, youthfulness, and is often portrayed as protective against everything from bone loss, dementia, to heart disease.

But from a bioenergetic perspective, estrogen isn't always the feminine superhero she's made out to be. In fact, when it becomes excessive or unopposed, estrogen can act more like a metabolic chokehold than a healthy and longer life promoting hormone. This is why excess estrogen is known as the fourth energy block.

Estrogen doesn't just influence the reproductive system; it interferes with how your cells generate and regulate energy. It can slow thyroid function, inhibit mitochondrial respiration, increase stress hormones, raise prolactin, and promote gut permeability and endotoxin absorption. In doing so, estrogen doesn't *burn* through energy like a workout would, it blocks the body's ability to *make* it.

It's like having a power plant with plenty of fuel, but the control room is dimmed, the machinery is jammed, and the operators are overwhelmed. The energy is there, but the system is too disorganized to use it efficiently.

Now, here's another way to look at it:

Imagine estrogen as a glamorous interior designer who shows up with vision and flair. She softens your figure, adds fullness to your curves, and casts a warm, romantic glow over everything she touches. But if she arrives without her project manager, progesterone, and your cellular infrastructure isn't ready for a remodel, things get out of hand. She starts knocking down support beams to "open up the space," rewiring the lighting without checking the voltage, and installing hot tubs on the roof just because they feel luxurious.

Before long, you're running extension cords through the bathroom, the energy bill is maxed out, and the plumbing is leaking into the basement. It is chaos dressed as glamour. Instead of maintaining balance, she creates dysfunction, bloating, fatigue, edema, and inflammation. And in the worst cases, she stops redecorating and starts building unauthorized additions, like fibroids, cysts, even cancer.

Now, to be clear, estrogen isn't the enemy, but she needs oversight. Without balance from progesterone, a healthy liver, a responsive thyroid, and a resilient gut, estrogen becomes a beautiful form of chaos your energy system can no longer afford.

In the next two chapters, we'll explore what estrogen is, how you make it, the different types of estrogen your body produces throughout life, and how it interacts with other hormones. Then we'll dive into how estrogen disrupts energy production, the signs and symptoms of estrogen excess, and most importantly, what you can do to avoid the excess estrogen traps and restore your metabolic balance.

What Is Estrogen (And Where Does It Come from?)

Estrogen is a steroid hormone often referred to as "the female hormone," and for good reason. Remember, it shapes hips, breasts, curves, and cycles. It orchestrates puberty, prepares the uterus for pregnancy, and regulates the monthly ebb and flow of a woman's reproductive life. But despite its glamorized role in femininity, estrogen is far more complex, and not exclusive to women (1).

In men, estrogen is produced primarily in the testes by converting testosterone into estrogen via aromatase. Aromatase is an enzyme that converts androgens into estrogens. This process is called aromatization, and without it, estrogen wouldn't exist. While present in much smaller amounts, estrogen still plays key roles in libido, erectile function, and sperm development (2).

In women of reproductive age, most estrogen is produced in the ovaries, where it's made from cholesterol through a series of carefully coordinated steps. The dominant form is estradiol (E2), the most potent type of estrogen, and its levels ebb and flow throughout the menstrual cycle.

During the first half of the cycle (the follicular phase), estradiol rises to prepare the uterine lining for pregnancy. After ovulation, progesterone takes the lead in the luteal phase, but estradiol still plays a supporting role (3).

Now, here's where it gets interesting (so play close attention ladies): estrogen production in the ovaries depends on a team effort between two types of cells—the theca cells and granulosa cells—and two key pituitary hormones, LH (luteinizing hormone) and FSH (follicle-stimulating hormone).

LH stimulates the theca cells to convert cholesterol into androgens, mainly androstenedione and testosterone. These androgens then diffuse into neighboring granulosa cells, where FSH triggers the production of aromatase (4, 5, 6). Aromatase is the enzyme that converts androgens into estrogens: testosterone becomes estradiol (E2), and androstenedione becomes estrone (E1). Both contribute to the body's estrogen pool, with estradiol being the more potent form (7). In short, women make estrogen the same way men do, by converting androgens, but they simply produce much more of it, especially before menopause.

In postmenopausal women, estrogen production from the ovaries declines sharply, but that doesn't mean estrogen disappears. Instead, the body shifts to peripheral production, where tissues like body fat, adrenal glands, skin, and brain convert circulating androgens (such as DHEA, androstenedione, and testosterone) into estrogens via aromatase.

After menopause, the dominant estrogen becomes estrone (E1). It's often labeled "weaker" than estradiol (E2), but it still has biological effects. And it doesn't always stay weak—estrone can be converted back into estradiol through the enzyme 17β-hydroxysteroid dehydrogenase type 1 (17β-HSD1), which tends to be elevated during inflammatory or stressed states (8).

This widespread, tissue-based estrogen production is called peripheral aromatization, and it becomes especially significant in:

- Postmenopausal women

- Men and women with higher body fat

- People dealing with chronic stress, inflammation, or hypothyroidism

Unlike the beautifully choreographed rise and fall of ovarian estrogen, peripheral estrogen is more like an uninvited houseguest who shows up, overstays her welcome, and refuses to leave. She's poorly regulated, rarely opposed by progesterone, and sticks around when your liver and gut aren't clearing hormones well. Add stress, junk food, medications, and nutrient gaps, and estrogen takes the lead—sparking inflammation and symptoms like bloating, breast tenderness, puffiness, irritability, stubborn weight, poor sleep, and cranky skin.

And it's not just where estrogen is made that matters, it's also which kind you're dealing with.

Types of Estrogen

Estrogen isn't one singular hormone, it's a whole family, and not all members behave the same. Some are made naturally inside your body (endogenous), while others come from outside sources (exogenous). They vary in strength, source, and effect, and understanding which kind is dominating your system can help you make sense of your symptoms and better support your metabolism (9).

Endogenous Estrogens (Made by Your Body)

1. **Estrone (E1):** Produced primarily in the adrenal glands and peripheral tissues (like fat, liver, and skin), estrone becomes the dominant estrogen after menopause. It's considered "weaker" than estradiol, but it lingers longer and is more likely to accumulate in tissue. Estrone can be reconverted into estradiol in inflamed or stressed environments and is often involved in fibroids, bloating, and estrogen-sensitive cancers when not properly cleared.

2. **Estradiol (E2):** The most potent and active form of estrogen, estradiol is produced by the ovaries in women and the testes in men. It's also created in peripheral tissues via aromatase. Estradiol is 10x stronger than estrone and 100x stronger than estriol. It regulates the menstrual cycle, fertility, and secondary sex characteristics, but in excess, it can interfere with energy production, thyroid function, and mitochondrial health.

3. **Estriol (E3):** Known as the "pregnancy estrogen," estriol is produced in high amounts by the placenta. It's much weaker than E1 and E2, and some believe it may have protective effects due to its low binding affinity and short half-life. However, outside of pregnancy, estriol plays a minimal role.

4. **Estetrol (E4):** The least understood of the estrogens, estetrol is produced only during pregnancy by the fetal liver. Research is ongoing into its potential roles and

therapeutic uses, but it's not a major player in non-pregnant adults.

Exogenous Estrogens (Coming from the Outside World)

1. **Hormone therapy (HRT / ERT / MHT):** These are pharmaceutical estrogens given to manage menopausal symptoms or hormonal imbalances. Some are bioidentical, others are synthetic or derived from equine sources (like Premarin, which is high in estrone). While often touted as "natural," these therapies can elevate systemic estrogen levels and overwhelm detox pathways when not carefully balanced.

2. **Hormonal birth control:** Oral contraceptives and implants often contain synthetic estrogens, designed to suppress ovulation. These estrogens don't cycle naturally, can deplete key nutrients, suppress natural hormone production, and create long-term endocrine disruption for some women.

3. **Phytoestrogens:** Found in soy, flax, legumes, seeds, and some grains, these plant estrogens can mimic estrogen in the body by binding weakly to estrogen receptors. While often marketed as "gentle" or "protective," their effects depend on gut health, liver function, and overall estrogen burden.

4. **Xenoestrogens:** The sneakiest of them all, these are man-made chemicals that act like estrogen in the body. Found in plastics (like BPA), pesticides, personal care products, detergents, mold, alcohol, polyunsaturated fats, and industrial toxins, xenoestrogens are a major contributor to estrogen excess, especially in modern environments. They're hard to break down, often stored in fat, and can disrupt hormonal balance for years.

Now that you've met the estrogen family, from the potent estradiol to the sneaky xenoestrogens, it's time to meet estrogen's counterpart—progesterone.

You can't talk about estrogen without talking about progesterone, because progesterone is the hormone that helps "balance" out the effects of estrogen. Again, I want to be abundantly clear that estrogen is not bad. You need it, and it serves many reproductive and metabolic functions. However, when there is excess estrogen to progesterone, you can start to have problems.

Meet Progesterone: Estrogen's Balancing Counterpart

You can't fully understand estrogen without also talking about progesterone, because progesterone isn't just a "balancing hormone," it's estrogen's metabolic counterweight. Estrogen builds and amplifies; progesterone refines, stabilizes, and protects. When the two work together, they create a healthy rhythm of growth and restoration. But when progesterone is too low, or absent, estrogen becomes a one-woman show that can get a little reckless and out of control.

Progesterone, also a steroid hormone, is produced by the adrenal glands and gonads—ovaries in women and testes in men. Progesterone's main function is to support menstruation and pregnancy in women and spermiogenesis and androgen production in men (10). It also positively affects bone mineralization and supports the smoothness of blood vessels and myelin sheaths in both men and women (11). For reference, during menopause and pre-ovulation, men and women have similar progesterone levels. It's only after ovulation and during pregnancy that women's progesterone levels rise significantly (12, 13).

Women produce progesterone primarily in the second half of their menstrual cycle (the luteal phase) and during pregnancy, hence the term "pro-gestation hormone" During a woman's cycle, progesterone is produced in the corpus luteum, the temporary endocrine structure that forms in the ovary after ovulation. In a healthy cycle, estrogen rises during the follicular phase, peaking just before ovulation to help stimulate the release of the egg.

After ovulation, progesterone takes the lead in the luteal phase, while estrogen rises again, just not as dramatically. Progesterone should now dominate the hormonal environment, preparing the uterus for implantation, calming the nervous system, and supporting thyroid and energy metabolism.

While estrogen production in the luteal phase typically hovers around 100–200 pg/mL, progesterone can reach 10,000–20,000 pg/mL, a ratio of 100:1 or more (14). This is a huge difference. It reflects progesterone's vital role in opposing and modulating estrogen's effects, not by matching estrogen in amount, but by buffering its impact. When this ratio is disrupted due to stress, inflammation, gut dysbiosis, or anovulation, estrogen's activity becomes excessive, even if its actual levels haven't changed. That's when symptoms emerge: PMS, breast tenderness, anxiety, migraines, edema, heavy cycles, PCOS, varicose veins, even fibroids and cancer.

It should be noted that progesterone is usually measured in nanograms per milliliter (ng/mL) on blood labs, while estrogen is measured in picograms per milliliter (pg/mL). There are 1,000 pg/mL in one ng/mL. So, if you have 10 ng/mL of progesterone and 100 pg/mL of estrogen, you still have 100 times more progesterone than estrogen.

Yet, many would look at this and mistakenly believe they have more estrogen than progesterone, because that's how the labs report them. Progesterone is fat-soluble and circulates in much higher concentrations, while estrogen, also fat-soluble, is potent in very small amounts. Unless you convert them to the same unit, it's like comparing teaspoons to gallons.

So why do so many women experience PMS during the luteal phase, when progesterone is supposed to be highest? Because that "peak" only happens if ovulation is strong. If ovulation is weak, delayed, or doesn't occur at all, which is common with stress, under-eating, overtraining, or perimenopause, progesterone stays low or flatlines completely. Even if estrogen levels are "normal," they become unopposed. And when estrogen runs the show without its calmer counterpart, things get messy: bloating, migraines, insomnia, mood swings, and hormonal chaos.

Unlike estrogen, which stimulates tissue growth, fluid retention, and stress signaling, progesterone is anti-inflammatory, anti-catabolic, and pro-metabolic. It:

- Supports thyroid hormone action and metabolic rate
- Boosts GABA, the calming neurotransmitter, improving sleep
- Protects against cortisol's tissue-wasting effects
- Reduces aldosterone and fluid retention
- Promotes blood sugar stability and regulates glucose oxidation *see side bar

---

Progesterone Therapy, Glucose Oxidation, and Blood Sugar

Progesterone helps regulate glucose metabolism by supporting glucose uptake (15). Unlike estrogen, progesterone therapy encourages glucose oxidation over fat oxidation (16). In simpler terms, if glucose is available, progesterone enhances your cells' ability to absorb and burn it. When your cells increase glucose uptake and oxidize it, stress hormones like cortisol and adrenaline fall, and you feel calmer, more relaxed, and metabolically stable. This is a major reason why many people report better sleep and reduced anxiety on progesterone therapy (17,18).

But not everyone has that experience. Some people, particularly women (although men can use it), report feeling worse after using progesterone: more anxious, more nauseated, and more wired.

So, what gives?

If you take something that ramps up glucose uptake, but you don't have enough glucose available (because you're not eating enough, restricting carbs, or have sluggish energy metabolism), your blood sugar can crash. And low blood sugar equals a stress response. In my experience, people who are underfed, under-carbed, or metabolically compromised often don't tolerate progesterone therapy well, at least not initially.

British physician Katharina Dalton, who pioneered progesterone therapy for PMS from the 1950s through the early 2000s, believed regulated blood sugar was essential before starting progesterone. She recommended eating starch (complex carbs) every three hours to ensure steady blood sugar. Why? Because when blood sugar drops due to increased glucose uptake, cortisol and adrenaline rise (19). And when adrenaline is high, it counteracts the calming effects of progesterone.

This is why I always recommend building a strong food foundation before experimenting with any hormone therapy, especially those like progesterone that can accelerate your metabolism.

And just like estrogen, progesterone's reputation is clouded by confusion between natural progesterone and synthetic progestins. Both are lumped under the label of "progestogens," but they are not the same. Natural progesterone is identical to what your body makes. Progestins are synthetic, structurally different, and can act very differently in the body, sometimes with unwanted effects.

Context matters. A hormone's effect depends on the health of the body it's working in. That's why the same hormone can calm one person while making another feel worse.

Bottom line: In a well-fed, low-stress body, progesterone is an anti-stress superstar. It can reduce hot flashes, support deep sleep, ease anxiety, balance blood sugar, and may even help prevent certain cancers. But in a poorly nourished or stressed-out system, progesterone might backfire. The key is to understand what form of progesterone you're using (natural vs. synthetic), and whether your body is ready to receive it. Always talk to your health care provider to tailor a plan that fits your needs and your current metabolic state.

It should be noted, since this comes up often in health circles, progesterone doesn't block estrogen; it guides it. It's the project manager to estrogen's creative director: making sure growth has structure, timing, and purpose. Without enough progesterone, estrogen's natural flair turns into fatigue, fluid retention, mood instability, and systemic inflammation.

And because ovulation is the only reliable way to make meaningful amounts of progesterone, anything that disrupts ovulation, whether stress, illness, inflammation, or xenoestrogens, can leave estrogen unopposed. Estrogen becomes the loudest voice in the room, but no one's around to manage the consequences.

In short, estrogen builds and designs your tissues, while progesterone keeps the blueprints in check and makes sure, you're not building a hot tub over the electrical panel. Progesterone's effects aren't about suppression, they're about supervision.

From Counter Partner to Psycho: When Estrogen Blocks Energy Production

While estrogen plays essential roles in growth, development, and reproduction, when left unopposed or poorly metabolized, it can quietly sabotage your metabolic engine. I want to be clear (again); estrogen is not inherently bad. You need it—for puberty, fertility, bone growth, collagen production, neurotransmitter regulation, and more. But when estrogen becomes excessive, unopposed by progesterone, or poorly cleared by the liver and gut, it starts to act more like a metabolic saboteur than a supportive partner.

Essentially, estrogen doesn't just make you curvier, it can interfere with how your cells generate energy. Estrogen can lower thyroid output, impair T4-to-T3 conversion, weaken the gut lining, and raise cortisol, nitric oxide, aldosterone, and prolactin, all of which drain your energetic reserves.

Unfortunately, estrogen's negative effects don't stop at hormones. Estrogen directly interferes with mitochondrial function; the very process your cells use to convert fuel into usable energy. It inhibits key enzymes in the energy cycle, increases oxidative stress, and chokes off clean glucose oxidation. Even when nutrients and oxygen are present, the cell struggles to burn fuel efficiently.

In other words, excess estrogen doesn't just throw off your hormonal balance, it body slams your metabolic machinery.

Let's break down how.

Estrogen and Thyroid—When "SHE" Hinders Thyroid Function

Estrogen doesn't just affect your mood or menstrual cycle, she can hijack your thyroid, one of the main engines driving your metabolism. Whether it's coming from your ovaries, fat tissue, birth control, or hormone replacement therapy (HRT), excess or unopposed estrogen can interfere with how your thyroid produces, activates, and delivers energy to your cells.

One of the key ways that estrogen does this is by increasing levels of thyroxine (thyroid)-binding globulin (TBG), a protein made by the liver that latches onto thyroid hormones in your bloodstream. The more TBG you have, the more thyroid hormone gets "bound," meaning it's inactive and can't be used by your cells. So even if your labs show normal total T3 and T4, your free (active) hormone levels might be low, and you can be left with classic hypothyroid symptoms like fatigue, brain fog, cold hands, and stubborn weight gain (20, 21).

Estrogen also interferes with your brain's ability to regulate thyroid output. It can suppress both TRH (thyrotropin-releasing hormone) and TSH (thyroid-stimulating hormone), the signals your brain uses to tell your thyroid to make more hormone (refer to the thyroid chapter for a refresher). Lower stimulation = lower output = lower energy (22).

Then there's the issue of conversion. Estrogen can block the enzymes (especially type 1 deiodinase) that convert inactive T4 into active T3, mostly in the liver and kidneys. So even if you're making enough T4, your cells might not be getting the message they need to keep metabolism humming (23).

And finally, excess levels can alter immune function and increase your risk of autoimmune thyroid disease, like Hashimoto's. In people with a genetic predisposition, this immune activation can tip the scales toward self-attack, and your thyroid becomes collateral damage (24).

All of this might help explain why women, who experience 10 to 20 times more estrogen exposure than men, a number that can go up to 1000 times more during pregnancy, are up to 8 times more likely to be diagnosed with hypothyroidism (25, 26). Between monthly hormonal fluctuations, birth control, pregnancy, HRT, and menopause, estrogen exposure is practically nonstop. And that means more opportunity for thyroid interference.

Bottom line: Excess estrogen can put your thyroid in a metabolic chokehold, restricting production, blocking activation, and disrupting endocrine communication. If you're dragging through the day, freezing under three blankets, gaining weight despite your efforts, or feeling moody and off, and you're on estrogen therapy or suspect estrogen excess, your thyroid might be caught in the crossfire.

Estrogen, Endotoxins, and Serotonin– When "She" Wrecks the Gut

Earlier you met endotoxin, those charming bacterial fragments (LPS) that sneak past the intestinal lining and light up the immune system like a Christmas tree. They're potent metabolic disrupters, and the gut barrier is supposed to keep them in check. But under certain conditions, particularly when estrogen is high or unbalanced relative to progesterone, the gut may become more vulnerable.

While estrogen does many beneficial things, shapes curves, supports fertility, influences brain chemistry, and can even be protective in certain tissues, its relationship with the gut is complex. In experimental and mechanistic studies, estrogen signaling has been shown *in some contexts* to alter intestinal tight-junction proteins such as ZO-1, potentially weakening the barrier and increasing permeability (27). This isn't universal, there are models where estrogen appears protective, but it suggests that, especially in inflamed or stressed systems, estrogen may tip the gut toward "leakier" rather than "tighter."

Estrogen also interacts with mast cells, which carry estrogen receptors and can become more active under estrogenic influence. Activated mast cells release histamine, and histamine increases inflammation and intestinal permeability (28). Clinically, many women notice more bloating, reactivity, and food sensitivity in high-estrogen states (PMS, certain contraceptives, perimenopause swings), and mast-cell activation is one very plausible mechanism.

Then there's serotonin. About 90% of the body's serotonin is produced in the gut, and estrogen can influence serotonergic signaling in the intestinal lining. Excess serotonin has been shown to downregulate tight-junction proteins like occludin and impair gut integrity (29). The takeaway isn't "serotonin is bad," but that excessive serotonergic signaling in the gut can contribute to permeability, an idea Dr. Ray Peat emphasized long before mainstream researchers caught up.

And the human evidence? It's emerging. A 2020 JCI Insight study following women in the SWAN cohort found that markers of gut permeability and microbial translocation (including FABP2, LPS-binding protein, and soluble CD14) increased during the menopause transition as hormones began fluctuating (30). These increases were associated with higher inflammation and lower bone mineral density.

That doesn't prove estrogen "causes" permeability, menopause comes with aging, stress, metabolic shifts, thyroid changes, and falling progesterone, but it strongly suggests that hormonal instability is linked to a weakening gut barrier.

So instead of the simplistic narrative that "low estrogen causes all bad things," a more nuanced perspective is that hormone imbalance, estrogen fluctuations, lack of progesterone support, thyroid suppression, stress physiology, and metabolic dysfunction may drive gut permeability, inflammation, endotoxin exposure, and ultimately bone loss and systemic decline. Estrogen is not inherently the villain, but in the wrong environment, or without progesterone's stabilizing influence, she can definitely add fuel to the fire.

Estrogen may still be the hormone that gives curves, confidence, and vitality, but when the system is stressed and regulation breaks down, she can contribute to gut chaos, open the door for bacterial toxins, and leave your immune and energy systems scrambling to cope. More human studies are needed to untangle this fully, but the mechanistic and emerging clinical evidence point in a direction worth paying attention to.

Estrogen and Cortisol—Stress Hormones Gone Wild

Estrogen doesn't just influence thyroid and gut health, it also exerts powerful effects on the hypothalamic-pituitary-adrenal (HPA) axis, which, if you remember from Chapter 6, is your body's primary stress response system. One of the ways that estrogen does this is by stimulating the release of corticotropin-releasing hormone (CRH) from the hypothalamus. This kicks off a hormonal domino effect: CRH signals the pituitary to release ACTH (adrenocorticotropic hormone), which then instructs the adrenal glands to churn out cortisol (31).

As you've already learned, cortisol is one of your main stress hormones. In small, well-timed bursts, it's lifesaving, it helps you respond to danger, reduce inflammation, and mobilize energy. But when cortisol stays elevated chronically (thanks to persistent stress or high estrogen levels), it becomes deeply catabolic and anti-metabolic.

Estrogen, especially in its most active form, estradiol, can influence how the body reacts to stress by acting on the brain's main stress pathway, the HPA axis. It does this by increasing the release of stress-signaling hormones like CRH and ACTH, which tell the adrenal glands to produce more cortisol. Estrogen may also make it harder for the brain to shut down the stress response, leading to longer-lasting effects. This is especially true with oral estrogen therapies, which have been shown to raise both free and total cortisol levels (32).

In a 2008 study, researchers studied the effects of estrogen and estrogen plus progestin therapy on cortisol levels. Women were randomized to one of three treatment arms: estrogen (as E2), estrogen plus a progestin, and a placebo. They found that those given estrogen-only had elevated cortisol levels, the levels were slightly mitigated by adding a progestin (a synthetic progesterone) (33).

It should be noted, transdermal estrogen (the patch) does not show any increases in total or free cortisol or CBG. More research needs to be done to show its impact on CRH and ACTH (34). I'll dive more into hormone replacement therapy a bit later in this chapter.

What can we learn from these studies? That estrogen doesn't just quietly alter cortisol by increasing cortisol-binding globulin, it can actively ramp up your entire stress response system. As you learned already, elevated cortisol impairs thyroid function by lowering TSH, impairing T4-to-T3 conversion, and increasing reverse T3, all of which slow down your metabolic rate.

In addition, blood sugar regulation can also take a hit. As I discussed earlier, cortisol will raise glucose levels, while simultaneously increasing lipolysis, which can inhibit glucose utilization and optimal energy production. At the same time, cortisol breaks down muscle tissue to convert amino acids into glucose, weakening the body's structure and draining a key driver of a healthy metabolism.

In short, estrogen can elevate cortisol, but the true effects may depend on the dose and the delivery system (exogenous over endogenous over oral vs patch). More research needs to be done to further explore the effects of exogenous estrogens on cortisol levels. Unfortunately, research on women's health issues, particularly those involving hormonal issues, has historically been underfunded and deprioritized due to systemic bias in medical research, where male physiology was often considered the default. This gap has left many female-specific concerns insufficiently studied.

Estrogen and Prolactin: Possible Bone Implications

You may remember prolactin from the chapter on stress (no judgment if you don't, I'll give you a quick review), where I introduced it as part of the Hypothalamic-Pituitary-Prolactin (HPP) axis. Back then, we talked about how prolactin, while best known for stimulating milk production, also ramps up in response to stress, contributing to immune regulation, tissue repair, and even bone metabolism.

Remember, prolactin has a beneficial purpose, until it remains high for too long. When prolactin stays chronically elevated, whether from stress or excess estrogen, it starts shifting from helpful to harmful. As we saw earlier, stress and prolactin can suppress the HPG axis (lowering estrogen), while increasing aromatase (which boosts peripheral estrogen). Yes—prolactin can decrease ovarian estrogen, while increasing peripheral estrogen, and this estrogen can increase prolactin. Welcome to the hormonal feedback loop from hell.

Estrogen stimulates prolactin directly by acting on lactotroph cells in the pituitary, and indirectly by lowering dopamine (which normally keeps prolactin in check). In pregnancy, this works beautifully; prolactin helps draw calcium from bones to make milk for the baby. But outside of pregnancy, when both estrogen and prolactin remain elevated for too long, that same mechanism can turn destructive. This can not only lead to energy issues, but also to bone break down (35).

Interestingly, a similar pattern can emerge in non-lactating, chronically stressed women. Just like in lactation, chronically high prolactin can suppress ovarian function, lowering estrogen and progesterone at the source, while simultaneously increasing peripheral estrogen through upregulated aromatase. It's a redistribution, not a deficiency. Ovaries slow down, but peripheral tissues (like fat) keep pumping out estrogen. What is the result? You might feel you have excess estrogen (sore boobs, clotting, heavy bleeding, edema, etc.) even with "normal" or even low blood levels.

So yes, prolactin serves a purpose, but it's a double-edged sword. It can be adaptive in acute situations (stress, lactation), but when chronically elevated, especially in the presence of high estrogen or low dopamine, it becomes a signal that your body is prioritizing survival over optimal function.

Ray Peat often said prolactin was a reliable proxy for excess estrogen. Even when estrogen levels appear "normal" on a lab test, high prolactin may indicate that estrogenic activity is still high at the tissue level. This makes prolactin a valuable, yet underused marker in understanding estrogen's broader effects on the system.

Estrogen and Bone Health—Mainstream Theory vs. Bioenergetic Theory

Estrogen is widely prescribed to postmenopausal women to prevent bone loss and reduce fracture risk. Since estrogen levels drop after menopause and bone loss tends to accelerate, hormone replacement is often framed as the go-to solution.

Studies like the Women's Health Initiative (WHI) and other large-scale trials have shown that estrogen therapy can reduce the risk of hip and vertebral fractures, particularly during the first 5 to 7 years of use (37, 38, 39).

Research has also shown that estrogen slows bone resorption by reducing osteoclast formation and activity, these are the cells responsible for breaking down bone (40, 41). That's why many doctors recommend MHT (menopausal hormone therapy) for osteopenia and osteoporosis.

But here's what the mainstream doesn't talk about...

While estrogen clearly reduces bone breakdown, it doesn't stimulate new bone growth. In fact, high or unopposed estrogen can inhibit osteoblast differentiation, the very cells responsible for building bone. A 2012 review in *Trends in Endocrinology and Metabolism* described estrogen's action as "not solely inhibitory or stimulatory but [involving] a balance of actions on different bone cells" (42). In other words, estrogen slows both resorption and formation, putting bone turnover on pause. That might make bones appear denser on a scan, but it doesn't mean they're functionally stronger.

And then there's the hormonal stress triangle we've talked about before: estrogen, prolactin, and cortisol. When these stay chronically elevated, calcium is pulled from the bones to meet other physiological demands, especially under long-term stress. Unlike the temporary bone loss that happens during lactation (which typically rebounds after weaning), this stress-induced depletion has no built-in recovery phase. It slowly chips away at bone integrity.

Estrogen may also misdirect calcium. Instead of sending it neatly into the bones, it can promote calcification of soft tissues like arteries and joints, especially when unbalanced or poorly metabolized. That means you could end up with stiff joints and hardened arteries, not exactly the protective picture we're often promised.

But Kate...how do you explain all the studies showing improved bone outcomes in women on HRT?

Great question. Some of the benefits attributed to estrogen might come from the type of woman who uses hormone therapy. Studies show that women on HRT often have healthier diets, higher education levels, more consistent medical care, and more active lifestyles (43, 44), this is referred to as healthy user bias.

Even though randomized trials (RCTs) eliminate health user bias, they cannot eliminate all indirect effects that arise because of the treatment. Hormone replacement therapies can often improve quality of life, reduce hot flashes and improve sleep. Better sleep enhances everything from insulin sensitivity to inflammation regulation and yes, even bone remodeling (45, 46). So, even in quality RCTs, it's entirely plausible that some of the bone benefit is indirectly rooted in better sleep and lifestyle, not solely from estrogen's direct action on the bone.

FUN FACT: Men have significantly stronger bones than women yet carry far less estrogen throughout their lives. That alone should make us pause before crowning estrogen as the holy grail of bone health. (Hint: testosterone helps build strong bones too.)

All of this suggests that estrogen's relationship with bone health is not one-size-fits-all. It can be beneficial in small, well-regulated doses, but it's not a magic solution. Protecting your bones takes more than just boosting estrogen.

The Bioenergetic View: What Really Builds Strong Bones?

Bone health isn't just about preventing loss—it's about supporting *regeneration*. A healthy metabolism drives that regeneration. That means:

- Activate osteoblasts (stimulated by thyroid hormone, progesterone, and vitamin D and K2) (47, 48, 49, 50).

- Plenty of dietary calcium and magnesium (51, 52).

- Strength training and movement (mechanical stress) (53, 54).

- Adequate fuel, this includes consuming enough glucose and protein to support adaptive remodeling (55, 56).

The bottom line: Don't just suppress bone loss. Support the system that builds new bones.

Estrogen—Nitric Oxide, Histamine, and Aldosterone

By now, you've seen how estrogen interferes with nearly every system that regulates energy, slowing thyroid function, increasing cortisol, increasing endotoxin absorption, upregulating serotonin, and elevating prolactin. But this fiery lady is not stopping here. Estrogen also teams up with a trio of biochemical disruptors, nitric oxide, histamine, and aldosterone, each of which adds more friction to your metabolism and pulls even more energy away from vital functions.

Take nitric oxide (NO), for instance. As a vasodilator, NO can be lifesaving in acute situations, helping to open blood vessels and improve circulation during times of stress. Like cortisol, it's designed to rise in response to threat and help the body adapt. But when nitric oxide is chronically elevated, as it often is under the influence of excess estrogen, it can backfire. When NO reacts with superoxide (a common byproduct of mitochondrial respiration), it forms peroxynitrite, a highly reactive molecule that damages mitochondrial membranes, enzymes, and even DNA. The result? Slower electron transport, reduced ATP production, and increased oxidative stress, especially in tissues already struggling to meet their energy demands (57, 58, 59).

In addition, estrogen increases mast cell sensitivity and upregulates histidine decarboxylase, the enzyme that converts histidine into histamine, leading to increased histamine production. As discussed in Chapter 7, histamine plays important roles in digestion, brain signaling, and immune defense. But like most biological messengers, too much of it creates problems. Elevated histamine contributes to inflammation, increased vascular permeability, and heightened stress signaling, including the ramping up of nitric oxide, which further disrupts cellular respiration. This may help explain why women with excess estrogen often experience headaches, bloating, anxiety, insomnia, and histamine intolerance, especially around ovulation or during perimenopause (60, 61, 62).

And finally, there's aldosterone, the hormone that tells your body to hold on to salt and water. Estrogen increases aldosterone both directly and indirectly by activating the renin-angiotensin system (if you've read *How to Heal Your Metabolism*, you'll recognize this pathway). When aldosterone goes up, your body holds onto more sodium, which pulls in water, leading to fluid retention and tissue swelling, also known as edema (63).

At first glance, this might sound like a good thing. A little extra fluid in the skin can give you that soft, plump, youthful look. But underneath the surface, it can cause problems. That fluid doesn't just sit there looking pretty, it creates congestion in the tissue, making it harder for oxygen and nutrients to reach your cells. It's like trying to deliver supplies through a crowded hallway, things move slower, and the cells on the other end may not get what they need. Studies have shown that even mild tissue swelling can make it harder for cells to breathe and produce energy, especially in tissues already under stress (64, 65).

So, while that estrogen-induced "glow" might look nice for a moment, it can come at the cost of efficient metabolism and long-term cellular health.

Estrogen and Glucose Oxidation: How it Directly Blocks Energy Production

Estrogen can interfere with your ability to make energy from glucose, and one of the key places it causes trouble is at an enzyme called pyruvate dehydrogenase (PDH). PDH acts like a gatekeeper that helps move glucose into the mitochondria so it can be burned efficiently for energy. When PDH is working well, glucose is converted into acetyl-CoA and smoothly enters the energy cycle, producing plenty of ATP.

But when estrogen levels are high, especially during times of stress, inflammation, or gut dysfunction, this gatekeeper becomes less cooperative. Estrogen indirectly raises cortisol, inflammatory cytokines, and a protein called PDH kinase (PDK), which flips the "off switch" on PDH. As a result, glucose can't enter the mitochondria, so your cells switch to backup generators: anaerobic glycolysis. As discussed earlier, this pathway is inefficient and produces lactic acid instead of an abundance of ATP (energy). The result? Less ATP, and more sluggishness, brain fog, and fatigue (66).

In addition, estrogen, particularly at high or unbalanced levels, has also been shown to impair cytochrome c oxidase (Complex IV), the final step in the electron transport chain. This enzyme transfers electrons to oxygen and drives most of your ATP production. When Complex IV is inhibited, mitochondrial respiration slows, ATP drops, and reactive oxygen species (ROS) start to build up (67).

And finally, estrogen disrupts the very nutrients your cells need to generate energy. Magnesium, for example, is essential for ATP synthesis, and estrogen increases its excretion through the kidneys. Thiamine (vitamin B1), a critical cofactor for PDH and the TCA cycle, becomes harder to retain under estrogen excess, especially during stress. Zinc and selenium, both vital for thyroid function and antioxidant defense, can be displaced or underutilized, while CoQ10, the molecule that shuttles electrons through the respiratory chain, may also be reduced. Without these micronutrients, even a well-fueled cell can't operate efficiently. Estrogen creates a scenario where fuel is available, but the engine is missing its spark plugs and workers, leading to poor energy production, low ATP, and a feeling of tired-and-wired (68, 69, 70, 71, 72).

It should be noted, that while estrogen therapy is often praised for its ability to lower blood glucose, it's crucial to understand that not all reductions in blood sugar are metabolically beneficial. Estrogen doesn't lower glucose by improving mitochondrial oxidation or increasing insulin sensitivity at the cellular level, instead, it tends to suppress appetite, slow gastric emptying, and increase peripheral glucose uptake into tissues like fat and muscle without fully oxidizing it for energy.

In fact, as covered earlier, estrogen inhibits pyruvate dehydrogenase (PDH), the very enzyme that allows glucose to enter the mitochondria and be burned efficiently. So even though blood sugar may drop, the body is often just shuttling glucose out of the bloodstream and into storage or alternative pathways, like lactate production, not using it to generate ATP. It's like sweeping a dirty floor and hiding the dust under the rug. The numbers may look better on a lab report, but underneath, the energy system remains compromised (73, 74, 75, 76).

In short, estrogen isn't just tweaking hormone levels, it's directly interfering with the body's ability to produce energy at the cellular level. Even when glucose is present and insulin is doing its job, estrogen can hinder the final steps of energy production, leaving the body stuck in a low-energy, stress-driven state.

When estrogen interferes with energy production at every level, from blocking thyroid signals, to increasing stress hormones, jamming up mitochondrial enzymes to draining key nutrients and fueling inflammation, it doesn't just make you tired. It rewires your entire physiology to prioritize survival over vitality. Over time, this low-energy state creates ripple effects across your entire system. The gut gets leakier, the brain gets foggier, metabolism slows down, and the stress response stays on high alert. And while all of this might be happening slowly under the radar, your body starts sending signals—

they are quiet at first but tend to get louder over time. So how do you know when estrogen has gone from helpful to harmful? In the next section, we'll look at the real-life signs and symptoms of estrogen excess, what they mean, and eventually, what you can do about them.

Signs and Symptoms of Excess Estrogens

Excess estrogen doesn't just show up as heavy periods or PMS, it affects nearly every system in your body. Because estrogen interacts with the reproductive system, nervous system, thyroid, digestive system, immune system, cardiovascular system, and skeletal system, its symptoms of excess can be widespread and confusing. When unopposed by progesterone, excessively produced due to stress, or poorly cleared due to gut dysfunction, estrogen can behave less like a feminizing beauty hormone and more like a "girls gone wild" party girl hormone, overstimulating tissues, disrupting energy flow, and leaving inflammation in its wake.

Reproduction and Menstrual Disruption

The most obvious symptoms of estrogen excess often show up in the menstrual cycle, but even these can be misdiagnosed or misunderstood. This excess can lead women to feel awful, unsupported, and stressed due to not understanding what is happening to them.

Excess estrogen can look like:

- Heavy bleeding with clots
- Short cycles or spotting before periods
- Severe PMS (mood swings, anxiety, cravings, fatigue)
- Breast tenderness, swelling, and fibrocystic changes
- Cramps, pelvic pain, painful ovulation
- Endometriosis, fibroids, adenomyosis
- PCOS and Anovulation
- Miscarriage risk and infertility

- Uterine, ovarian, and breast cancer

Estrogen stimulates endometrial tissue growth, while low progesterone (due to anovulation or luteal phase defect) fails to keep it in check, which can lead to overstimulation of the uterine lining and a multitude of different symptoms.

Client Story: Mary

Mary was a 29-year-old professional, recently married, who came to me with a list of frustrating symptoms: debilitating menstrual cramps, heavy bleeding with clots, bloating, and an ongoing struggle with infertility. At the time, she was working 50 hours a week, studying for her CPA exam, and training for a half marathon, all while restricting calories to get her "summer body" back.

I explained to Mary that menstruation and fertility are highly energetic biological processes. When the body is under stress and undernourished, it shifts into survival mode, making a symptom-free cycle (let alone a pregnancy) nearly impossible.

Our first step was simple, but powerful: more nourishment. We increased her intake of nutrient-dense proteins like steak, eggs, seafood, and dairy, along with easy-to-digest carbohydrates like fruit, honey, potatoes, and rice. We added in more healthy fats to support hormone production and brought in the famous Ray Peat carrot salad to help support estrogen detox and reduce endotoxin load. With more fuel and nutrients, the body can downregulate stress hormones and prioritize sex hormone production again.

I also encouraged Mary to delay the CPA exam and postpone marathon training for a year. Our goal was to create a body that felt safe, well-fed, and supported, not one constantly running on empty. Less stress meant more available energy for procreation.

Mary was deeply motivated to start her family, and she committed to the process fully. Within 60 days, her period shortened from 7 days of heavy bleeding to 5 days of moderate flow. Cramps eased, bloating subsided, and her sleep improved, an added bonus. After three more months of consistency, Mary became pregnant. Forty weeks later, she gave birth to a healthy baby boy.

Sometimes the fix for hormonal chaos isn't more medications or synthetic hormones, its food, rest, and an environment that tells the body, "You're safe to thrive."

Brain, Mood & Cognitive Function— Does Estrogen Protect the Brain?

Women are statistically twice as likely to develop Alzheimer's disease and dementia than men. While this is often blamed on their longer lifespan, emerging research suggests that hormonal differences, especially estrogen's influence on brain energy and stress regulation, may play a major role.

Excess estrogen ramps up brain signaling chemicals like serotonin, histamine, nitric oxide (NO), and even corticotropin-releasing hormone (CRH), the hormone that kicks off your stress response. In small doses, these compounds help with mood, focus, and alertness. But when estrogen is high and energy production is low (as it often is during stress, poor sleep, or under-eating), these chemicals don't get processed efficiently, and instead of helping, they start hurting.

That's because your brain needs energy (ATP) to properly recycle and regulate these compounds. When your cells' mitochondria aren't keeping up, these messengers build up, triggering a storm of neuroinflammation, oxidative stress, and what I call "wired but tired" brain chemistry.

Here's what that can look like:
- Migraines, especially around ovulation or before your period

- Racing thoughts, panic, or anxiety that feels out of proportion

- Depression or low motivation

- Brain fog, forgetfulness, poor word recall

- Early waking insomnia, where your brain is buzzing at 3 a.m.

- Mood swings or irritability that feel unpredictable

- Increased dementia risk, especially when estrogen therapy is started late in life or poorly metabolized

When estrogen increases CRH production, which kicks off the HPA-axis and makes more cortisol, you initially feel better. As you have learned earlier in Chapter 6, cortisol isn't always bad, it can heighten focus and alertness, especially in the short term. Estrogen itself also has a mildly excitatory effect on the brain, which is one reason many women feel sharper or more mentally "on" when they start estrogen therapy.

But that initial mental clarity can come at a cost. Both cortisol and estrogen boost glutamate, the brain's main excitatory neurotransmitter, which stimulates neurons to fire. That's great when energy production is strong, but when mitochondrial function is low, that stimulation becomes neurotoxic. Over time, this overactivity depletes calming neurotransmitters like GABA and creates a brain that's wired, overstimulated, and eventually exhausted. It's like running your nervous system into overdrive and then slamming it into a wall.

Although estrogen has been studied for potential neuroprotective effects, timing and context matter. Research from the Women's Health Initiative Memory Study (WHIMS) found that starting estrogen therapy after age 65 was associated with an increased risk of dementia and cognitive decline (77).

A large 2019 observational study from Finland compared MHT users with non-users and found an increased risk of Alzheimer's disease (78). The researchers also observed that risk increased the longer duration of hormone use. Several more recent large observational studies reported similar findings (79, 80, 81).

Additional animal studies suggest that excessive or unopposed estrogen, especially when thyroid hormone or progesterone are low, may worsen mitochondrial function and increase neuroinflammation (82).

In other words, estrogen isn't automatically protective, it can impair cognition when delivered in the wrong environment (i.e., a stressed, under-fueled brain), particularly if progesterone and thyroid hormones (both brain protective) are lacking. Currently, no major medical organization approves of estrogen therapy for cognitive function or protection.

The Gut, Gallbladder, and Estrogen's Effects on Digestion

Estrogen excess doesn't just influence menstruation and cognition; it can affect digestion too. When estrogen becomes excessive, poorly cleared, or unbalanced relative to progesterone, it may disrupt several aspects of gastrointestinal function, contributing to bloating, food sensitivities, sluggish digestion, and even gallbladder issues.

To recap from earlier, mechanistic and animal research suggests that estrogen signaling can reduce tight-junction proteins such as ZO-1 in certain inflammatory or stressed environments. When these junctions weaken, the gut becomes more permeable ("leaky"), allowing bacterial fragments such as lipopolysaccharides (LPS) to slip into circulation. These endotoxins fuel inflammation, stress energy production, and place additional strain on digestion.

Meanwhile, estrogen also interacts with mast cells, which carry estrogen receptors and can become more reactive under estrogenic influence. That increases histamine signaling in the gut. While histamine is normal and necessary in digestion, too much, especially in a compromised gut, can trigger bloating, nausea, itching, flushing, and that anxious, wired feeling after meals. It helps explain why many women notice digestive flare-ups during hormonally turbulent times.

Then there's bile. Estrogen slows gallbladder contractions and increases cholesterol saturation of bile. Together, this can thicken bile, impair bile flow, and set the stage for sluggish digestion and gallstones. That matters, because bile isn't just for fat digestion, it also helps eliminate estrogen and keeps bacterial overgrowth in check in the small intestine. When bile stagnates, digestion slows, bacteria thrive, and estrogen clearance suffers — a vicious cycle.

It's no surprise that women are roughly twice as likely as men to develop gallbladder disease and have their gallbladder removed, with risk rising in pregnancy, perimenopause, oral contraceptive use, and some forms of HRT (83). These are times when hormones fluctuate dramatically or estrogen exposure is relatively high.

Common symptoms in this estrogen-digestion loop include:

- Bloating (especially mid-cycle or after meals)
- Food sensitivities or histamine intolerance
- Nausea or heaviness after fatty meals
- Constipation or sluggish digestion
- Right-sided abdominal or shoulder tension
- Skin flushing or rashes after food
- Anxiety, fog, or fatigue after eating
- History of gallstones or gallbladder removal

Whether it's increased gut permeability or poor bile flow, estrogen excess or imbalance can leave the digestive system inflamed, overworked, and underperforming. Supporting gut integrity, improving bile flow, lowering stress physiology, and helping estrogen clear efficiently can improve far more than digestion.

Let's take a quick pause.

Despite everything I've said about the downsides of excess estrogen, estrogen itself is not the villain. I don't want you thinking, "How do I get rid of every trace of estrogen?" because that's not the goal.

Estrogen is essential; the key is understanding how and when it helps — and when it can create problems.

Estrogen is making a comeback in many pro-HRT circles. Some newer evidence is promising, but much of it comes from observational research, which can show associations — not cause and effect. At the same time, many of the mechanisms and potential risks we've been exploring in this book rarely get discussed. Context matters. Hormones don't work in isolation. And the gut, stress physiology, thyroid health, progesterone balance, bile flow, and metabolism all determine how estrogen behaves in your body.

Okay — now let's keep going.

Cardiovascular, Vascular & Clotting Risk—Heart Protection or NOT?

Estrogen's influence on the vascular system is often painted as protective, but that's not always the case, especially when levels are too high or unopposed by progesterone. One of the more overlooked issues is that estrogen increases clotting factors, tipping the balance toward a hypercoagulable state. It stimulates the liver to produce more coagulation proteins like Factors VII, X, and fibrinogen, while simultaneously reducing anticoagulant proteins like protein S and antithrombin III. In other words, estrogen shifts your blood chemistry toward clotting.

This is one reason why oral birth control pills and estrogen replacement therapies (specifically oral forms) are linked to a higher risk of deep vein thrombosis, pulmonary embolism, and even stroke (84, 85).

Did you know, young women aged 25 to 44 are more likely than young men to suffer strokes? In fact, women aged 35 and younger are 44% more likely to have an ischemic stroke than men of the same age. The American Heart Association points to estrogen-containing contraceptives, estrogen-induced migraines, and pregnancy-related hormonal shifts as contributing factors (86).

Then there's estrogen's effect on vascular tone. While it's often said that estrogen "relaxes" blood vessels, and it does, via stimulation of nitric oxide (NO), this isn't always a good thing in the long run. Chronic or excessive NO doesn't just open vessels. It increases vascular permeability, meaning the walls of your blood vessels become weaker and leakier.

In certain contexts, estrogen has also been shown to disrupt tight junctions in endothelial cells, the very cells that keep your blood vessels strong and intact. Mechanistic research found that estradiol increased permeability by reducing key structural proteins like claudin-5 and occludin, both of which help maintain barrier integrity (87).

Add in the fact that estrogen raises histamine, serotonin, and prostaglandins, all of which increase vascular leakiness, and you've got the perfect storm for puffiness, low-grade swelling, and poor circulation. Not surprisingly, many women experience cold hands and feet, palpitations, or fluid retention mid-cycle or premenstrual when estrogen levels are high.

And finally, let's talk about cholesterol. Yes, estrogen lowers LDL, which also drops your total cholesterol, and mainstream medicine treats that like a gold star. But here's what that means: estrogen increases the number of LDL receptors in the liver, pulling more cholesterol out of the bloodstream (88, 89). Sounds good, right? Maybe, but this doesn't solve the underlying issue.

Cholesterol tends to rise under stress. And if your thyroid function is low, which blocks the conversion of cholesterol into your steroidal hormones (like pregnenolone, progesterone, and cortisol), then cholesterol will remain elevated. So yes, your cholesterol numbers may drop, but that doesn't mean estrogen is fixing the problem. In many cases, it's just covering up a deeper metabolic slowdown.

**Common Symptoms of Estrogen Excess
in the Cardiovascular System:**

- Edema and fluid retention (especially before ovulation or menstruation)
- Cold extremities or poor circulation
- Spider veins or varicose veins
- Palpitations or heart flutters
- Increased stroke risk (particularly in women on oral HRT or birth control)

Bottom line: Estrogen has vascular effects that can seem beneficial in isolation, like relaxing blood vessels or lowering cholesterol, but context is everything. When estrogen is excessive, unopposed, or chronically elevated, those same "benefits" can backfire.

Estrogen and the Bone Paradox

While estrogen is often prescribed to "protect bones," the relationship isn't as straightforward as the medical establishment might make you think. Yes, estrogen can slow bone loss, but it doesn't necessarily build stronger, more resilient bones. In fact, unbalanced or prolonged exposure to estrogen, especially alongside high cortisol and low thyroid hormone can quietly erode bone integrity. This kind of stress-driven bone depletion doesn't show up overnight, but over time it increases the risk of fractures, even if bone density scans look reassuring (90, 91, 92, 93).

**Common Symptoms of Estrogen
Excess with Bones and Tissue**

- Loss of bone flexibility or microarchitecture
- Joint stiffness or tightness
- Early osteopenia or mineral loss in thin women
- Soft tissue calcification (e.g. arteries, joints)

For a deeper dive into this debate, refer to the sidebar on estrogen and bone health.

The FDA, Estrogen Therapy, and the Removal of the Black Box Warnings

At the end 2025, the US FDA announced updated recommendations to remove the long-standing "black box" warning from estrogen-containing hormone therapies for most women, excluding those with clear contraindications (such as breast cancer, history of estrogen-sensitive cancers, or prior blood clotting events).

The rationale for this change centers on the idea that earlier warnings may have overstated risks and discouraged women from using hormone therapy that could improve quality of life during perimenopause and menopause.

To support this decision, the FDA references several older observational studies suggesting benefits of MHT, particularly for cardiovascular health, cognitive decline, and bone density (94).

What is confusing about their recommendations is that the studies the FDA cites are older, observational research. This includes a 1996 observational study reporting a 35% lower incidence of Alzheimer's disease in women using estrogen therapy (95); a 1991 observational study suggesting a 50% reduction in coronary heart disease among estrogen users (96); and a 1980 observational study linking estrogen use to reduced fracture risks (97).

Now, I have nothing against older research, but when you have numerous, more comprehensive studies since then, it seems odd that you would leave them out. In addition, as stated before, observational studies on estrogen have a healthy-user bias: women who take estrogen therapies are typically healthier, wealthier, better educated, and more medically engaged than non-users. That alone makes risk reduction appear exaggerated in non-randomized research.

When researchers moved beyond observational data and examined these same health outcomes using large, modern databases and randomized controlled trials, the story became far more complicated.

On cognitive health, several large, well-designed studies published between 2019 and 2023, including research from Finland (98), Denmark (99), Taiwan (100), and the United Kingdom (101), found either no protective effect of menopausal hormone therapy, or in some cases, higher dementia risk in certain user groups. Additionally, the WHIMS randomized trial (part of the Women's Health Initiative) found no cognitive protection, and in older postmenopausal women, showed an increased risk of dementia.

On cardiovascular health, the earlier observational paper the FDA references suggested a dramatic 40–50% reductions in heart disease risk among estrogen users. But when true randomized trials were finally conducted, those benefits did not hold. The landmark HERS trial in women with established heart disease found no reduction in heart attacks or cardiac deaths with hormone therapy (102). The large WHI estrogen-plus-progestin trial actually showed higher coronary events, along with increased stroke and blood-clot risk (103).

Even estrogen-alone trials failed to demonstrate reliable heart protection (104). Yes, a few smaller studies in very recently postmenopausal women suggest potential benefit, but the absolute effect size is modest (a few fewer cardiovascular events per thousand women per year) and must still be weighed against clear increases in stroke and clotting risk (105). In other words: the dramatic cardiovascular protection once assumed from early observational research was not confirmed when tested in rigorous randomized trials.

When it comes to bone health, estrogen therapy does reliably reduce bone loss while it is being used. However, bone protection gradually diminishes once therapy stops (106, 107). More importantly, estrogen is not the only, nor necessarily the most fundamental tool for bone resilience. Adequate nutrition, strength training, sufficient protein intake, vitamins D and K2, appropriate mineral status, thyroid balance, sleep quality, and overall metabolic health all play critical roles in maintaining strong, resilient bone tissue.

Now, here's an important point of clarity.

It *does* make sense that the FDA would ease warnings for low-dose vaginal estrogen. This form is minimally absorbed systemically and primarily acts locally on vaginal and urethral tissues. For women dealing with severe vaginal atrophy, dryness, painful intercourse, or urinary symptoms, vaginal estrogen can be extremely effective, with far fewer systemic risks compared to oral or transdermal systemic estrogen. So, acknowledging its safety profile and therapeutic benefit in this specific context is reasonable and a decision many clinicians agree with.

What feels especially disappointing, however, is that the FDA's broader messaging appears to be built on half the story. By elevating older observational evidence while giving far less weight to newer randomized trials and larger more comprehensive datasets, the public message becomes incomplete at best and misleading at worst.

And this doesn't just matter academically; it shapes women's fears and decisions. We're already seeing a growing wave of messaging suggesting that if a woman cannot take, or chooses not to take, hormone therapy, she is somehow doomed to dementia, heart disease, frailty, and brittle bones. That simply isn't true. None of those outcomes have been conclusively proven to be prevented by hormone therapy, and framing estrogen as a magical shield against aging is neither scientifically honest nor emotionally fair.

So, what does this mean for women?

Hormone therapy can be an appropriate and helpful tool for some women, especially for managing severe hot flashes, sleep disruption, and supporting bone density in the right context. But it is not a universal solution, and it should not be framed as a cure-all, particularly for protection against cardiovascular disease or dementia based solely on older observational studies.

From my clinical perspective, this is important to say out loud. In over 15 years of working with perimenopausal and menopausal women, I've seen most symptoms improve with a bioenergetic nutrition approach, thyroid optimization, progesterone support when appropriate, and targeted lifestyle strategies, often without the need for systemic estrogen therapy.

Women deserve the entire picture so they can make truly informed decisions.

There is a huge difference between symptom relief and disease prevention—and between observational findings and randomized controlled evidence. Sadly, we don't have nearly enough long-term RCTs in women's health. So, we make the best decisions we can with existing data and right now, we do not have strong enough evidence to recommend hormone therapy as a blanket strategy for heart or brain protection.

Estrogen and Autoimmunity

Autoimmune diseases disproportionately affect women, with approximately 80% of all autoimmune cases occurring in females

(108). Conditions such as Hashimoto's thyroiditis, systemic lupus erythematosus (SLE), and rheumatoid arthritis (RA) are significantly more prevalent in women than in men. For example, lupus affects women at a rate of 9:1 to 11:1, and Hashimoto's thyroiditis occurs in women 4 to 9 times more often than in men (109, 110, 111).

Knowing this, it's fair to ask: could estrogen play a role?

Estrogen plays a complicated role in the immune system. In small, balanced amounts, it can be protective. But when estrogen levels are too high, or out of sync with progesterone or thyroid hormone, it may cause the immune system to become confused and overly reactive.

Here's what that can look like:

- It over-stimulates immune cells, which can lead to the body mistakenly attacking its own tissues (112).

- It throws off the balance of inflammation, sometimes keeping the body in a low-grade "flare" state (113).

- It disrupts immune tolerance, making the body more likely to overreact to everyday things, including foods, stress, or even your own cells (114).

This kind of hormonal miscommunication can set the stage for autoimmune diseases to develop, or existing conditions to worsen.

Can Hormone Therapy Impact Autoimmune Issues?

Hormone replacement therapy (HRT) is widely promoted for easing menopausal symptoms, but its relationship to autoimmune risk is far less discussed. Emerging research suggests that, in some women, adding estrogen into an already sensitive immune environment may increase the likelihood of autoimmune or inflammatory conditions.

What we have right now are large observational studies. These don't prove cause-and-effect the way randomized controlled trials do, but they still matter, especially because observational HRT research often suffers from healthy-user bias (a reminder that people who use HRT are typically healthier, more health-conscious, and have better access to medical care). So when outcomes look worse, not better, that deserves attention.

Here's what the current evidence shows:

- A large Swedish study found that women on menopausal hormone therapy had a 30% increased risk of developing lupus, and those using both systemic and local estrogen had nearly double the risk (115).

- The same study showed a 40–80% increased risk for systemic sclerosis among MHT users (115).

- A UK Biobank study tracking over 220,000 women reported that HRT use was associated with a 46% higher risk of developing rheumatoid arthritis (116).

- For women who already have autoimmune diseases like lupus, HRT has been linked to increased rates of mild to moderate flares, though not necessarily major flares (117).

- A Korean nationwide cohort study found that women using estrogen-only or estrogen—progestogen therapy had a 12–24% increased risk of developing osteoarthritis compared to non-users, especially in joints other than the hip (118).

- A 2022 meta-analysis of over 2.5 million women showed that HRT users had a 24% increased risk of knee osteoarthritis and a 30% higher likelihood of undergoing knee joint replacement (119).

- The Million Women Study also found that HRT users had a 38% higher risk of knee replacement and a 58% higher risk of hip replacement (120, 121).

We do not currently have large randomized controlled trials specifically testing whether hormone therapy causes autoimmune or inflammatory diseases. But when large, carefully conducted observational studies repeatedly show higher risk signals, and in groups that typically should have *better* outcomes, we shouldn't ignore that pattern.

To be clear, this does not mean women on MHT should automatically stop treatment. For some women, the benefits will outweigh the risks. What it does mean is that we need a far more nuanced conversation about estrogen, especially when it is being added to bodies that may already have metabolic stress, thyroid suppression, chronic inflammation, or immune hyper-reactivity.

This is a side of the estrogen story rarely acknowledged in pro-HRT circles, but it matters. Millions of women struggle with fatigue, joint pain, thyroid symptoms, mystery inflammation, or autoimmune tendencies. Hormone therapy may help some of those women, but in others, it may amplify the very problems it's meant to relieve if the underlying energy and immune system aren't supported first.

Common Signs and Symptoms of Estrogen-Driven Immune Dysregulation

- Flaring joint pain or stiffness (especially in small joints)
- Skin rashes or new sensitivities (especially to sunlight or skincare products)
- Swelling in fingers, wrists, knees, or ankles without injury
- Worsening of autoimmune conditions during mid-luteal phase or estrogen surges
- Migrating pain, fibromyalgia-type symptoms, or general achiness
- Hashimoto's flare-ups or rising thyroid antibodies despite medication

Understanding how estrogen interacts with immunity isn't about demonizing the hormone, it's about recognizing the tipping point. Remember, the goal isn't to eliminate estrogen, but to create an internal environment where it can manage the positive effects of estrogen without pushing it over.

Thyroid, Energy, and Metabolic Slowdown

As you've probably noticed by now, estrogen doesn't just dabble in one system, it meddles everywhere. And when it comes to your metabolism, it can pull the brakes hard.

Earlier we talked about how estrogen affects thyroid hormone production and conversion. It increases thyroxine-binding globulin (TBG), which ties up free T3 and makes it unavailable. It also suppresses TSH output from the pituitary and blocks the enzymes (deiodinases) that convert T4 into active T3, your body's real metabolic driver.

Interestingly, estrogen doesn't just influence metabolism on paper. You can feel its influence. Across a woman's life and menstrual cycle, when estrogen is higher and progesterone is lower (like in the follicular phase), core body temperature naturally runs lower. Estrogen shifts thermoregulation in a way that promotes heat loss and lowers the internal "set point," while progesterone does the opposite and raises temperature (during the luteal phase) (122). So, if you've ever noticed feeling cooler, more chilled, or less thermally "robust" during estrogen-dominant phases, that's estrogen showing you her physiological powers.

But estrogen doesn't stop at the thyroid. Inside the cell, it inhibits key enzymes like pyruvate dehydrogenase (which funnels fuel into your mitochondria) and cytochrome c oxidase (Complex IV of the electron transport chain). Translation? Less ATP, more oxidative stress, and a sluggish system that feels like it's running on fumes.

Classic Signs Include:
- Cold hands and feet
- Fatigue and sluggishness
- Poor recovery from exercise
- Weight gain despite "doing everything right"

So, if your body feels like it's stuck in low gear, it might not just be your thyroid, or your cells. It could be estrogen quietly throwing a wrench into both.

But Kate, doesn't taking estrogen *help* some women feel better?

Yes, it can, especially at first. Many women report feeling more energized, mentally clear, and emotionally stable after starting estrogen therapy. And for good reason; estrogen can reduce hot flashes, night sweats, and the sleep disruption that often comes with them. And when you start sleeping better, everything feels better, including mood, energy, life.

But here's an important distinction, feeling better doesn't always mean you're *functioning* better at a cellular or hormonal level. Estrogen can improve symptoms, but it doesn't necessarily restore the deeper systems behind energy production, like thyroid function, mitochondrial efficiency, or the cortisol response. In fact, excess or prolonged estrogen exposure can quietly suppress those very systems over time.

So, while estrogen may feel like a miracle fix in the short term, for some women it's more of a well-wrapped band-aid. The root causes of fatigue, brain fog, and hormonal imbalance still need to be addressed at the source.

Why Estrogen Reduces Hot Flashes and Why It Matters

It's true that hormone therapy, whether it's HRT, ERT, or MHT, can relieve some of the most uncomfortable symptoms of menopause. Estrogen is particularly effective at reducing hot flashes, improving sleep, and lifting mood. And when those symptoms ease, women often feel like they've gotten their life back. They sleep better, think more clearly, and feel less irritable. When quality of life improves, other systems follow.

So how does estrogen help with hot flashes?

Hot flashes are thought to originate in the hypothalamus, the brain's temperature control center and chief of your stress alarm. When estrogen drops, as it does in menopause, the hypothalamus becomes hypersensitive. Minor stressors in your body are suddenly treated like emergencies. Blood vessels dilate, sweat glands activate, cortisol surges, and you're left sweating like a pig, for no apparent reason, every 30 minutes.

Estrogen calms this alarm system. It makes the hypothalamus less reactive, less jumpy. It doesn't fix the underlying reason why the system is on edge; it just desensitizes the stress response. It tells the brain, *"Everything is fine. No need to overreact."* And when the alarm stops blaring, symptoms improve.

But it's important to understand this is symptom relief, not a fix-and-repair. Estrogen is dampening the siren, not restoring the wiring. The deeper factors, like blood sugar swings, thyroid dysfunction, and excess cortisol, remain until they're addressed directly.

Another way to think of this is:

We all know alcohol has negative effects on the body. It can damage the liver, impair sleep, and mess with brain function. And yet, multiple studies show that people who drink moderately often live longer than those who don't. Why? It's probably not the alcohol itself. It's what alcohol does for some people; it relaxes them, makes them more social, helps them laugh. In other words, it improves their quality of life. And sometimes, that net gain of less tension and more connection can outweigh the negative effects the substance may have on your body.

But here's the deal:

If you drink beyond what your body can handle (and that dose is different for everyone), the benefits don't just disappear, they can flip on you. The same alcohol that once helped you relax can start interfering with your sleep, increasing inflammation, and worsening anxiety or hormone imbalances. As with anything, the outcome depends on your individual health and the dose.

Hormones can work similarly.

Even if estrogen isn't restoring deep metabolic health, it may still help you feel better, because it's calming the alarm. And that matters. When you sleep better and feel better, a huge amount of internal and external stress drops away. That reduction alone can tip the scale in favor of better overall health outcomes.

So yes, estrogen therapy can work, especially when it comes to improving quality of life. That's why so many women on hormone therapy report better sleep, better mood, and fewer disruptive symptoms. And it's also why so many observational studies show women on hormone therapy having better health outcomes overall.

But here's the question we need to keep asking:

Is it the estrogen itself that's improving your health?

Or is it what estrogen does to your experience of life?

If a woman sleeps better, feels more like herself, laughs more, moves more, eats better, and has more energy to care for herself, all because she's no longer battling a furnace in her body at 3 a.m., then of course her health markers will look better. These changes are not just about perception. They create real physiological benefits. Better sleep improves blood sugar regulation and lowers inflammation. Reduced stress supports immune balance and hormonal stability. More movement improves cardiovascular health and metabolic function.

But that still doesn't mean estrogen is fixing the underlying system. It may be helping her feel and function better by muting the internal alarms, but unless those alarms are investigated, the deeper issues may remain unaddressed.

So yes, estrogen can help. But if we want lasting resilience, we must ask a different question: What turned the alarm on in the first place? Which, as you've already learned, is an energy issue—not an estrogen issue.

Estrogen excess doesn't look the same in every person, and that's part of what makes it so tricky. For some, it shows up as heavy periods or joint pain. For others, it's migraines, gallbladder issues, or varicose veins. But underneath the symptoms, the story is the same: a hormone that's out of balance, energy systems under strain, and a body trying to stay above water.

The good news? There's a lot you can do to help improve estrogen status, without needing to shut it down or fear it entirely. In this next chapter, I'll go into some practical steps you can take to support detox pathways to improve estrogen clearance, mitigate peripheral estrogen production, support progesterone production, restore energy production, and create an environment where estrogen can do its job, without making your body go into chaos.

CHAPTER 9

THE BOTTOM LINE

Estrogen Unmasked—From Feminine to Frazzled

1. Estrogen isn't evil, but excess is an energy block. When unopposed or poorly cleared, it slows thyroid function, disrupts mitochondria, and drives a stressed metabolism.

2. Ovaries/testes are your primary sources for estrogen, but after menopause and under stress (men and women), peripheral aromatase creates "background" estrogen that's rarely opposed.

3. Excess estrogen can lower thyroid action, increase gut permeability/endotoxin load, activate the HPA axis, raise prolactin, alter vascular tone, and increase clotting risk. It can also inhibit PDH and Complex IV, lowering ATP and pushing inefficient energy production.

4. Estrogen therapy often eases hot flashes and improves sleep, but relief does not equal restored metabolic function; context, dose, and delivery route matter.

5. Support progesterone and thyroid, improve gut and bile flow, lower chronic stress, and nourish well, so estrogen can do its job without running the show.

CHAPTER 10

HOW TO SUPPORT ESTROGEN EXCESS (AND THE SYMPTOMS THAT FOLLOW)

When estrogen is produced (or you are exposed) in excess, poorly detoxified, or left unchecked by low progesterone, it can wreak havoc on everything from metabolic function to mood and digestion.

The good news? These issues are fixable, not by trying to erase estrogen entirely, but by managing it more intelligently. Estrogen is powerful, and when it's supported and its effects are kept in check, it can work *with* your body instead of against it.

There are four key ways to support estrogen excess:

1. **Support estrogen detoxification** – through the liver and intestines.

2. **Reduce peripheral estrogen production** – by reducing aromatase, 17β-HSD1, and STS activity. Each of these enzymes is involved in estrogen production, intensity, and activity.

3. **Minimize total estrogen exposure** – including exogenous sources like xenoestrogens, hormonal birth control, MHT, and HRT.

4. **Support progesterone production and thyroid function** – to counterbalance estrogen and restore optimal hormonal signaling.

Let's take a closer look at each of these.

Estrogen Detoxification – How It's Done and What You Need to Support the Process

Once your body makes estrogen and uses it, it needs to break it down and get rid of it. That job falls mostly to your liver and intestines—and both need to be working well to keep estrogen in check.

Estrogen detox happens in three phases, each relying on a mix of enzymes, nutrients, and a healthy gut. When any of these steps slow down, estrogen can linger too long and start causing symptoms—like mood swings, weight gain, or heavy periods.

Let's break it down.

STEP 1: Phase I Liver Detoxification: Hydroxylation

In this first step, estrogen is hydroxylated, a small chemical group (a hydroxyl group) is added to prepare it for removal. This process takes place in the liver, where a family of enzymes called cytochrome P450 gets to work.

Think of this step like your liver's "workers" opening a package, scanning what's inside, and tagging it with a note that says, "handle with care." Sometimes this tag helps the body move estrogen out efficiently. Other times, the modification creates something more reactive, or even risky. For example, one of the metabolites produced during this phase, 4-hydroxyestrone (4-OH), can be damaging if it's not handled quickly in the next step.

The type of metabolite your liver produces depends on the state of your liver health. A well-fed liver with plenty of B vitamins and magnesium will steer estrogen down the 2-hydroxyestrone (2-OH) pathway, generally considered safer. But if your liver is overworked or undernourished, it may favor the more inflammatory 4-OH or 16-OH routes (1).

To keep this first phase moving along, your liver needs nutrients like B2, B3, B6, magnesium, iron (but not too much), and high-quality protein. That's why I'm always nudging you toward a weekly serving of beef liver for the B vitamins, iron, and protein, and daily servings of dairy, fruit, potatoes, chocolate, coffee, or well-cooked greens for ample magnesium (a magnesium supplement can also work). These foods naturally support the enzymatic machinery your liver needs to do its job.

Once estrogen is hydroxylated, it's ready for Phase 2, where the real packaging happens.

STEP 2: Phase II Liver Detoxification

Now it's time to make these estrogen metabolites safe to move. This second phase is called conjugation, and it's where your body takes those tagged estrogen molecules and wraps them up for shipping. You can picture this like adding bubble wrap and a bright red sticker that says "FRAGILE. Dispose of Immediately."

Conjugation makes estrogen water soluble, neutralizing the hormones into an inactive state. This makes estrogen safe to leave your body through urine or bile. Without this step, estrogen can recirculate, linger too long, and create more problems.

Estrogen is conjugated in three main ways:

- **Glucuronidation** – adds glucuronic acid (via UGT enzymes). The primary conjugation pathway

- **Sulfation** – adds sulfate groups (via SULT enzymes)

- **Methylation** – adds methyl groups (via COMT enzyme), especially important for detoxifying 2-OH and 4-OH estrogens

Each pathway attaches a different chemical group to the estrogen molecule, a glucuronic acid, a sulfate, or a methyl group, all with the same end goal: make it water-friendly and get it out.

These processes rely on very specific nutrients. B6, B12, folate, choline, magnesium, glycine, and taurine are the big players here. And, of course, you will cover a lot of these with a nutrient-dense diet. Beef liver (you knew it was coming) delivers B6, B12, and choline. Coffee and cooked greens help with magnesium. Bone broth, collagen, or gelatin are rich in glycine. And taurine shows up in shellfish, turkey, beef heart, and lamb.

Once conjugated, estrogen is ready for elimination, either filtered out by your kidneys into urine or secreted into bile and carried out through your stool.

It should be noted that both Phase I and Phase II detoxification pathways depend on adequate thyroid hormone, particularly T3. T3 is essential for the expression and activity of cytochrome P450 enzymes involved in Phase I detox, as well as for supporting key Phase II processes like sulfation and glucuronidation. Without sufficient thyroid hormone, these detox pathways slow down, impairing the body's ability to clear estrogen efficiently (more on this later).

Step 3: Phase III: Taking Out the Trash – Elimination

At this point, estrogen has gone through the liver's assembly line, it's been tagged, modified, wrapped up in water-soluble packaging, and sent off to be eliminated. Now it's time for the final step: getting it out of the body.

There are only two exit pathways: urine and stool.

Conjugated estrogen metabolites either get filtered out by your kidneys and flushed through urine, or they're packaged into bile, sent into the intestines, and eliminated through stool. When everything's working well, this process is seamless. But when it's not? Estrogen can boomerang right back into circulation, increasing the total estrogen load on your body, which, if it gets excessive, can make symptoms appear.

Exit Route #1: Urine (via the Kidneys)

Once estrogen has been conjugated in the liver, especially through sulfation and glucuronidation, it becomes water soluble and can be filtered by the kidneys. From there, it's excreted in your urine. Urine is your primary excretion path.

This route is especially important for smaller, more polar conjugated estrogens, such as estrone sulfate, estradiol glucuronide, and 2- or 4-hydroxy estrogens (once they've been methylated or conjugated). When liver detox and kidney filtration are functioning well, these conjugates are removed efficiently.

This is also the pathway measured by most urine hormone tests, like the DUTCH test, but as we'll see below, this test has its limitations.

Is the Dutch Test an Accurate Measurement of Your Hormones?

If you have worked with a functional doctor or practitioner, you've probably heard of the DUTCH test (Dried Urine Test for Comprehensive Hormones). It's marketed as a cutting-edge way to assess hormone levels, especially for estrogen, progesterone, testosterone, and cortisol, using dried urine samples collected over 24 hours.

And yes, it does measure estrogen metabolites (like 2-OH, 4-OH, and 16-OH estrone), as well as how much estrogen is methylated or excreted in urine.

Sounds useful, right? Well, there are a few issues.

The DUTCH test only shows what's leaving the body through urine. But estrogen is also eliminated via the bile and stool, which the test doesn't capture. Only about 50-60% of estrogen metabolites are excreted via the urine. The rest is removed via the bile or enters enterohepatic circulation and is reabsorbed.

And here is the biggest issue, there's no established baseline for what "normal" estrogen metabolite levels look like in urine. The ranges on DUTCH test reports are based on limited population studies, not gold-standard clinical endpoints. In other words, we don't know if high 2-OH is good, bad, or meaningless, especially outside the context of symptoms or clinical history. And if we don't know the true meaning of a test, in my opinion, the test is meaningless.

Although the DUTCH test can offer some insights, it doesn't provide the full hormone picture. It can be pricey, not covered by health insurance, and without agreed-upon reference ranges, interpreting the results often raises more questions than it answers.

The best way to get accurate hormone levels?

Use a combination of symptom tracking and blood tests (especially serum estradiol, progesterone, prolactin, a full thyroid panel, and cholesterol). No single test tells the whole story, but when paired with your symptoms, these labs can offer a solid starting point.

Back to your urinary exit route: once estrogen moves through the liver, it travels via the bloodstream to the kidneys, where it's filtered out and excreted in the urine. This process relies on a handful of nutrients to work well, including magnesium, potassium, vitamin B6, vitamin C, taurine, glycine, zinc, sodium, and CoQ10, plus, of course, plenty of water.

As a quick reminder, food sources for the above nutrients are:

- **Potassium:** orange juice, potatoes, apricots, coconut water

- **Sodium:** salt is your friend here (don't fear it)

- **Magnesium:** Cooked greens, mushrooms, coffee, and supplements
- **B6:** Beef liver, turkey breast, tuna, chicken breast, salmon, eggs
- **Vitamin C:** Orange juice, red peppers, cherries, guava, papaya, kiwi
- **Zinc:** Shellfish, oysters, milk, beef
- **Taurine:** Turkey, shellfish, beef heart, and lamb
- **Glycine:** bone broth, gelatin, and collagen
- **CoQ10:** beef heart, chicken liver, beef liver, sardines, and tuna

Exit Route #2: Stool (Via Bile)

The other major exit route is via bile, which carries conjugated estrogens from the liver to the gut. And here's where your gut plays a much bigger role in hormone regulation than most people realize.

Once estrogen is dumped into the gut via bile, it should head straight for the exit, in your stool. But if your digestion is sluggish, your gut is inflamed, or your microbiome is giving you the middle finger, that estrogen might not leave as planned.

Why? Because certain gut microbes produce an enzyme called beta-glucuronidase. Gut dysbiosis, stress, leaky gut, sluggish bile, lack of fiber, and even estrogen itself can increase beta-glucuronidase. Its job is to *undo* what your liver just did, by removing the glucuronic acid "label" that marked estrogen for elimination. Once that label is gone, the estrogen can be reabsorbed through your intestinal wall, sent back to the liver, and put right back into circulation.

We call this enterohepatic recirculation, a loop gone rogue. It refers to substances that were *supposed* to be excreted but end up boomeranging back into the bloodstream.

That's different from enterohepatic circulation, discussed in chapter 8, which is the normal recycling loop of bile acids and other molecules between the liver and intestines. Recirculation is when estrogen hijacks that system and slips back in through the back door.

What helps stop the recirculation loop and supports proper estrogen detox?

A healthy, well-energized bowel with good motility, enough dietary fat to stimulate bile release, and with a daily gut "sweeper" like the raw carrot salad, cooked white button mushrooms, or bamboo shoots.

For more on this, flip back to Chapter 8 on colon health and endotoxins.

Even if all three detox phases are firing—tagging, neutralizing, and taking out the hormonal trash, it's still only part of the estrogen story. If your body is making too much estrogen to begin with, not just from your ovaries (or testes), but from peripheral tissues, you'll always be playing catch-up. Reducing estrogen overload isn't just about breaking it down. It's about slowing the supply chain at the source. And as you age, that source often shifts from your gonads to your fat tissue, muscles, bones, skin, and even your brain.

Let's talk about how to reduce peripheral estrogen production and start easing the estrogen load upstream.

Peripheral Estrogen Production: The Estrogen Your Sex Glands Didn't Make

Estrogen isn't just made in the ovaries or testes. In fact, after menopause, or during times of chronic stress or inflammation in either sex, a significant amount of estrogen is produced outside the reproductive organs. This is known as peripheral estrogen production, and it happens in tissues like fat, skin, muscle, bone, and even the brain.

Unlike ovarian or testicular estrogen, this kind of production isn't governed by a tidy feedback loop like the HPG axis. Instead, it operates under the radar, often driven by inflammation, stress, and certain enzyme activity, and it comes with very little oversight.

When left unchecked, this silent estrogen engine can fuel symptoms like weight gain, brain fog, blood clots, bloating, fluid retention, hypothyroidism, and autoimmune issues, while also raising the long-term risk of cancer, heart disease, and dementia.

What most people don't realize is that blood levels of estrogen are a poor reflection of what's happening in tissues, especially in postmenopausal women and aging men. Peripheral estrogen is made and acts locally, so it often doesn't show up in blood tests. In fact, research shows that in postmenopausal women, circulating estradiol (E2) levels have little physiological correlation with actual estrogen activity at the tissue level (2). Which means just because your blood levels of estrogen are low, does not mean your total estrogen exposure is low.

If we want to understand someone's true estrogen burden, we need to look beyond lab values. In this next section, we'll dive into how peripheral estrogen is produced, who is most prone to making it, and what you can do to turn the dial down.

How Peripheral Estrogen Is Produced— and the Enzymes Behind It

Once estrogen production shifts away from the ovaries or testes, it doesn't disappear, it simply relocates into your tissues. Peripheral estrogen production is your body's plan B for keeping some estrogen around, whether you need it or not. You see, your body still has the raw materials (androgens like testosterone and androstenedione), and it still has the biochemical tools to convert them into estrogen. Those tools are enzymes, and certain ones are especially good at doing this job outside the reproductive system.

The Main Enzymes Driving Peripheral Estrogen Production

So, what's stirring up all this extra estrogen in your body tissues? It mainly comes down to three big enzyme players—aromatase, 17β-hydroxysteroid dehydrogenase (17β-HSD), and steroid sulfatase (STS).

Let's break it down.

First up is aromatase, the most famous of the bunch. Aromatase takes androgens like testosterone and androstenedione and flips them into estrogens (specifically estradiol and estrone). You'll find aromatase in fat cells, skin, your brain, and even in your blood vessels. And here's the thing, aromatase ramps up when you're under stress. Cortisol, insulin, leptin, inflammation, and even estrogen itself can dial it up. It's like throwing fuel on an estrogen bonfire, the more stress or fat tissue you have, the more aromatase you get, which means more estrogen, which then keeps feeding the loop.

Next is 17β-HSD, which comes in different types, but two are key here: 17β-HSD1 and 17β-HSD2. Think of these like a seesaw. 17β-HSD1 pushes estrone (a weaker estrogen) toward estradiol (the more potent one), while 17β-HSD2 does the opposite, helping tone it down. These enzymes show up all over your body: in fat, skin, breast tissue, brain, bone, liver, kidney, the uterine lining, and if you're pregnant, the placenta is loaded with them.

When 17β-HSD1 is in overdrive, you get more powerful estrogen floating around, especially in places like the breast or uterine lining, which can lead to increased risks of hormone-sensitive cancers (3, 4). That's why scientists are studying 17β-HSD1 inhibitors as potential cancer treatments (5). Unfortunately, chronic inflammation, obesity, stress, insulin, IGF-1, prostaglandins, and even estrogen itself can crank up this enzyme too.

Then there's steroid sulfatase (STS), which adds another layer of complexity. This enzyme has the power to reactivate estrogens your liver had already tagged for removal by adding a sulfate group (sulfation). Instead of leaving your body, estrone sulfate (ES-1) can circle back, get reabsorbed through your gut, and hang out in fat, skin, muscle, and brain. From there, STS can pop the sulfate tag right off, turning it back into the active estrone. This creates a hidden "reserve pool" of estrogen, especially after menopause.

When STS activity is high, more of this backup stash gets converted into active estrogen, often right in fat or breast tissue. Unfortunately, inflammation, obesity, and stress tend to ramp up STS while also suppressing its counter-enzyme, estrogen sulfotransferase (SULT1E1), which normally helps deactivate estrogen by sulfation.

So, you can see how this becomes a perfect storm. In one little spot like belly fat or breast tissue, you could have androgens being turned into estrogen, weak estrogen made stronger, and stored estrogen getting reactivated, all at the same time (6). If your liver and detox systems can't keep up, this local estrogen buildup can fuel bloating, mood swings, hypothyroidism, blood clot risk, and even cancer. And because so much of it acts locally, your blood tests might still look "normal" or even low, while inside your tissues, estrogen is throwing an out-of-control rager!

Alright—enough of the doom and gloom. Let's get to the part where we talk about how to fix it.

How to Reduce Peripheral Estrogen Production

Once you understand that a significant portion of estrogen, especially in men and postmenopausal women, is produced outside of the ovaries and testes, it becomes clear that managing peripheral estrogen isn't just about detoxification or ordering lab tests. It's about cutting off the excess production at its source. And that means supporting your whole system, particularly metabolism, thyroid, and the enzyme activity happening within your tissue.

Here are four things you can do to reduce peripheral estrogen production and its downstream effects:

1. Lower stress

I know I keep coming back to this, but for good reason: chronic stress is one of the most powerful drivers of peripheral estrogen production. Elevated cortisol ramps up aromatase, 17β-HSD1, and STS, the key enzymes that either convert or reactivate estrogen inside tissues. At the same time, stress suppresses thyroid function and slows metabolism, which only adds to the estrogen burden. If you're stuck in a stress loop, your body is probably making more estrogen and struggling to clear it.

Action steps: Support your parasympathetic nervous system. Think: deep breathing, sun exposure, journaling, quality sleep, and balanced meals. Don't underestimate the power of a walk in the sun, a glass of milk, and some well-salted orange juice. (For more, jump back to the chapter on stress.)

2. Support mitochondrial energy production

Energy-deprived tissues tend to rely more on compensatory survival pathways, including estrogenic signaling. Estrogen can act like a growth signal in damaged or stressed tissues. But when you increase cellular energy production, your body no longer needs to lean so hard on estrogen or stress hormones to keep things functioning.

Action steps: Prioritize bioavailable carbohydrates like fruit and root vegetables, get enough protein, and support key mitochondrial nutrients: B vitamins, magnesium, selenium, zinc, copper, and iron. If needed, use exogenous thyroid hormone to boost cellular respiration. This might be a great time to re-read my first book, *How to Heal Your Metabolism*.

3. Reduce body fat

Fat tissue is one of the main sites of aromatase activity. More fat = more estrogen. So, losing excess body fat can significantly reduce peripheral estrogen production. But here's the kicker: how you lose fat matters even more than how much.

Crash diets, chronic fasting, and overtraining can all backfire. They increase stress, slow thyroid function, and impair mitochondrial efficiency. When your mitochondria aren't making enough energy, your body flips into survival mode, raising cortisol, lowering metabolic rate, and storing more fat. This becomes a vicious cycle: poor energy = more fat = more estrogen = more dysfunction.

Action steps: Aim for sustainable fat loss through nourishment, not restriction. Eat enough to support thyroid and liver function. Reduce endotoxin exposure. Lift weights to build muscle and support metabolism. (See the fat loss chapter for a deeper dive.)

4. Utilize natural inhibitors of peripheral estrogen enzymes.

There are some nutrients that can reduce the production of estrogen, by inhibiting the enzymes that are needed to make peripheral estrogen.

Apigenin, a flavonoid found in citrus peels, chamomile, and celery, has been shown in vitro to directly inhibit aromatase and 17B-HSD activity (7, 8).

Naringenin, another flavonoid also abundant in orange and citrus peels, similarly targets aromatase and 17B-HSD (7, 8). Apigenin and naringenin are a great argument for adding a serving of marmalade into your daily diet.

Zinc, present in beef, oysters, and milk, can play a role in estrogen synthesis. Zinc-deficient rats showed increased testosterone-to-estradiol conversion; zinc repletion reversed it (9).

Vitamin D, whether via sun exposure or D_3 supplementation, is linked to reduced aromatase activity in some tissues. Vitamin D is needed for thyroid hormone production, and optimal thyroid levels lower estrogen production.

Aspirin doesn't just fight headaches; it lowers aromatase activity. That's why studies have found that people who regularly take low-dose aspirin often have lower estrogen levels and a lower risk of estrogen-related cancers, like certain types of breast cancer (10, 11).

Progesterone directly suppresses aromatase activity, especially in ovarian and breast tissues. In childbearing years, women produce adequate progesterone production to protect against the effects of ovarian estrogen production. Yet, later in life, they don't have this protection due to lack of ovulation, thus, supplementation may be necessary. Both animal studies and human breast cancer cell assays show progesterone reduces enzyme expression and activity in granulosa and epithelial cells (12, 13).

Thyroid hormone (T3), by increasing cellular respiration and metabolism, you can reduce the activity of aromatase. Improved energy production always mitigates the stress cycle, which lowers the enzymes needed for peripheral estrogen production. T3 is also needed for proper liver detoxification, which can help break down and remove estrogens.

It should be noted, for T3 to work properly, optimal fuel and nutrition must also be present. Which means that taking T3 medication without a proper nutritional foundation may not produce the same result.

By addressing both systemic factors (stress, thyroid, energy metabolism) and local enzyme activity (aromatase, STS, 17β-HSD1), you're no longer just reacting to estrogen overload, you're cutting it off at its source. And that, in the long run, is what keeps the hormonal tidal wave from rising in the first place.

Unfortunately, peripheral production is only one side of the estrogen exposure equation. The other major contributor? Xenoestrogens, from plastics, personal care products, food additives, hormone replacement, and even tap water. These compounds may not be produced inside your body, but they can still act like estrogen once they get in. The next section will walk you through how to identify, reduce, and avoid the most common sources of environmental estrogens so you can stay ahead of the curve and lighten your estrogenic load.

Hidden Sources of Estrogenic Burden: Exogenous Estrogens and Endocrine Disruptors

Not all estrogen overload comes from inside your body. Every day, we're exposed to environmental estrogens, better known as xenoestrogens (foreign chemicals that mimic or disrupt estrogen) and endocrine-disrupting chemicals (EDCs). These compounds can bind to estrogen receptors, increase aromatase, slow estrogen clearance, or sabotage the organs that regulate hormones, like the liver and thyroid. And they're everywhere.

Let's look at the worst offenders:

Mycotoxins (Mold Toxins)

It's not the moldy wall, it's what the mold releases. Mycotoxins like zearalenone and alternariol can sneak into your system and act like estrogen, binding to receptors and kicking off hormonal chaos from the inside out. Studies show high levels of these mold toxins are linked to early puberty, disrupted menstrual cycles, and fertility challenges. So yes, living in a moldy house can *literally* raise your estrogen load (14, 15).

Pesticides and Herbicides

Weed killers and bug sprays don't just take out pests, they mess with your hormones too. Chemicals like atrazine, DDT, and glyphosate have all shown estrogenic effects. Atrazine increases aromatase and has been shown to feminize male frogs. Glyphosate, meanwhile, activates estrogen receptors in breast cancer cells, mimicking estrogen's effects almost perfectly (16, 17).

Plastics and Food Packaging

BPA and BPS (found in water bottles, food storage, and canned goods) are textbook xenoestrogens. They bind to estrogen receptors and promote estrogen-responsive gene activity. Translation: these plastics can turn on the same cellular machinery as estradiol, with none of the nuance (18, 19).

Industrial Chemicals

Alkylphenols like nonylphenol are added to detergents because they're amazing at lifting grime. The downside? They're also great at activating estrogen receptors. Chronic exposure has been shown to interfere with the endocrine system. These chemical imposters weren't designed to mess with your hormones; they were just *really* good at cleaning your socks (20, 21).

Environmental Pollutants

It's not just your air quality that's suffering. Dioxins (from exhaust and incineration), PCBs (old paint, caulking), flame retardants (PBDEs in foam and furniture), and PAHs (from combustion and pollution) have all been shown to disrupt estrogen balance. Some bind directly to estrogen receptors; others jack up aromatase or slow detox in the liver. These pollutants build up in fat tissue and stick around for years, quietly adding to your hormonal burden (22, 23).

Birth Control

Birth control pills replace your natural hormonal rhythm with a flat-line dose of synthetic estrogen, specifically ethinyl estradiol, which is far stronger and harder to clear than the real thing. So even though ovulation is suppressed, your total estrogen exposure usually goes up (24).

Menopausal Hormone Therapy (MHT)

Whether you call it HRT, ERT, or MHT, it's still more estrogen, and it adds to your lifetime load. That's why doctors often advise using the lowest effective dose for the shortest necessary time. Prolonged MHT can significantly increase cumulative estrogen exposure (24).

Individually, each of these exposures may have a minimal effect. But they can layer on top of each other, building a chronic, low-grade estrogenic burden that your body must manage. You may not feel it day to day, but over time, it can fuel symptoms of estrogen excess— weight gain, edema, digestive issues, low thyroid hormone, etc.

I am sure you are asking by now, what can I do to help myself?

Well, the good news is you're not powerless. There are plenty of simple, evidence-based steps you can take to reduce your exposure, and I am about to go there next.

How to Reduce Exogenous Estrogen Burden

If you've just read through that list of estrogenic landmines and feel like you need to move to a deserted island and only eat natural, home-grown foods—breathe. The point isn't to panic. It's to get savvy. You don't need to eliminate every trace of synthetic or environmental estrogen exposure (good luck with that), you just need to lower your total load, so your body has a fighting chance to rebalance.

1. Detox your home like you would your diet. Your skin is not a force field. What you breathe in, slather on, and wash with matters.

- Switch to fragrance-free or essential-oil–based cleaning products.

- Use natural soaps, baking soda, or vinegar instead of conventional cleaners loaded with alkylphenols.

- Ditch dryer sheets and scented detergents—they're often endocrine-disruptor bombs in disguise.

- Vacuum frequently (especially with HEPA filters)—dust is a major carrier of phthalates and flame retardants.

2. Eat (and store) smarter. Estrogen isn't just in your cleaning products, it can be in the plastic lid, the bottle, and the microwavable tray.

- Store food in glass, not plastic.

- Never microwave food in plastic containers (even "BPA-free" ones can leach other estrogenic chemicals).

- Prioritize organic, when possible, especially for produce high in pesticide residue.

- Scrub fruits and veggies or use a vinegar rinse to reduce pesticide load.

- Choose fresh or frozen over canned, when possible, particularly high fat or acidic foods, which leach more BPA from can linings.

3. Mind your mold. If your home smells musty, don't just light a candle.

- Fix leaks, improve ventilation, and consider a professional mold inspection if symptoms persist.
- Use air purifiers with activated carbon and HEPA filters to trap airborne spores and VOCs.
- And if your orange juice smells like a forgotten gym sock, toss it.
- Mold on shredded or soft cheeses should go in the trash, not in your mouth.

5. Upgrade your body products. Your lotion shouldn't double as a hormone disruptor.

- Look for paraben- and phthalate-free on the label.
- Avoid products with "fragrance" listed (it's often code for dozens of hidden chemicals).
- Use mineral-based sunscreens instead of chemical ones, especially those with oxybenzone. Refer to the website www.katedeering.com for my go-to choices.

6. Rethink hormone-based medications (if appropriate)

If you're using hormonal birth control or menopausal hormone therapy, work with a practitioner who understands the pluses and negatives of hormone use. Hormone therapy does not come without negative effects. You need to take into consideration your overall health, exposure length, and personal risks. Refer to the side bar on estrogen and hot flashes earlier in this chapter, for my take on hormone therapies.

When it comes to improving estrogen exposure, the goal isn't perfection, it's reduction.

Even a 10–20% drop in exogenous estrogen exposure can lift strain from your liver, lower aromatase activity, and reduce estrogen receptor stimulation throughout your body. In short, this can mean fewer migraines, less bloating, fewer PMS blowups, and a whole lot more energy.

We've already tackled the three big levers for lowering estrogen excess: improving detoxification, decreasing peripheral estrogen production, and reducing exogenous estrogen exposure. Each of those strategies helps lighten the load. But to truly keep estrogen in check, you also must strengthen your hormonal counterparts. That means restoring the body's natural defenses, especially progesterone and thyroid hormone. These two don't just buffer estrogen's effects, they actively support healthy energy production, which reinforces hormonal function at every level.

In this final section, we'll focus on how to support the production and function of these two essential hormones, particularly in their relationship to estrogen.

Supporting Progesterone Production

Progesterone plays a critical role in keeping estrogen in check. It doesn't just oppose estrogen, it helps shape, time, and refine its actions. Where estrogen builds, stimulates, and expands, progesterone anchors, regulates, and buffers.

Without enough progesterone, even normal estrogen levels can feel like too much. That's why boosting progesterone production is one of the most important things you can do to protect against estrogen excess. It's not just about managing estrogen symptoms; it's about restoring balance and guiding estrogen's influence in the right direction.

If progesterone is the project manager to estrogen's eccentric creative direction, then ovulation is the ride that gets her to the job site. No ovulation means no corpus luteum, and no corpus luteum means no meaningful progesterone production. So, supporting ovulation is step one.

Here's the issue: ovulation is one of the first things to go when a woman is overstressed or undernourished. The hypothalamic-pituitary-gonadal (HPG) axis shuts down under stress, while the hypothalamic-pituitary-adrenal (HPA) axis ramps up. This shift disrupts or halts ovulation, lowering progesterone and allowing estrogen to run unchecked.

This hormonal imbalance may result in skipped periods or chaotic ones, heavy bleeding, cramps, breast tenderness, clots, sugar cravings, anxiety, and other classic estrogen-excess symptoms. But here's the part most women don't know: your period isn't supposed to feel like a bloated, weepy, chocolate-seeking, angry tornado. A healthy cycle should arrive quietly and leave with barely a whisper, more like a breeze than hurricane.

To restore ovulation, start by supporting the body's readiness to ovulate. That means fueling it, not depriving it. The hypothalamus tracks stress signals, energy, and nutrient availability. If it senses scarcity or chaos, ovulation gets skipped. Eat enough calories, prioritizing carbs, nutrient-dense protein, and saturated fats. Reduce unnecessary stressors. Signal safety, not survival.

Proper rest and nutrition also support adrenal health. The adrenals can produce small amounts of progesterone, especially important after menopause or in men—but only in a calm, well-nourished environment. Chronic fight-or-flight physiology always favors cortisol over progesterone, survival over restoration.

Thyroid hormone plays a key role, too. It's required for follicle development and for the hormonal surge that triggers ovulation (128). Without adequate T3, ovulation becomes erratic or absent, dragging progesterone down with it. (See the thyroid chapter for optimizing your T3 status.) T3 is also needed to convert cholesterol into steroid hormones, including progesterone.

Micronutrients matter as well. Vitamin A, B6, magnesium, zinc, and copper all help the enzymes inside the ovaries and adrenals do their job. Food sources like beef liver, oysters, eggs, milk, fruit, and root vegetables can help restore and sustain progesterone production.

What About Exogenous Progesterone?

This comes up a lot, and the answer isn't a simple yes or no.

If you're not ovulating or experiencing irregular ovulation (think perimenopause, PCOS, or hypothalamic amenorrhea), you're probably not making much progesterone. In that case, bioidentical progesterone therapy can be incredibly helpful. It can ease symptoms, support thyroid function, stabilize blood sugar, reduce inflammation, and protect tissues from unopposed estrogen.

But it's not magic. If your metabolism is struggling and you're under-eating or overstressed, taking progesterone before building your foundation can backfire. You might experience blood sugar crashes, anxiety, or insomnia. That's why food comes first: adequate calories, frequent meals, enough carbs, and micronutrient density. Once that foundation is in place, exogenous progesterone (oral or transdermal) can work beautifully.

And a word of caution; not all "progesterone" is created equal. Synthetic progestins are not the same as bioidentical progesterone. They bind differently to receptors and carry very different risk profiles. Make sure to ask your health care provider about what you're being prescribed.

Progesterone Types and Dosage

- **Oral micronized progesterone (prometrium):** 100–300 mg/day. This is the most studied form, especially for use in menopausal hormone therapy (MHT) and hormone replacement therapy (HRT). It is metabolized in the liver into allopregnanolone, a neurosteroid that supports calm and sleep. Often used for perimenopausal symptoms,

PMS, or as endometrial protection in women on estrogen therapy.

- **Transdermal progesterone (creams, oils):** 10–100 mg/day. Bypasses liver metabolism, offering smoother absorption. Often used in functional medicine for PMS, anxiety, menopause relief, and blood sugar regulation. However, absorption can be variable, and mainstream providers may not consider it adequate for endometrial protection.

- **Injectable progesterone:** 25–50 mg every 3–4 days. Used primarily in fertility settings or for women who don't absorb progesterone well by other methods. Typically delivered in sesame or peanut oil for slow release.

- **Vaginal progesterone:** 100–200 mg/day. Comes as suppositories, capsules, or gels. Common in fertility protocols and menopause, especially when local tissue support is needed.

- **Synthetic progestins:** Structurally different from natural progesterone. Found in birth control pills and older HRT formulas. While easier to absorb and longer lasting, they carry higher risks of side effects like blood clots, mood disruption, and breast cancer.

If you're not on estrogen therapy, it's best to cycle progesterone (e.g., 14 days on, 14 days off or 21 days on, and 7 days off) to maintain receptor sensitivity and prevent liver enzyme induction. Liver enzyme induction occurs with continuous use of progesterone, this can train the liver to metabolize it fast over time, the liver gets good at breaking it down, which means you feel it less, require more, and/or worse become desensitized to its positive effects.

What About Men and Progesterone?

Men don't ovulate, obviously, but they do produce small amounts of progesterone, mainly in the testes and adrenal glands. In men, progesterone helps regulate cortisol, supports brain health, acts as a precursor to testosterone, and buffers excess estrogen and DHT. Stress, inflammation, and hypothyroidism can all suppress it.

Which means men can support progesterone in the same way women can; by supporting metabolic health, eating enough carbs and protein, and lowering chronic stress.

Bridging Progesterone and Thyroid Support

Before we move fully into thyroid, it's important to understand how deeply interconnected these two hormones are. Progesterone and thyroid hormone don't work in isolation; they operate as a team. While progesterone helps modulate estrogen's impact at the receptor level, thyroid governs how estrogen is detoxified and cleared. If progesterone is the one keeping estrogen's behavior in check, thyroid is the one keeping her from overstaying her welcome.

The Unsung Role of Thyroid Hormone in Estrogen Regulation

Thyroid hormone is one of the most underappreciated regulators of estrogen activity, and T3 is the star of the show. Think of it like your body's metabolic traffic controller, directing where estrogen goes, how fast it's processed, and when it's cleared. Without enough T3, that traffic backs up, and estrogen builds up like rush-hour congestion.

Specifically, T3 fuels both phase I and phase II liver detox pathways, including cytochrome P450, sulfation, and glucuronidation. These are the biochemical detox routes estrogen relies on to be safely broken down and eliminated. When T3 is low, those routes get sluggish, and estrogen starts to overstay its welcome.

Thyroid hormone also keeps aromatase in check, the enzyme that converts androgens into estrogen in peripheral tissues like fat and skin. In a hypothyroid state, aromatase ramps up, especially in fat tissue, leading to more local estrogen production. That means even if blood estrogen looks "normal," tissue levels can be higher, and more inflammatory.

And let's not forget that progesterone depends on thyroid hormone too. Without sufficient thyroid function, progesterone production drops, leaving estrogen unopposed and free to stir up lots of trouble: bloating, mood swings, PMS, tender breasts, fibroids—the entire PMS storm.

So, while thyroid is often framed as the hormone for energy and metabolism, it's also an estrogen regulator. It helps regulate, detoxify, and oppose excessive estrogen activity.

How to support your thyroid (refer to the chapter on thyroid for more detail)

1. Eat enough food
2. Carbs are essential
3. Consume nutrient rich foods
4. Reduce stress
5. Support liver and kidney function
6. Reduce exogenous estrogen exposure
7. Check for medications that interfere with thyroid hormone production
8. Take exogenous thyroid hormones if needed

If you've made it this far, you now understand that managing estrogen excess isn't about waging war on estrogen, it's about making sure estrogen is kept in check. Estrogen, in its right place and proportion, is essential for health. But like any strong force, it needs boundaries, context, and support.

We've explored how to improve detoxification, slow down peripheral production, limit environmental exposure, and amplify your body's natural buffers, progesterone and thyroid hormone. Each one of these pillars plays a role in not just managing symptoms, but in restoring a system that works. A system where hormones don't feel like chaos, but an extraordinary well-coordinated dance.

Because that's what hormonal health is, a dynamic dance, not a fixed formula. And when you support estrogen from all sides, you stop reacting to symptoms and start creating resilience. Fewer migraines, calmer cycles, steadier moods, stronger bones, and more energy. This isn't about chasing perfect labs, it's about giving your body what it needs to feel safe, nourished, and supported.

Estrogen isn't the enemy. But unchecked, unregulated, and over produced estrogen can be. Luckily, you know you have the insight and understanding to restore yours.

Next up, we'll shift our focus to another double-edged nutrient: iron. You need it to survive, but too much, especially in the wrong place, can quietly sabotage your metabolism, increase oxidative stress, and block energy production. In the next chapter, we'll unpack the often-overlooked problem of iron overload, and how to strike the right balance between deficiency and excess.

CHAPTER 10

THE BOTTOM LINE

How to Support Estrogen Excess (And the Symptoms that Follow)

1. Support estrogen *detox* with macro and micronutrients. Prioritize B-vitamins (liver), magnesium (cooked greens/coffee), protein, glycine/taurine (collagen, shellfish).

2. Improve elimination so estrogen leaves via urine/stool—hydrate, salt/potassium balance, gut cleaners (carrot salad, bamboo shoots, cooked mushrooms), have daily bowel movements—use cascara sagrada or magnesium supplements.

3. Reduce peripheral estrogen by lowering aromatase/17β-HSD1/ STS activity: manage stress, lose fat sustainably, support thyroid, and use food-based inhibitors (citrus peel flavonoids like apigenin/naringenin, zinc, vitamin D); aspirin/progesterone may help where appropriate.

4. Reduce exposure. Cut xenoestrogens/EDCs: swap plastics for glass, avoid "fragrance" and harsh cleaners, mind mold, choose cleaner body/home products, and use the lowest effective dose/ shortest duration if on HRT/HC. Please check with your health provider.

5. Support progesterone production (by restoring ovulation, calories, carbs, protein, micronutrients) and thyroid (fuel, minerals, stress reduction) so estrogen is guided, not running the show.

6. Support over all metabolic rate to mitigate the stress response. Best to favor glucose availability, adequate protein, and micronutrients (B's, Mg, Se, Zn, Cu, iron as needed) to shift cells from stress chemistry to efficient oxidation. This creates less of a need for stressed-induced estrogen production

CHAPTER 11

IRON: THE DOUBLE-EDGED SWORD
HOW EXCESS IRON CAN SABOTAGE
YOUR ENERGY PRODUCTION

Iron has already earned plenty of praise in the pages in this book, rightfully so. It's essential for making energy, delivering oxygen, and keeping your metabolism running like a 20-year-old rock star on tour. Without iron, you'd be a sluggish, breathless, brain-fogged mess.

But like most biological rock stars, iron has a less glamorous side. Under the wrong conditions, it can be downright destructive. Too much iron, especially when it's hanging around where it shouldn't, can flip from life-giving to life-draining, choking off your mitochondria, triggering oxidative chaos, and sabotaging the very energy production it's supposed to support.

This is a big deal, because many people today have this exact problem; iron loading into places it doesn't belong, which can drive inflammation and block their ability to produce abundant, efficient energy. It's one of those hidden energy blocks that rarely gets blamed, yet it often sits right at the center of fatigue, metabolic slowdowns, and even accelerated aging.

Researchers such as Dr. Ray Peat highlighted iron's darker potential decades ago. He connected it to everything from oxidative stress, fibrosis, and age spots, to the way excess iron and chronic stress mess with energy production. And today, we're still playing catch-up (1).

In this chapter, I'm going to look at both sides of iron's personality. I'll start by introducing iron, its functions, and your daily needs. Then I'll revisit why your body depends on it so much, because perspective matters, and nothing in health is ever black or white. After that, I'll flip on the flashlight and expose how excess iron becomes one of the most overlooked energy blockers out there. And finally, I will give insight on what you can do to prevent excess iron, and how to improve it.

What You Need to Know About Iron

Although I've already touched on iron numerous times in this book, I want to give you a complete and comprehensive review of what iron is, how much you need, and what affects its absorption and utilization.

First, you must remember iron is more than just the stuff that makes up your favorite skillet. It's an essential trace mineral and your body absolutely relies on it to stay alive.

Men have about 4 grams, and women have about 3 grams of total body iron. About 70% of your body's iron is found in your red blood cells and muscle cells. Another 5-6% is tucked into certain enzymes involved in respiration and energy metabolism. The remaining 25% gets stored in the protein ferritin, your iron warehouse. On average, men store about 1,000 mg of iron, while women average closer to 300 mg (thanks to regular monthly menstrual losses) (2, 3).

Most non-menstruating people only lose about 1-2 mg of iron daily through shedding intestinal cells, skin, and tiny blood losses, so that's all you typically need to absorb to stay balanced. Considering we only absorb about 5-30% of the iron we eat, you generally need to consume 10-18 mg of iron each day to replace what you lose. Pregnant women may need up to 27 mg/day, due to the needs of the growing child (2).

Unlike certain minerals (like magnesium, potassium, or sodium) that your kidneys flush out daily, your body doesn't have an active system for getting rid of excess iron. Once absorbed, it's basically recycled forever by your reticuloendothelial system (RES), the network that breaks down old red blood cells and salvages the iron (more on this below) (4).

Because your body can't easily get rid of iron, it relies on your small intestine to tightly control absorption. If you're low on iron, absorption ramps up. If you have plenty, the hormone hepcidin steps in, lowering absorption by telling your gut to pull back. Yes, your body is damn amazing and has numerous protective mechanisms to keep you safe and regulated.

Essentially: if you're depleted, you'll soak up more; if you're full of iron, you'll soak up less.

Things that Can Increase Iron Absorption:

1. Heme iron (found in animal foods) is far more absorbable than non-heme iron (found in plants). Heme iron glides through your gut's specialized transporters with little interference (5).

2. Ascorbic acid (vitamin C) increases non-heme iron absorption. So that OJ with your spinach salad can help iron absorption, but it won't make much difference with the iron in your steak, because heme iron already gets absorbed well on its own (5).

3. Alcohol boosts iron absorption by increasing gut permeability and blunting hepcidin. That's partly why chronic drinkers often have higher iron stores (6).

4. Estrogen suppresses hepcidin and can increase gut permeability, driving more iron uptake (because remember: less hepcidin means more iron absorption). This is why oral contraceptives and menopausal hormone therapy can increase iron absorption. In general, women can absorb up to three times as much iron from food

as men. Yet, thanks to their menstrual cycles, women typically store far less, at least until menopause (7, 8, 9) *.

5. Disrupted microbiome. Studies in germ-free and antibiotic-treated mice demonstrate that a disrupted microbiome lowers hepcidin levels and increases gut iron absorption. Anything that lowers hepcidin, will increase iron absorption (9).

*Once women hit menopause, they tend to store more iron, leading to levels as high as men. This increase may explain the rise in metabolic and cardiovascular risks seen in women post-menopause (10).

Things that Can Decrease Iron Absorption:

- Phytates, found in grains, legumes, nuts, and seeds (11).
- Polyphenols, like the tannins in coffee, tea, and cocoa (12).
- Certain minerals, calcium, copper, manganese, and zinc all compete with iron absorption (13, 14).
- Low stomach acid, which reduces iron's conversion into the absorbable ferrous form (15).
- Small intestine inflammation, SIBO, and IBD can all disrupt normal absorption pathways for iron (16, 17).
- Hepcidin, your main iron-regulating hormone, increases when iron levels increase. It increases, so that your body decreases iron absorption (18).

So yes, some things crank up your iron absorption, and others slow it down. I'll dive deeper into how to use these to your advantage, especially if you suspect you're carrying too much iron, which we will get to later in this chapter.

The Reticuloendothelial System: Your Iron Regulator and Recycler

When most people think about iron balance, they picture the things they eat, liver, red meat, spinach, or maybe that nasty iron supplement. But the truth is, about 90% of your daily iron needs don't come from food at all, they come from your body's internal recycling system, known as the reticuloendothelial system (RES) (19).

The RES is a network of specialized immune cells, primarily macrophages, scattered throughout your liver, spleen, lymph nodes, and bone marrow. Think of it as your body's clean-up crew and scrap yard, rolled into one. Each day, these macrophages quietly patrol for old, damaged, or worn-out red blood cells.

Your worn-out blood cells are the ones that have lived their typical 120-day lifespan and are ready to be retired. The macrophages engulf these aging cells, break them down, and carefully harvest their iron. This reclaimed iron is then either stored safely inside the macrophages, locked up in ferritin, or released back into circulation when new red blood cells need to be made.

FUN FACT: Every day your body recycles about 200 billion red blood cells. A typical adult has about 20-30 trillion red blood cells. Which means about 1% of your RBC turn over every single day. Crazy!

Your RES isn't just important; it's your primary regulator of your iron warehouse and janitorial system. Without it, your body would either lose iron too rapidly or let it float freely in ways that drive oxidative stress. The RES keeps iron under tight control, ensuring it's available for critical processes like making hemoglobin and fueling mitochondria, while minimizing its potential to spark harmful free radicals.

And, if you remember back when we talked about iron in the oxygen chapter, the efficiency of your RES doesn't just depend on iron. The management of iron hinges on a whole symphony of other nutrients that keep this recycling and regulatory machinery running smoothly.

Copper is perhaps the most crucial. It's needed for ceruloplasmin, the enzyme that oxidizes iron so it can be loaded onto transferrin and safely transported through your blood. Without enough copper, iron gets stuck inside macrophages, leading to poor recycling and functional iron deficiency, meaning your cells can't get what they need, even when total iron stores are high (20).

Vitamin A is another major player. It works alongside copper to regulate the release of iron from storage and influences the genes that drive erythropoiesis (the creation of new red blood cells). A lack of vitamin A can disrupt this balance, causing iron to pile up in storage sites while your bloodstream runs low (21).

Zinc also indirectly supports this system by modulating immune activity and helping maintain the structural integrity of the RES cells themselves. And B vitamins, especially B2 and B6, are needed for proper red blood cell maturation and for running the enzymes that process recycled iron (22).

A shortage of any of these can negatively impact the RES, leading to iron being dysregulated and creating functional iron deficiency (FID). FID occurs when iron is present but trapped. The macrophages decide to hold onto iron, producing high ferritin, instead of releasing it, so the rest of the body (bone marrow, thyroid, mitochondria) can't access it. This produces symptoms that feel just like iron deficiency (fatigue, poor recovery, low blood iron), but this is not a problem of too little iron overall, but rather of iron trapped in the wrong place, a problem of utilization, not supply.

So, while iron often hogs the spotlight, it's this broader nutrient orchestra, copper, vitamin A, zinc, and B vitamins, that makes sure your RES can keep iron safely circulating where it's needed most. Without them, your body's most amazing recycling system starts to falter, paving the way for energy problems, oxidative stress, and that paradox of being simultaneously overloaded with iron yet starved for it where it counts.

The Bright Side of Iron: Why Your Body Can't Live Without it

Before we dive into iron's dark side, let's not forget all the reasons your body loves, and needs, this mineral. Iron is one of those nutrients that's completely non-negotiable. It's the butter to your bread, the ice cream to your cake, the cheese to your pizza. You get the point.

When it comes to energy production, iron wears multiple hats. It helps power your mitochondria, hauls oxygen around like a loyal delivery truck, and supports your thyroid hormone's production and conversion so your metabolism can keep up with all its daily demands.

Inside every cell, your mitochondria crank out ATP, your body's energy currency. Iron is needed to produce and transport electrons through the electron transport chain. It builds iron-sulfur clusters and cytochromes, which, if you remember from Chapter 3, act like wires and electrical relays that keep energy flowing. Without them, your "delivery trucks" NADH and $FADH_2$ would have nowhere to drop off their electrons, and ATP production would screech to a halt (23, 24).

Iron also plays a huge role in hemoglobin production and oxygen transport. It's like a tiny hook, grabbing onto oxygen so your red blood cells can carry it from your lungs to every corner of your body. Without enough iron, you make less hemoglobin and fewer red blood cells. That means less oxygen delivery, less energy production, and feeling exhausted, even after ten hours of sleep (25).

And finally, there's iron's role in thyroid hormone. Iron is a cofactor for TPO, the enzyme that helps produce thyroid hormones. It's also needed by the deiodinase enzymes that convert inactive T4 into active T3. Without enough iron, active thyroid hormone production slows down, which means you slow down, too (26).

What I want you to remember is that iron is essential. It supports your mitochondria to produce energy, binds oxygen so your cells can breathe, and keeps your thyroid from putting your entire system in slow motion.

So yes—iron is vital. Without it, your energy tanks.

But...(Why does there always have to be a "but"?) iron, with all the wonderful things it does, can quickly become your worst nightmare if you end up storing too much.

How Excess Iron Can Hinder Energy Production

We've established that iron is critical for making energy. But too much iron? That's like overloading your electrical system until the wires fry and the lights go out. It can quickly flip from essential to downright destructive.

The reality is, many people today carry excess iron that's quietly wrecking their metabolism, without them even knowing it.

Here is how this happens on a cellular level.

Excess Iron Fuels Oxidative Stress that
Burns Out Your Mitochondria

Iron is also a bit like fire: safely contained, it powers your system; left loose, it can burn the house down.

Inside your bloodstream, most of your iron is safely chaperoned. It's either stored in ferritin or hitches a ride on transferrin, a transport protein. Your serum iron is iron that is attached to transferrin. Picture transferrin like a fleet of trucks, each with two seats for iron. Your transferrin saturation (TSAT) on labs tells you how many of these seats are filled.

- A healthy TSAT (around 25–35%) means plenty of seats are still open—there's a built-in safety buffer.

- But when TSAT climbs over 45–50%, your trucks are nearly maxed out. With no more seats, excess iron is forced to float around unbound. This is called non-transferrin bound iron (NTBI). (I'll explain how this happens below.)

This is where the real problems start.

NTBI is rogue iron, loose in your bloodstream, unescorted and hyper-reactive.

It collides with hydrogen peroxide (H_2O_2), a normal byproduct of your mitochondria, through the Fenton reaction, generating hydroxyl radicals, the most destructive, DNA-wrecking free radicals in biology (27).

Think of the Fenton reaction like tossing gunpowder into a fireplace. The mild smoke (H_2O_2) plus heat suddenly becomes an explosive reaction (producing hydroxyl radicals), damaging the fireplace itself (that's you).

These hydroxyl radicals attack mitochondrial membranes, enzymes, and even mitochondrial DNA. Over time, this oxidative storm damages your electron transport chain, causing electrons to leak, which creates even more ROS (reactive oxygen species). It's a vicious cycle that slows ATP production, leaving you fatigued, brain-fogged, and inexplicably worn down (28, 29).

And here's the unfortunate truth.

NTBI isn't picked up on standard blood labs. Your regular "serum iron," "TSAT," and even "ferritin" give indirect clues, but they don't measure this dangerous, free-floating iron directly. That's why people can look "normal" on paper while iron is quietly fueling oxidative chaos at the cellular level.

It should be noted that although NTBI isn't measured in your standard iron labs, research shows it's detectable in most people when looked for, and it strongly correlates with oxidative stress (30). This means many of us may carry small but biologically significant amounts of rogue iron that routine tests completely miss.

Your body's high-tech system of transferrin trucks and ferritin warehouses is designed to keep iron safe. But when these systems get overwhelmed, whether from too much intake, poor recycling due to low copper or vitamin A, or inflammation hijacking hepcidin, iron spills into NTBI form. That's the iron gasoline that torches your mitochondria from the inside out.

Excess Iron Disrupts Thyroid Hormone Activation, Slowing Energy Production

Iron overload doesn't just hammer your mitochondria; it can mess with your thyroid gland too. Your thyroid needs iron, but like so many things in the body, it's a Goldilocks deal; too little, and you struggle to even make thyroid hormones. Too much, and it becomes a different kind of problem.

Research shows that excess iron can accumulate in endocrine tissues, including the thyroid, leading to oxidative stress and cellular damage (31). In people with hereditary hemochromatosis, where faulty genes cause iron to pile up year after year, scientists have found hemosiderin (iron "rust") lodged inside thyroid tissue. One study even estimated that thyroid disorders are up to 80 times more common in men with hemochromatosis than in the general population (32).

It's even more striking in people who receive regular blood transfusions, like patients with severe anemia or beta thalassemia major (a genetic disorder that slashes hemoglobin production). Each unit of blood delivers 200–250 mg of iron, and unlike dietary iron, transfused iron skips your gut's regulatory checkpoints, flooding directly into circulation. Over time, this iron loads into tissues with rich blood flow, including your liver, heart, pituitary, pancreas, and yes, the thyroid, raising the risk of damage.

Studies have found that up to 12–30% of transfusion-dependent thalassemia patients develop hypothyroidism, with the frequency climbing alongside higher ferritin levels and more cumulative transfusions (33). A large meta-analysis of 382 patients pinned the prevalence of hypothyroidism at 16.2% in those who were regularly transfused, compared to 7.2% in less transfused individuals, with overt hypothyroidism found in about 12.5%, strongly linked to rising ferritin (34).

So yeah, while low iron is famously bad for thyroid function (and it absolutely is), the flip side can happen too; too much iron can blunt thyroid activity by building up in the gland and potentially interfere with local hormone activation.

Now, before any of you panic and start eliminating all things iron, let me reassure you; these more dramatic effects are mostly seen in people with genetic iron-loading conditions or those who receive frequent transfusions. For the average person with balanced iron intake and a healthy recycling system, there's little evidence that normal dietary iron will push the thyroid into dysfunction.

That said, because iron does tend to accumulate quietly over decades, especially after menopause or in men, it's smart to stay aware of this double-edged sword. Knowledge is not about fear; it's about being informed so you can keep all your metabolic functions running smoothly well into your later years.

Iron Encourages Mitochondrial "Cellular Jams" by Promoting Lipofuscin

Okay, this one gets a bit messy but stick with me. When your mitochondria are constantly battling iron-driven oxidative stress, they start to accumulate something called *lipofuscin*. Think of lipofuscin as a stubborn, rusty sludge made up of damaged fats (like PUFA), proteins, and metals like iron. It's literally cellular junk, the stuff that ends up forming those brown age spots (or liver spots) on your skin. But the real problems happen inside your cells, where you can't see it (35, 36).

Imagine lipofuscin-like gunk piling up in your kitchen trash. Now picture that gunk overflowing into the neighborhood recycling center, that's basically what happens in your body. Your cells' recycling centers are called *lysosomes*. Their job is to clean out old, broken mitochondria and other worn-out parts so new, efficient ones can take over.

But when lipofuscin builds up, it clogs the lysosomes, slowing down the cleanup crew.

Damaged mitochondria start sticking around way too long, pumping out less ATP (energy) and more harmful reactive oxygen species (ROS). It's like a recycling plant where the conveyor belts jam. Instead of old, broken parts getting cleared out to make way for new, efficient ones, the junk keeps piling up. Your cells are forced to run on outdated, glitchy machinery that leaks toxins and waste at every turn (37, 38).

What Causes Lipofuscin—The Bioenergetic Prospective

From a bioenergetic perspective, lipofuscin is a telltale sign that your cells have been under chronic stress, and it's not just about getting older. Lipofuscin is that brownish-yellow pigment that builds up inside cells when your mitochondria and lysosomes can't keep up with damage. Under the microscope, it's literally oxidized clumps of fats, proteins, metals (like iron and copper), and other cellular leftovers.

So why does this happen?

Polyunsaturated fats (PUFAs) are especially prone to oxidation. They're like unstable firewood; too many double bonds make them eager to react with free radicals. When your mitochondria are stressed (or overloaded with iron), these PUFAs get peroxidized (lipid oxidation), producing toxic byproducts like aldehydes that damage proteins and DNA, which then end up trapped in lipofuscin (I will talk more about this in the next chapter) (39, 40).

Iron makes this exponentially worse. Free iron catalyzes the Fenton reaction, turning mild oxidative byproducts into savage hydroxyl radicals. This is why tissues that accumulate iron often show more lipofuscin (41).

Excess estrogen indirectly fans the flames too. It tends to promote iron uptake and retention, increases polyunsaturated fat deposition, suppresses thyroid hormone (reducing protective CO_2), and can heighten oxidative stress, all of which set the stage for more lipofuscin (42).

What you need to know is that lipofuscin is more than a harmless pigment of aging. It's a cellular scar left by years of oxidative imbalance, a combination of too much iron, too many unstable fats, and hormonal states that push metabolism toward stress.

So, in the end, too much iron doesn't just sit there quietly. It's actively stirring up oxidative chaos, slowing down thyroid hormone activation, and jamming up your cellular recycling systems. The result? Less energy, more cellular damage, and a vicious cycle that leaves you feeling like a city where the garbage trucks stopped running, trash piles up, and the whole system starts to stink.

What Does Iron Overload Look Like?

When most people hear "iron overload," they think of the hereditary genetic condition hemochromatosis. This is caused primarily by a mutation in the HFE gene, which disrupts how your body senses iron levels and controls hepcidin production. The mutation keeps hepcidin chronically low, so iron absorption stays high, pulling in more iron from food, year after year, with no real off switch (41).

In hereditary hemochromatosis, this excess iron piles up everywhere it shouldn't: the liver, pancreas, heart, joints, and even your skin (hello, bronze skin and age spots). People can end up with cirrhosis, heart arrhythmias, arthritis that makes you feel 80 at age 35, and a telltale bronzing of the skin, not from a healthy tan, but from excessive iron storage. There's also a 30–60% chance of developing diabetes (nicknamed "bronze diabetes"), thanks to iron damaging the pancreatic beta cells and accelerating insulin resistance (43).

Classic symptoms of full-blown hemochromatosis are:

- Fatigue and weakness. The most common, but easiest to dismiss. It comes from iron-driven mitochondrial stress.

- Joint pain and stiffness (often the knuckles, hands, hips, knees). This is sometimes mistaken for early arthritis.

- Skin bronzing or hyperpigmentation. This gives a tanned or grayish look, especially on sun-exposed areas.

- Diabetes ("bronze diabetes"). From iron damaging pancreatic beta cells, leading to insulin resistance.

- Liver enlargement (hepatomegaly). This can progress to cirrhosis over time.

- Heart rhythm problems (arrhythmias) or heart failure. This happens if iron deposits in cardiac tissue.

- Hormonal issues. Loss of libido or impotence in men, irregular periods or early menopause in women, from iron affecting the pituitary gland.

- Abdominal pain. This can be due to liver congestion.

- Cancer. Iron is a powerful pro-oxidant producing excessive free radicals. These free radicals can damage DNA, proteins, and cell membranes. Plus, tumors love iron.

Hereditary hemochromatosis is often first suspected based on elevated ferritin and transferrin saturation levels and is typically confirmed through genetic testing for mutations in the HFE gene, most commonly the C282Y and H63D variants.

But here's the good news: full-blown hereditary hemochromatosis is rare.

Even though 1 in 200 to 300 people carry two copies of the faulty gene, most stay asymptomatic. Only about 1–5% develop serious complications, while another 10–30% might accumulate enough iron to run into problems down the road. Many more people carry just one copy of the gene, which might slightly raise their tendency to store iron but usually doesn't cause the runaway train wreck of full disease (44).

So, if hemochromatosis is what most people think of as iron overload, what about everyone else? Well, here's where it gets interesting, and frankly way more relevant to most people.

You don't need faulty genes to slowly accumulate too much iron. Plenty of men, women on hormones, postmenopausal women (who've stopped losing iron monthly), and those consuming excessive amounts of iron supplements or even foods with iron, can quietly build up iron over decades.

How Does This Happen?

A dysregulated RES. Eating iron-rich foods is perfectly healthy, but if your RES isn't recycling properly (due to low copper, vitamin A, or zinc) that iron starts to stockpile.

Alcohol consumption. Alcohol lowers hepcidin and increases gut permeability, so your gut pulls in more iron.

Estrogen. Estrogen from birth control, hormone therapy, xenoestrogens, peripheral estrogen, and even ovarian estrogen can blunt hepcidin too, nudging iron absorption higher.

Excessive iron supplementation, without proper copper, vitamin A, and zinc consumption. Iron supplements can work temporarily but without copper and vitamin A, to help regulate iron, iron can sequester into the tissue, rather than be used by cells.

So, while hereditary hemochromatosis might look like a runaway train smashing through your liver, this milder iron overload is more like a slow leak in your plumbing, barely noticeable at first, but over the years it can still flood your basement.

Symptoms of Iron Overload Without the Genetic Markers of Hemochromatosis:

- Mild fatigue that doesn't improve with rest or iron supplements

- Brain fog or trouble concentrating

- Slightly elevated blood sugar

- Hypothyroid-like symptoms (cold hands/feet, slow metabolism)

- Recurrent infections (some pathogens thrive on excess iron)

What Iron Overload May Look Like on a Blood Lab

You might expect iron overload to jump off the page on your labs, but it's often sneakier, showing up as patterns that look "pretty normal" until you know what to watch for.

- Ferritin often sits over 200–300 ng/mL, especially in men and postmenopausal women. But there are a few caveats, ferritin can also rise with inflammation, infections, or even after a tough workout. In addition, you can have overloaded tissues with ferritin that looks perfectly average.

- Transferrin saturation (TSAT) tends to climb above 45–50%, sometimes soaring into the 60–80% range. This means your transport proteins (shuttle buses) are getting maxed out.

- Serum iron might be high-normal or mildly elevated, but it fluctuates from day to day, so it's easy to miss.

- TIBC (Total Iron Binding Capacity) often drops, since your transferrin buses are already full, there's not much extra room to grab more iron.

- You might also see slightly elevated fasting glucose or A1c, since iron can interfere with energy production and insulin signaling.

- Liver enzymes (ALT, AST) can run a bit high too, hinting that your liver is taking on extra strain as it tries to manage the iron load.

Even if your numbers are only slightly out of range, or your doctor reassures you everything is "fine," I would still watch for blood lab and symptom changes. When ferritin starts to elevate, TSAT creeps past 45%, and liver enzymes and blood sugar start moving north, it can be a sign your system is trying to handle more iron than it knows what to do with.

Pair this with skin changes, stubborn joint aches, or fatigue that will not go away, and you might be looking at the metabolic slow leak of iron overload, which can happen long before it ever looks like classic hemochromatosis.

Looking back, I believe I suffered from this exact pattern of iron overload, even while being repeatedly told I was "iron anemic."

Like I told you earlier, for years, I took iron supplements, chasing lab numbers that never seemed to stay up and symptoms that never seemed to improve. I finally realized I was starving my body of copper-rich foods. Without enough copper to keep my RES recycling system humming, my body began hoarding iron in all the wrong places.

Meanwhile, during this time, life was piling on stress (bad break up, adverse reaction to Botox, negative thoughts). My cortisol was high, which likely lowered my hepcidin further, pulling in even more iron from my gut. I started developing skin changes, age spots and a bronzy tint that no amount of exfoliating would fix. I became achy, stiff, and felt a fatigue that just wouldn't go away.

Eventually, all that excess iron (paired with low copper and sky-high stress) took its toll on my nerves too. I developed small fiber neuropathy, a burning, tingling reminder that my mitochondria and nerves had been under siege.

It took a lot of research, stopping the iron supplements, loading up on copper-rich foods like beef liver, and making myself my number one priority (reduced work, brain retraining, breath work, eating enough), before my body could begin to rebalance. Even then, it's been years of slow improvement. But in hindsight, the pattern couldn't be clearer: I wasn't just low on iron. I was drowning in it, metabolically speaking, and paying the price for a system that couldn't regulate it properly.

So, while you might think, *"Whew, I don't have hemochromatosis, I'm in the clear,"* the truth is a bit murkier. Many people can carry milder iron load that never gets flagged by routine labs, yet it's still enough to slow down your mitochondria, age your tissues, and leave you feeling like sh#t.

Which, I am sure, is making you ask the question, "How do I keep my iron in check?" In other words, you want to make sure you have enough for optimal function, but not too much for iron overload.

How You Keep Your Iron in Check

So, you've seen how iron overload can creep up, what it feels like, and what it might look like in your labs. Now comes the million-dollar question:

How do you keep your iron levels in that metabolic Goldilocks zone? Enough to fuel your thyroid, mitochondria, and oxygen delivery, but not so much that it's rusting your tissues from the inside out.

Well, it turns out, you don't have to become iron-phobic or avoid every piece of steak for the rest of your life. It's about supporting your body's iron recycling system, maintaining gut and liver health, practicing some basic lifestyle habits, and utilizing specific supplements if necessary.

Support Your Iron Recycling System

Remember, about 90% of your daily iron needs are met by recycling old red blood cells. Only 10% comes from what you eat. This means the health of your reticuloendothelial system (RES) is incredibly important.

Your RES runs best when it has all its supporting nutrients, including copper, vitamin A, and zinc. These nutrients help load iron onto transferrin, keep it circulating properly, and support red blood cell turnover. Without these supportive nutrients, iron can sequester into the tissue, producing functional iron deficiency, a situation where you have plenty of iron, yet it's stored in the wrong places.

As discussed earlier, the best way to get enough iron and all the nutrients that regulate iron is to consume foods that contain all these nutrients. These include beef liver, beef, eggs, oysters, dairy, and even well-cooked leafy green vegetables.

Support Gut Health (So You Don't Swing into Anemia or Overload)

Your gut plays a surprisingly complex role in iron balance. Inflammatory gut issues like SIBO, IBD, or celiac disease often end in iron deficiency anemia because inflamed or damaged intestines simply can't absorb iron well. Chronic bleeding from irritated tissues adds to the problem, draining iron faster than you can replace it.

But here's the paradox; the same gut dysfunction can sometimes lead to unregulated iron absorption, especially if the lining becomes "leaky." When your gut barrier breaks down and hepcidin regulation gets disrupted (due to stress, estrogen, or alcohol), more iron slips through in ways your body wouldn't normally allow. Meanwhile, a disturbed microbiome means fewer friendly bacteria competing for iron, further tipping the scales.

Since I have already written extensively on gut health, I'll leave you with some quick refreshers:

- **Avoid chronic gut irritants** - excess alcohol, hard to digest foods—nuts, seeds, raw vegetables, ultra-processed foods, unnecessary antibiotics.

- **Consume plenty of nutrient-rich foods** to support gut motility and energy production. Whole fruits, juices, animal proteins, dairy, honey, roots, cooked vegetables, and even white sugar.

- **Manage stress** - stress increases intestinal permeability and lowers hepcidin, allowing the body to absorb more iron.

- **Gut cleansers** - carrot salad, cooked mushrooms, bamboo shoots, activated charcoal, soil-based probiotics.

- **Reduce endotoxins** - limit alcohol, estrogen exposure, PUFA.

- **Support motility** - coffee, cascara sagrada, magnesium, movement.

In short, a healthy gut does far more than just digest your food, it acts like a smart gatekeeper for iron, deciding how much to let in and when. Keep your gut lining strong, reduce irritants, and keep your digestion moving, and you'll naturally avoid swinging into hidden overload or running dry into anemia. It's one of the simplest ways to let your body regulate iron exactly as it was designed to, without all the additional micromanagements.

Keep Hepcidin in Check

Hepcidin, a small peptide hormone produced mainly by your liver, is your body's iron gatekeeper. When hepcidin levels are high, iron absorption drops; when hepcidin is low, more iron pours in.

Alcohol and estrogen are two of the biggest factors that suppress hepcidin.

- Alcohol lowers hepcidin, while making your gut more permeable, both of which drive more iron absorption. In addition, it does not help that alcohol damages your liver, the very organ that produces hepcidin and serves as your biggest iron warehouse (6). If you suspect iron overload, cutting back or giving up alcohol is one of the smartest first moves.

- Estrogen, whether from birth control, MHT, xenoestrogens in plastics, or just your own ovarian production can blunt hepcidin, letting more iron slip through. This helps explain why cardiovascular disease rises so dramatically after menopause, when women lose their monthly way of shedding iron (7, 8). (For more on mitigating estrogen's effects, see the estrogen chapter.)

On the flip side, inflammation and infections ramp hepcidin up.

Your immune system uses hepcidin as a defensive strategy; during infections or chronic inflammation (like autoimmune conditions, insulin resistance, diabetes, or even dental infections), your body raises hepcidin to tuck iron safely into storage, away from bacteria and pathogens that thrive on it. That's why high ferritin, especially when paired with low serum iron and low transferrin saturation, is a hallmark for inflammation and a sign of anemia of chronic disease.

Yes, you can absolutely feel "anemic" while your ferritin is high. In this case, your body is keeping iron locked away on purpose. The real fix isn't more iron but treating the root of the infection (sometimes with antibiotics) or lowering inflammation by resting, managing stress, and making sure you're eating enough to support recovery.

Understand the Effects that Certain Foods Have on Iron Absorption.

If you suspect your iron levels might be out of balance, too high or too low, it helps to know which foods and supplements can nudge iron absorption up or down.

Animal Foods vs. Plant Foods:
Animal foods like beef, liver, fish, and poultry contain heme iron,
iron already bound to a porphyrin ring, which makes it far easier to
absorb. Heme iron absorption is less influenced by hepcidin, dietary
inhibitors, or even your body's existing iron stores. This means you'll
take in a steady amount, regardless of your feedback loops or current
ferritin levels.

By contrast, plant foods like grains, legumes, vegetables, and most
iron supplements contain non-heme iron. This form is highly
regulated by hepcidin, meal composition, and your existing iron
stores. So, when ferritin is high, absorption drops dramatically; when
iron is low, absorption ramps up.

On average, heme iron is absorbed at 2–3 times the rate of non-heme
iron. That's incredibly helpful if you're battling anemia, but it can be
risky if you already have iron overload. People with elevated iron
often need to limit or avoid heme iron, unless it's consumed alongside
nutrient-dense foods that help regulate iron (like those rich in copper
and vitamin A). Even then, it's wise to keep portions small, roughly
2–3 ounces a week.

Coffee, tea, and cocoa:
These are rich in polyphenols that significantly reduce absorption
of non-heme iron (the type found in plants and supplements). They
have little effect on heme iron (from meat), so your dark roast won't
block the iron in your steak.

Calcium-rich foods:
Dairy, fish bones (like in sardines), and well-cooked leafy greens all
reduce absorption of both heme and non-heme iron. That means if
you have high iron, enjoying cheese or a glass of milk with your liver
or steak can blunt some of that uptake. On the flip side, if you're low
on iron, you'll want to keep calcium-rich foods away from your iron-
heavy meals (45).

Vitamin C (ascorbic acid):

This is the superstar for boosting non-heme iron absorption. It helps by reducing ferric iron (Fe^{3+}) to the more soluble ferrous form (Fe^{2+}) in your gut, making it easier to absorb. So yes, your OJ with spinach will help, but pairing orange juice with liver won't change much, because heme iron already sails through its own absorption route.

Phytate-rich foods:

Grains, legumes, nuts, and seeds contain phytates that can strongly inhibit non-heme iron absorption. However, they also block zinc, calcium, and magnesium. So, if you're dealing with iron overload, I wouldn't rely on phytates as your primary defense, they might starve you of other crucial minerals too.

Lactoferrin:

This iron-binding glycoprotein is found abundantly in human breast milk (especially colostrum) and in cow's milk. It's fascinating because it acts like a smart iron buffer. Low iron levels? Lactoferrin can boost absorption by reducing gut inflammation and hepcidin (46, 47). But if you're overloaded, it helps bind up free iron, reducing oxidative stress and keeping excess iron from damaging tissues (48, 49).

Lactoferrin vs. Colostrum, What's Better for Iron Regulation?

If you're aiming to keep your iron in that Goldilocks zone, not too high, not too low, you might wonder whether to reach for colostrum (the "first milk" loaded with immune goodies) or a purified lactoferrin supplement.

Here's the scoop:

Lactoferrin supplements

- These are like the sniper version: precise, targeted, and consistent.

- They're standardized to give you 100–200 mg of lactoferrin, the exact doses used in human studies to raise iron when you're deficient or help regulate iron and cut down oxidative stress if you're overloaded.

- Think of it as a straight shot of your body's own natural iron chaperone.

Colostrum powders

- These are more like the fancy form of lactoferrin, with the price that follows.

- Yes, they contain lactoferrin, but usually only 5–10% by weight, and it can vary wildly by brand, processing, and how soon it was harvested after calving.

- You'd have to take big scoops (5–10 grams) to get into the ~250 mg lactoferrin range. But you're also getting growth factors and immunoglobulins that support gut repair and immunity.

Essentially, if your goal is targeted iron regulation, purified lactoferrin is your best bet.

If you're after wider gut-healing support, colostrum has its perks, but you will pay the price, as most quality brands are expensive.

Cut Back on Iron Supplements and Fortified Foods

If you're dealing with iron overload (or even suspect your levels are creeping up), the simplest starting point is to scale back iron supplements and watch for heavily fortified foods (like many cereals, granola bars, or "enriched" flours).

Most people don't realize that many processed foods are loaded with added iron, often in a metallic form that isn't well-regulated by your body's normal absorption controls. If your hepcidin is already low (from stress, estrogen, or genetics), you could be absorbing more of these irons than your tissues can safely handle.

But here's an important caveat:

Even if you have low iron, it's still best to rely on food sources rather than jumping straight to supplements or fortified foods. The iron in fortified foods and supplements are cheap, stable, and designed to meet RDA guidelines, but your body does not regulate them as well as it does iron in whole foods.

Foods like beef, liver, eggs, and leafy greens come packaged with co-factors (like copper, vitamin A, and zinc) that help your body regulate and use iron properly.

That said, some people genuinely need iron supplements, especially if they have increased blood losses (heavy periods, GI bleeding), are pregnant, or have very low hemoglobin that diet alone can't fix quickly. In these cases, short-term targeted supplementation under medical supervision makes perfect sense.

Move and Sweat

Studies show you can lose anywhere from 0.2 to 0.5 mg of iron per liter of sweat. That means with high-volume sweating (from intense workouts or hot environments), you could lose 1–1.5 mg of iron per day.

If you're dealing with iron overload, sweating more, whether through exercise or sauna, can be a helpful strategy to gently reduce iron stores (50, 51). Just be mindful; forcing your body into high heat or intense workouts adds stress, so make sure you're healthy enough to handle it.

Start slow with 10-15 minutes of activity or sauna usage and increase daily if your body feels good and not overwhelmed. Signs you have done too much are fatigue, sleep issues, loss of appetite, and/or anxiety. Always pair intense activity or sweating with adequate fluids, sugars, and minerals to replenish electrolytes and protect circulation.

On the flip side, if you're a heavy sweater and prone to low iron, you might need to bump up your intake of iron-rich foods to offset these losses.

For perspective:

- In everyday life, most people lose about 400–700 mL/day through sweat and skin evaporation without even noticing.

- Mild activity or warmer temps can push this to ~1 liter/day, while heavy exercise or hot humid conditions can shoot it up to 1–2 liters *per hour*.

Sweating isn't the biggest tool for lowering iron, but it's a gentle, natural one, and when done safely, it can absolutely help.

Consider Donating Blood

Blood donation is hands down the fastest, most reliable way to lower excess iron.

Each standard donation is about 500 mL (1 pint) of blood. Since there's roughly 0.5 mg of iron per mL of blood, that means you'll drop about 250 mg of iron in one go. Most people see ferritin levels fall by 30–50 points after a donation.

The basics:

- You must be over 17, weigh at least 50 kg (110 lbs.), and have a minimum hemoglobin of 12.5 g/dL (women) or 13.0 g/dL (men) to ensure you're not already anemic.

- You can donate every 8 weeks for whole blood, or every 16 weeks for double red cell donations (which remove twice as many red cells, and twice the iron).

There's also some evidence that blood donors, who typically have lower iron stores, may have fewer heart events (52). That might be because less iron means less oxidative stress. Or it could just be "healthy donor bias," since people well enough to donate are generally healthier to start with. Either way, donating blood saves lives, possibly someone else's today, and maybe yours in the long run.

Keeping your iron in check isn't about fear, avoidance, or obsessing over whether you're eating too much or too little iron. It's about creating the right internal environment, with the proper minerals, vitamins, gut health, hormone balance, and simple daily strategies that keep iron moving where it should, not stockpiling where it shouldn't. When your system is supported, iron naturally stays in that sweet metabolic Goldilocks zone: enough to energize your mitochondria and oxygen delivery, but not so much that it's quietly rusting your tissues from the inside out.

So, there you have it, the double edges of iron. A critical nutrient when kept in check, but a sneaky oxidizing force when it piles up in all the wrong places.

But iron isn't the only player that can quietly sabotage your mitochondria, trash your thyroid, and age your tissues from the inside out. If iron is the match that can spark oxidative fires, then our next topic is the fuel that feeds them, the increasingly famous polyunsaturated fats.

In fact, you could have perfect gut health, beautifully balanced minerals, and flawless iron recycling, but if you're flooding your cells with unstable fats that oxidize at the first sign of stress, you're still setting your mitochondria up to struggle.

In this next chapter, we're going to tackle the final big energy block head-on: how polyunsaturated fats (PUFAs) quietly destabilize your metabolism, damage your cell membranes, and keep you stuck in low-energy mode, and more importantly, how to get them out of the way so your cells can finally breathe.

So, let's keep going and *iron-out* the issues over those unsaturated fats.

CHAPTER 11

THE BOTTOM LINE

Iron: The Double-Edged Sword
How Excess Iron Can Sabotage Your Energy Production

1. Iron is essential for ATP production, hemoglobin formation, oxygen delivery, and thyroid hormone synthesis and conversion.

2. Iron absorption increases with heme iron, vitamin C, alcohol, estrogen, and a disrupted gut microbiome.

3. Iron absorption decreases with phytates, polyphenols, calcium, copper, manganese, zinc, low stomach acid, small intestine inflammation, and elevated hepcidin levels.

4. 90% of daily iron needs are recycled through your reticuloendothelial system (RES), which breaks down aging red blood cells and reclaims their iron. This system relies on more than just iron, it needs copper, vitamin A, zinc, and B vitamins to function properly.

5. Iron overload impairs energy by driving oxidative stress through the Fenton reaction (via non-transferrin-bound iron), disrupting thyroid function, and increasing lipofuscin accumulation.

6. Iron overload can stem from genetic mutations (like hemochromatosis), excessive iron intake (via supplements or fortified foods), a dysregulated RES, alcohol use, or chronic estrogen exposure.

7. Regulating iron means eating nutrient-dense foods that support RES function, maintaining gut health, minimizing alcohol and estrogen exposure, understanding what increases or decreases absorption, avoiding unnecessary supplementation or fortification, staying active, and considering blood donation when appropriate.

CHAPTER 12

THE POLYUNSATURATED FATS: HEART HEALTHY OR ENERGY KILLER?

If you've read my first book, *How to Heal Your Metabolism,* you already know I have strong opinions about polyunsaturated fats, better known as PUFAs. These fragile fats, hiding in seed oils, vegetable oils, nuts, seeds, fatty fish, and just about all forms of processed foods (even the organic ones), have now stepped into the spotlight of one of the biggest nutrition debates of our time.

On one side, health practitioners and bioenergetic thinkers warn that PUFAs are ticking time bombs, unstable fats that disrupt mitochondria, inflame tissues, and accelerate aging. On the other, mainstream medicine continues to champion them, pointing to piles of research showing PUFAs lower cholesterol and additional evidence showing they are not harmful, and even heart protective.

Here's the frustrating part, both sides have data to back them up. Human short term and observational studies often show that replacing saturated fats with PUFAs improves blood markers and, in some cases, cardiovascular outcomes. The anti-PUFA camp counters that these studies are short, focus on the wrong endpoints, and fail to capture the slow oxidative damage PUFAs may cause over time. In addition, they point to additional animal studies and a few long-term human studies that show the harmful health effects of excessive PUFA exposure.

So yes, the PUFA debate is alive, loud, and confusing. Who's right? Who's missing the bigger picture?

In this chapter, we'll dig into both sides, the evidence that paints PUFAs as "heart healthy" and the research suggesting they may be inhibiting your cellular energy. You'll see how PUFAs interact with your mitochondria and why this interaction matters for energy, metabolism, and long-term health. Along the way, I'll challenge the mainstream belief that "PUFA oils are safe" and show you why I consider polyunsaturated fats to be the sixth and final energy block standing in the way of optimal health and metabolism.

First, What Exactly are PUFAs?

Since I don't expect anyone to have memorized my first book (*gold star if you have!*), let's start with a quick refresher on what PUFAs are, where they come from, and why they matter.

Polyunsaturated fats, or PUFAs, are fatty acids that contain multiple double bonds in their chemical structure. They're called "unsaturated" because they're not fully saturated with hydrogen, and "polyunsaturated" because they have more than one of these double bonds.

But here is the deal, those double bonds make PUFAs flexible in membranes (why they are liquid at room temperature) but also highly reactive to oxygen. While a double bond is stronger than a single bond, the double bond makes the surrounding structure weaker. This makes the fats more chemically unstable, making these fats prone to oxidation, the same process that causes oils to go rancid or metals to rust.

Where Do We Find Them?

PUFAs are everywhere in the modern diet. You'll find them concentrated in:

- Seed oils: soybean, corn, sunflower, canola, safflower
- Nuts and nut oils
- Vegetable oils: The backbone of almost every processed food, loaded with omega-6s
- Soy and corn-fed chicken and pork: Their fat composition mirrors their feed
- Fatty fish, naturally rich in omega-3 PUFAs

Unlike the stable saturated fats found in butter or coconut oil, PUFAs are fragile. They break down easily under heat, light, and stress, producing reactive byproducts that can damage cells.

Which makes you stop and ask:

If PUFAs are so unstable, why do we have them at all? Why would nature build something this delicate into our food and even into our cells if it serves no purpose? After all, PUFAs are also found in smaller amounts in nutrient-dense, pro-metabolic foods like liver, eggs, oysters, and milk. So, can they really be all bad? (I will get to this later.)

Like most things in nutrition, the answer is nuanced. There's a valid argument that some PUFA oils, particularly omega-3 and omega-6, are essential because the human body cannot make them on its own. There is also an argument that these oils have numerous health benefits, which is why they are so touted in most medical circles.

With that, let's get into the argument as to why polyunsaturated fats are seen as a health benefit vs. a metabolic energy burden.

The Mainstream Story: The "Heart-Healthy" Polyunsaturated Fats

For decades, mainstream science and nutrition have celebrated polyunsaturated fats (PUFAs), particularly omega-6 linoleic acid from seed oils and omega-3s from fish, branding them as heart-protective, anti-inflammatory, and even as shields against diabetes. And to be fair, they have an army of studies backing them up. According to this view, PUFAs are basically the Mack-daddies of dietary fat.

PUFAs Lower Cholesterol (Cue the Applause by Every Heart Doctor)

Yes, this one is true, PUFAs do lower LDL and total cholesterol. They pull this off by upregulating LDL receptors in the liver, which snatch LDL particles from the blood like a compulsive clothes hoarder raiding a 50%-off clearance rack, grabbing everything in sight without hesitation. They also inhibit HMG-CoA reductase, the same enzyme statin drugs target. Reduced enzyme activity means less cholesterol production (1,2). So, if the end game is simply lowering cholesterol numbers, the "eat more PUFAs" advice makes perfect sense. But whether that's the healthiest thing...well, that's the story we have yet to unfold.

Meta-analyses of dozens of RCTs have found that replacing saturated fats with PUFAs results in significant LDL reductions and, in some cases, a modest dip in heart attack incidence. A landmark 2010 review of eight RCTs found about a 10% reduction in coronary heart disease events per 5% of energy replaced with PUFAs (3). A 2014 meta-analysis echoed this, reporting a 9% lower risk of cardiovascular events and 13% fewer CHD deaths for every 5% of energy from dietary linoleic acid swapped in for saturated fat (4).

Observational studies also pile on the support. The NHANES cohort, which followed over 45,000 adults, found that every 5% increase in PUFA calories correlated with a 9% lower risk of heart-related death (5). On paper, this all looks pretty damn compelling.

PUFAs: Anti-Inflammatory and Diabetes-Friendly?

Mainstream science doesn't stop at the heart. It also claims PUFAs soothe inflammation and keep type 2 diabetes at bay. The reasoning goes like this: PUFAs, thanks to their flexible double bonds, slide into cell membranes, making them more fluid. This membrane upgrade supposedly improves insulin receptor function, helping glucose get where it needs to go. On top of that, some studies show PUFAs reduce low-grade inflammation, one of the villains in insulin resistance, and even lower liver fat, which can improve glucose control (6,7,8).

One of the strongest cases comes from a pooled analysis of nearly 40,000 adults across 20 observational studies. Those with higher blood levels of linoleic acid, the omega-6 star of seed oils, had a 35% lower risk of developing type 2 diabetes compared to those with the lowest levels (9). Cohort studies like the Nurses' Health Study and Health Professionals Follow-Up Study back this up, finding that people with higher linoleic acid blood levels tend to have lower inflammation markers, less diabetes, and fewer cardiovascular events (10). From this lens, linoleic acid isn't a villain at all, but rather a metabolic superhero.

So, case closed, right? Well, not so fast.

From the mainstream perspective, PUFAs come out looking squeaky clean, they lower cholesterol, improve inflammation markers, and reduce disease risk. This is why the official advice keeps telling you to swap butter for vegetable oil, eat more nuts, and throw some more salmon on the grill.

But before you start bathing in canola oil, know this, this is only half the story. These studies, while impressive, are often short-term, typically one or two years, or they are observational studies, which show correlation, not causation. They might also focus on easy-to-measure markers like cholesterol, which can be temporarily lowered even if underlying cellular health is tanking. A suppressed immune response can look like "low inflammation" on paper, but that doesn't necessarily equal better health.

When you shift the lens to energy production and how well your cells create energy, the narrative changes. The damage PUFAs may cause at the mitochondrial level doesn't always show up in these studies because it's a slow burn, the kind of thing that takes years or decades to fully manifest. So, while the mainstream celebrates improved lab results, the long game might tell a different story.

As we'll see next, the debate heats up when we stop asking, *"Do PUFAs lower cholesterol?"* and start asking, *"Do PUFAs make our cells healthier in the long run?"* That's when the PUFA debate really gets interesting.

Why the "Heart-Healthy" PUFA Story Might Be Misleading

On the surface, lowering cholesterol looks like a win, your labs look better, your doctor smiles, and everyone's happy. But dig a little deeper, and you'll see it's not that simple. Chasing lower numbers without context can do more harm than good.

Why Lower Cholesterol Isn't Always a Good Thing

For decades, cholesterol has been cast as the villain of modern medicine. The moment your total cholesterol creeps over 200, doctors reach for the prescription pad, ready to hand out statins as if they're candy. Butter? Eggs? Forget it, apparently, they are coming for your arteries, like a hairball clogs your sink. But the truth is lowering cholesterol isn't always the best thing for your health or your cells.

Your liver doesn't crank up cholesterol production because it has a statin deficiency. It makes cholesterol because your cells need it. Cholesterol is the raw material for every cell membrane, every steroid hormone (think cortisol, estrogen, testosterone, progesterone), bile salts, and even vitamin D. Which means less cholesterol could also result in less of all of these!

Cholesterol also rises under stress because it's part of your body's adaptive repair toolkit, helping build and restore tissues when things go sideways. The problem isn't high cholesterol itself; the problem is when cholesterol oxidizes. Under conditions of chronic stress, inflammation, smoking, or diabetes, cholesterol can be transformed by reactive oxygen species (ROS) into damaging oxysterols. These oxidized molecules can accumulate, forming plaques, injuring arteries, and triggering inflammation (11).

Another thing to think about is that under stress, thyroid hormone levels, particularly T3, drop. And what's T3's job? Among many things, it's needed to convert cholesterol into your steroidal hormones, vitamin D and even bile salts. Without enough T3, the production of these three things can lower, and cholesterol levels rise. This is why elevated cholesterol is a classic sign of hypothyroidism.

Then there's the issue of PUFAs (and statins) inhibiting the HMG-CoA reductase enzyme. This enzyme doesn't just make cholesterol, it also drives the production of Coenzyme Q10 (CoQ10), a crucial nutrient for mitochondrial energy and antioxidant defense (12). When this pathway is suppressed, CoQ10 levels can plummet, starving your muscles of the energy they need to function. The result is muscle irritation, damage, fatigue, and pain. This is one reason many statin users complain about muscle issues, and why some doctors pair statins with CoQ10 supplements (13,14).

Finally, let's talk about the cultures that completely blow up the "elevated cholesterol is bad" narrative. Traditional groups like the Maasai and Polynesian tribes such as the Tokelauans and Pukapukans (15,16) thrive on diets high in saturated fats and low in PUFAs. They often have higher cholesterol levels, yet heart disease is virtually absent. They weren't pounding seed oils or obsessing over LDL particles. Their cholesterol was doing its job, protecting, repairing, and supporting their cells, proving that higher-than-normal cholesterol doesn't automatically spell poor health.

So, before you throw a party over your plummeting cholesterol numbers courtesy of a PUFA-heavy diet or a statin, remember this, your body makes cholesterol on purpose. The goal isn't to shut it down; it's to keep it from oxidizing. That means reducing stress, sleeping well, eating nutrient-rich foods, and supporting your thyroid, so cholesterol can do what it's meant to do: protect your cells, and turn into hormones, bile, and vitamin D.

Statins: Context Is Everything

I'm going to say something that might irritate a few health influencers, but for the sake of context and nuance, it needs to be said.

It's easy to criticize doctors and statins when you're deep in the health world, reading bioenergetic theories and doing everything to optimize your metabolism. But let's flip the lens for a moment and see this from a doctor's perspective.

Doctors aren't trying to rob your husband or friend of their cholesterol; they're trying to keep them alive. Medical doctors work with patients who are overweight, stressed, inflamed, eating processed foods, and, let's be honest, are unlikely to completely overhaul their diets or lifestyles. For these high-risk individuals, statins lower LDL cholesterol and reduce cardiovascular events, at least in the short to medium term. In these cases, statins can absolutely be the right tool at the right time (17,18).

Despite what some health influencers may tell you, statins do work in populations that aren't changing anything else. They're not magic bullets, but they do reduce risk where risk is high. For someone unwilling or unable to make lifestyle changes, a statin may be the thing that keeps a cardiovascular event at bay, at least for a while.

The real problem is when medications create a false sense of security. Many people believe that because their lab numbers look better, they don't need to change their habits, so they don't. Statins lower cholesterol, but they do not fix the underlying reasons it's elevated in the first place.

Statins also come with potential risks and side effects including myalgia (muscle aches), myopathy (muscle inflammation), rhabdomyolysis (muscle breakdown), reduced CoQ10 levels, increased risks of diabetes, and liver injury (19, 20, 21). Yet, even knowing all of this, for some taking a statin is still a better option than doing nothing and facing higher risk.

At the same time, I want to be clear: dropping your statins and loading up on saturated fat because "the Maasai do it" is not the fix you think it is. These tribes eat whole foods, move daily, and live in strong communities, factors that likely protect against cholesterol oxidation, the real danger behind high cholesterol.

Your health choices matter. If you're supporting your metabolism, eating nutrient-rich foods, managing stress, staying active, reducing alcohol, avoiding smoking, and taking care of your thyroid, then eliminating your statins might be the right choice, but always talk to your doctor first. If you're tossing your medication just because a social media influencer told you statins are "bad," it's time to rethink that decision.

Essentially, don't ditch your statin because of something you read online. Work with your doctor, know your risk, and make changes thoughtfully.

But What About All Those Studies Saying PUFAs Are Heart-Healthy?

At first glance, the data does look convincing, higher PUFA intake seems to mean fewer cardiovascular events. If you stop there, PUFAs start to look like the superhero your doctor promised would save your heart and arteries. But much like statins, the story is more complicated.

For one, most of the randomized controlled trials (RCTs) showing a benefit from PUFAs were done on populations that were already quite sick. We're not talking about metabolically healthy, active adults who eat real food. These were mostly middle-aged or older men, overweight, stressed, diabetic, smoking, and often recovering from heart attacks.

When you start with a high-risk group, anything that lowers LDL cholesterol or reduces inflammation, whether it's statins or a jug of corn oil, will look protective in the short term. This is exactly what we saw in the Oslo Diet-Heart Study, men with previous heart attacks had fewer repeat events when they swapped butter for PUFA oils. If the only intervention is replacing one fat with another, short-term numbers could improve because these people were starting from a bad place (22).

Yet, here's the problem, most RCTs only run for a few years. That's long enough to count heart attacks but far too short to reveal the slow burn of oxidative stress or cellular damage that might show up decades later. The few longer-term studies we have tell a very different story:

The LA Veterans Trial (1959–1967): 846 male veterans, living in institutional settings were studied. Half continued a diet higher in saturated fat, while 1/2 swapped saturated fats for PUFA oils. While the PUFA diet lowered cholesterol and reduced certain heart events, it did not significantly extend life, due to an increase in non-CVD deaths. Essentially, as time went by, more people started to die of other things, including cancer (23).

The Sydney Diet Heart Study (1966–1973): 458 men at high risk of CHD disease. Half the men continued their high saturated fat diet, while half were instructed to replace saturated fat with PUFAs. The PUFA-arm didn't just fail to improve, these men died at higher rates from coronary heart disease, cardiovascular causes, and all causes combined. Not exactly the "heart-healthy" result researchers expected (24).

The Minnesota Coronary Experiment (1968–1973): Nearly 9,500 institutionalized men and women participated in one of the most tightly controlled dietary trials ever conducted (Institutionalized individual's diets can be controlled over long periods of time). Those in the PUFA group saw their cholesterol plummet. However, despite the dramatic drop in cholesterol, there was no reduction in deaths from coronary heart disease, and all-cause mortality went up. Even more striking, the data revealed that the lower the cholesterol fell, the higher the risk of dying, a finding that completely flipped the diet-heart hypothesis on its head (25).

Essentially, most short-term trials show benefits, like decreased cholesterol, and fewer CV events, but long-term trials start to show a different story.

Observational studies, like the Nurses' Health Study, cloud the water even further. This study found that people who ate more PUFAs also tend to exercise more, smoke less, and eat more fruits and veggies. Even with adjustments, it's impossible to completely strip out this "healthy-user bias." So, while these studies often show PUFAs as beneficial, the fats themselves may not deserve all the credit.

The benefit of observational research is that it can track people for decades, but it's a lot messier than RCT. There are simply too many variables to control, and none of these studies look at the deep, slow-moving effects of PUFAs on things like mitochondrial function or cellular energy production.

To summarize, PUFAs might reduce cardiovascular events in people who are already in poor health, but that doesn't make them harmless or beneficial when consumed in large amounts over decades. Essentially, what looks protective in the short term may not tell the full story of long-term health.

Do High Blood Levels of PUFA Really Mean Better Health?

There's a common finding in research that trips people up, studies often show that people with higher blood levels of linoleic acid (the primary omega-6 PUFA) have lower rates of cardiovascular disease. On the surface, it looks like more PUFA in the blood equals better health. But hold on, does this mean these people are guzzling seed oils?

Not necessarily.

Here's what is interesting, high blood PUFA levels don't always reflect high intake, they often reflect low oxidation. Healthy people tend to preserve their PUFAs; they don't burn through or damage them rapidly. Sick or inflamed individuals, on the other hand, experience more lipid peroxidation, meaning their PUFAs get chewed up by oxidative stress, leaving blood levels lower. In other words, it's not that the PUFA is making them healthy; it's that their health is protecting the PUFA.

I experienced this firsthand. After a decade on a low-PUFA diet, I had my fatty acids tested, expecting them to be low. Surprisingly, my levels were at the high end of normal. When I asked Dr. Ray Peat about it, he explained:

"PUFAs are very susceptible to oxidation, especially in red blood cells, so sick, inflamed people with lots of lipid peroxidation lose them first."

This concept is beautifully illustrated by research on the Maasai. The Maasai of Kenya eat a traditional diet rich in saturated fat and almost devoid of PUFAs, yet studies found they have surprisingly high levels of long-chain PUFAs in their red blood cells (26).

How?

Their lifestyle, nutrient-dense whole foods, minimal processed oils, constant physical activity, strong social bonds, and low chronic stress created a metabolic environment where PUFAs are protected from oxidation and used efficiently.

The bottom line is healthy blood PUFA levels are more a sign of a resilient metabolism than a reflection of how many seed oils you're pouring on your salad.

But Aren't Some PUFAs, Omega-3 and Omega-6, Essential?

Another great question...

For decades, nutrition science has labeled omega-3 and omega-6 as "essential fatty acids," implying that without them, our health would unravel. But as with many nutrition claims, the story is far more complicated. To understand their true role, we need to revisit the research that gave these fats their essential status in the first place.

That belief stems from the classic experiments by Mildred and George Burr in the 1920s and 30s. When rats were fed fat-free diets, they developed scaly dermatitis, poor growth, and infertility. These symptoms reversed when linoleic acid (an omega-6 PUFA) was added back, leading researchers to conclude that certain PUFAs were essential (27).

Later observations, however, revealed that these fat-free diets were also lacking other critical nutrients, particularly B vitamins, which are key to healthy metabolism. Additional studies showed that supplementing B vitamins corrected many of the same symptoms attributed to "EFA deficiency." This suggests the original findings were multifactorial rather than proof that large amounts of omega-3 and omega-6 are indispensable (28).

But here is the deal, when omega-3 and omega-6 intake is extremely low, the body doesn't just fail. It adapts by producing Mead acid, an omega-9 polyunsaturated fat synthesized from oleic acid. Mead acid can step in to perform many of the structural and signaling roles typically filled by omega-3 and omega-6, often with less inflammatory signaling. This adaptation makes you question whether these "essential fatty acids" are as essential as we've been told (29, 30).

In fact, research shows the actual requirement to prevent deficiency symptoms is tiny, around 1-2% of total calories for omega-6 and less than 0.5% or less for omega-3 (31, 32). For perspective, the modern diet supplies 6-10 times more omega-6 than necessary, mostly from industrial seed oils. Instead of protecting health, this overload may fuel oxidative stress, inflammation, and mitochondrial dysfunction.

So, are omega-3 and omega-6 PUFAs truly essential? Technically, yes, in the strict biochemical sense, a trace amount may be needed. But when the body is metabolically supported with a nutrient-rich diet, the need to add more becomes unnecessary. In a low-PUFA environment, humans can synthesize their own alternative (Mead acid) and maintain healthy tissues without relying on high dietary PUFA intake.

Ultimately, by meeting minimal needs through whole-food sources like eggs, liver, and seafood, while avoiding the flood of unstable fats from seed oils, you can support your mitochondria and sidestep the long-term risks of PUFA overload.

Knowing all this, let's get back to one of my original questions.

If PUFAs are so bad, why does mother nature add them to our food supply?

Polyunsaturated fats (PUFAs) aren't nature's mistakes. In nature, they absolutely serve important roles, just not necessarily ones that align with the modern human diet. One of their most critical natural functions is to protect seeds from the animals that might consume them. Seeds are the plant's genetic future, and plants have no interest in having animals destroy their chances of reproduction.

The PUFA-rich oils in seeds act as a built-in defense system. Because these oils are chemically unstable and prone to oxidation, they can cause digestive upset in animals that eat too many of them. Many seeds also contain bitter compounds and anti-nutrients alongside

PUFA, making them less appealing. To help protect themselves, seeds are usually packaged with vitamin E, a powerful antioxidant that helps offset some of the oxidative stress PUFA can cause (33).

In some species, containing enough PUFA is a matter of survival. Cold-water fish, such as salmon, naturally contain more omega-3 PUFA because these fats keep tissues flexible in cold waters. If salmon were made entirely of saturated fats, their cell membranes would become too rigid to function at those temperatures, and they simply couldn't survive. This high-PUFA content is an environmental adaptation, not necessarily a sign that humans should consume large amounts of these fats year-round.

Another advantage of consuming PUFAS is they are fattening agents. While this is not an advantage for you or me, it certainly is for farmers who want to fatten their cows, pigs, and chickens quickly. If you are selling your meat per pound, then a fatter animal is going to bring you more money, more quickly.

In a study of Brown Swiss bulls, six groups were fed a standard ration with 3% of dry matter replaced by various fats—rumen-protected crystalline fat, coconut oil, rapeseed, sunflower seed, or linseed. While the higher PUFA groups on rapeseed, and linseed groups gained about 1,240 g/day, the coconut oil group only managed 1,038 g/day, a significant drop in growth performance. Essentially, those on PUFA oils gained 20% more weight than those on the coconut oil (34). This makes sense because PUFAs can lower cellular respiration, slowing metabolism, so more calories get stored as fat.

PUFAs are also involved in creating signaling molecules called eicosanoids. These compounds help regulate inflammation, blood flow, clotting and immune responses. In the right (small) amounts, these signals are essential for healing and defense. In excess, like so many things, they can become stress-driven mediators, keeping you in a self-sustaining inflammatory loop (more on this later).

And finally, PUFAs are also still needed by the human body. In small amounts, they serve structural purposes. They are part of every cell membrane, helping maintain the right balance between fluidity, which comes from PUFA, and rigidity, which comes from saturated fat. They are concentrated in the brain and eyes, where a certain level of membrane fluidity is critical for nerve signaling and visual processing.

Essentially, PUFAs exist in nature for protection, survival, fattening animals, and structural balance, not because they are an ideal fuel for humans. Traditional diets contained PUFA in small amounts, naturally paired with protective nutrients like vitamin E, and packaged within whole foods. The problem comes when we extract, concentrate, and consume these unstable fats daily, in excessive amounts, replacing the more stable, energy-efficient saturated fats our bodies handle with greater ease.

Nature has its reasons for PUFA, and so do we, but those reasons have been twisted into a health story that leaves out the most important chapter. Yes, we need a trace amount, yet our plates are flooded with them in the name of "heart health" and cholesterol reduction. What the mainstream health advice ignores is the quiet, relentless way these unstable fats weave into your cell membranes, disrupt energy production, and set the stage for long-term metabolic damage. Now it's time to go into the nitty-gritty on what happens inside your cells when PUFA takes over, and why I believe they're the sixth and final obstacle in optimizing cellular energy production.

How Do PUFAs Interfere with Energy Production

Polyunsaturated fats (PUFAs) interfere with energy production at multiple levels, from damaging mitochondria to thyroid suppression, to disrupting digestion. In excess, PUFAs encourage the cells of the body to slow down, and live in a low-energy, stress adapted state.

PUFAs and Your Mitochondria

Remember that your mitochondria are the power plants of your cells. Each one is churning out energy (ATP) that keeps your body running. To work efficiently, these power plants need strong membranes, enzymes, and proteins, much like a power plant needs strong walls and well-working machinery. When PUFAs come along, due to their multiple double bonds, they are more prone to oxidation, a process that is a bit like metal rusting, but inside your cells (35).

When PUFAs oxidize, they break apart into harmful byproducts, including lipid peroxides and toxic fragments, called aldehydes, including malondialdehyde and 4-hydroxynonemnal (4-HNE). These toxic troublemakers act like vandals breaking into your power plant, punching holes in walls and messing up your machinery (36).

When you punch holes in the mitochondrial membrane, the protein gradients can't hold a strong charge, which is needed to make ATP. In addition, the toxic aldehydes gum up your electron transport chain by binding to key enzymes at Complex I and III. Both will lead to slower energy production, by damaging the system designed to make ATP.

The net effect is a metabolic system that produces less energy, while also generating more reactive oxygen species (ROS), creating a destructive feedback loop. In other words, PUFA not only decreases your energy output, but it also increases the metabolic "waste products" that age and inflame your tissues.

PUFAs and Your Thyroid

If you remember from Chapter 5, you learned your thyroid is your body's metabolic CEO, setting the pace for how fast or slow your cells turn fuel into energy. Which means it is pretty damn important when it comes to ATP production. PUFAs can interfere with thyroid activity, in not one, two, but three different ways, each of which can slow things down.

PUFAs Mess with Thyroid Hormone Transport

Once your thyroid releases T4 (the inactive form of thyroid hormone), most of it travels through your bloodstream bound to transport proteins like thyroxine-binding globulin (TBG). Think of

TBG as a fleet of taxis that safely carry thyroid hormone passengers to their destinations, keeping them stable and ready for delivery.

Unsaturated fats, especially PUFAs, can compete with T4 for those taxi seats. Numerous studies have shown that the more unsaturated the fat, the more it displaces thyroid hormone from its carrier (37, 38, 39). When that happens, it's as if PUFAs hop in and push T4 and T3 passengers out onto the street.

At first, more "free" or "unbound" hormone might sound good, but without a taxi, those passengers wander around and are quickly removed from circulation by the liver and kidneys. This means less hormone ultimately reaches your tissues. Over time, the loss of this protein-bound buffer shifts you from a steady, reliable hormone supply to a pattern of short-lived spikes followed by dips, a ride service that's more erratic and far less dependable, which may trend toward lower overall thyroid action at the tissue level (40, 41, 42).

PUFAs Slow the Conversion of T4 to T3

Your thyroid mostly produces T4, the inactive form of thyroid hormone, while T3 is the active form that keeps your metabolism humming. Most of the conversion from T4 to T3 happens in the liver and other tissues through enzymes called deiodinases, which depend on the mineral selenium to work (43).

When PUFAs oxidize, they create toxic byproducts like 4-hydroxynonenal and lipid peroxides. These trigger oxidative stress, and your body responds by diverting selenium toward making antioxidant enzymes such as glutathione peroxidase and thioredoxin reductase. While these enzymes are essential for damage control, they leave fewer resources for deiodinases to activate thyroid hormone (44, 45).

Think of selenium like a small team of skilled mechanics. Their main job is to tune up your "metabolic engine" by converting T4 into T3. But when PUFAs rust the system with oxidative stress, those same mechanics must drop their tools and start putting out fires.

With fewer hands on the engine, less T3 gets made, and your whole metabolic system slows down.

PUFAs May Reduce Thyroid Hormone Secretion

This is the most speculative piece of the puzzle, but it's still intriguing. Your thyroid gland responds to TSH from the pituitary, but it's also influenced by local chemical messengers within the gland itself. PUFAs, especially arachidonic acid, are precursors to prostaglandins and other eicosanoids that can dampen TSH's effect on the gland (46).

Inflammatory cytokines (which rise when PUFAs oxidize) can further blunt hormone release (47). Some animal studies have even shown drops in circulating T4 after PUFA exposure (48). While the human data is more indirect, the evidence suggests that PUFA metabolites and the inflammation they trigger can turn down the thyroid's output at the source.

In summary, PUFAs can affect your thyroid at every stage: transport, activation, and possibly secretion. The result is less active thyroid hormone reaching your cells, and a slower, less efficient metabolism.

PUFAs, Digestion, and Endotoxins

High-PUFA diets can set the stage for gut barrier breakdown, not because these fats literally become part of the intestinal lining, but because they alter the gut environment in ways that make the barrier more fragile. In the intestine, PUFAs are highly prone to oxidation, producing lipid peroxides and other reactive byproducts. These compounds, along with PUFA-derived inflammatory mediators such as prostaglandins and leukotrienes, can disrupt tight junction proteins like occludin and claudins, loosening the seal between intestinal cells and increasing permeability (49, 50).

Think of your gut lining like a tightly woven fishing net that keeps the bad stuff out of your bloodstream while letting the good stuff through.

PUFA oxidation is like tossing acid onto that net, the holes widen, the weave weakens, and before long, debris starts slipping through.

When this barrier becomes more permeable ("leaky"), the debris, bacterial endotoxin (lipopolysaccharide, or LPS) can slip into the bloodstream. Once there, endotoxin acts as a metabolic disruptor, triggering systemic inflammation, suppressing mitochondrial respiration, and pushing the cell toward less efficient glycolysis. This results in slower energy production and a dampened metabolic rate.

PUFAs, Your Pancreas, Insulin, and Blood Sugar

At first glance, high-PUFA diets can look like they *improve* insulin sensitivity. By making cell membranes more fluid, PUFAs can help insulin receptors and glucose transporters (GLUT4) move and signal more efficiently. On an early blood test, this may show up as "better" insulin sensitivity.

But this effect is deceptive and short-lived.

The same PUFAs are highly unstable and prone to oxidation, producing toxic byproducts such as 4-hydroxynonenal (4-HNE). Beta cells in the pancreas, the very cells responsible for releasing insulin, are especially vulnerable, since they have naturally low antioxidant defenses.

When PUFA byproducts reach the pancreas, they damage beta-cell mitochondria, cutting ATP production. That's a major problem, because ATP is the signal that tells beta cells: *"Glucose is here, release insulin!"* With less ATP, insulin release falters, and blood sugar lingers higher after meals (51, 52).

Chronic PUFA exposure doesn't just weaken signaling, it stirs up ongoing oxidative stress and inflammation in pancreatic tissue. Over time, this stress can push beta cells into apoptosis (cell death), steadily eroding the body's insulin-making capacity (53). As insulin regulation breaks down, blood sugar rises, and the body shifts into a stress-driven survival mode, relying on adrenaline and cortisol to mobilize fuel. But cortisol is catabolic and suppresses thyroid function, which throttles back energy production even further.

Besides affecting the pancreas, these unstable fats also interfere with the pyruvate dehydrogenase (PDH) complex, the critical enzyme that turns pyruvate into acetyl-CoA so glucose can fully enter the mitochondria (54). When PDH is inhibited, glucose can't be oxidized efficiently. Instead of cleanly burning glucose into 36 ATP and CO_2, the cell pushes toward glycolysis, the less efficient pathway that produces lactate, wastes glucose, and produces only 2 ATP. This creates the appearance of "low blood sugar," as the cells waste glucose, and produce less ATP (55).

Much like estrogen, PUFA flips this metabolic switch: glucose oxidation is blocked, glycolysis rises, and the body compensates by leaning harder on fatty acid oxidation. In the short term, this can make blood sugar tests look deceptively normal or even improved, since glucose is being pulled into cells (56). But underneath, the mitochondria are being starved of their cleanest fuel, while the body increasingly depends on PUFA oxidation and stress hormones, like cortisol and adrenaline, to keep energy flowing. The result is a vicious cycle: glucose "wasting," lactate buildup, and fatty acid reliance, all of which drag metabolism into the stressed, inefficient state I keep warning about.

In short, PUFA may look like a friend to blood sugar control in the beginning, but it quickly reveals its troublemaking, crazy self, undermining the pancreas, destabilizing metabolism, inhibiting cellular respiration, and forcing the body to lean on stress hormones instead of true energy production.

PUFAs and Eicosanoids: Too Much of a Good Thing

Most people haven't heard the word *eicosanoids*, but I'd bet good money most have *felt* them in action. Cramping? Blood clotting? Swelling? Inflammation? Yep, those are eicosanoids at work.

Eicosanoids are hormone-like signaling molecules made from polyunsaturated fatty acids (PUFAs), especially arachidonic acid (omega-6) and EPA/DHA (omega-3). The big three are prostaglandins, thromboxanes, and leukotrienes, each with critical roles in regulating inflammation, immune defense, and blood flow (57, 58).

In the right amounts, they're essential for survival:

Prostaglandins help the uterine muscles contract just enough to shed the lining during menstruation. In a balanced system (healthy progesterone-to-estrogen ratio, moderate PUFA load, nutrient-rich diet, and enough calories to meet energy needs), these contractions happen quietly, like a well-fed baby drifting off to sleep. You hardly notice they're there. But crank up the estrogen, load the diet with PUFAs, add stress or chronic inflammation, and prostaglandins go into overdrive. Suddenly, that baby is awake, screaming, and thrashing—ladies, you know this pain. Now you've got intense cramps, headaches, nausea, maybe even diarrhea (59, 60).

Thromboxanes are vital for blood clotting. They help you stop bleeding when you cut yourself. But in excess, say, in an inflamed, PUFA-rich environment (specifically Omega-6), they can promote unnecessary clotting, raising the risk of heart attack or stroke. It's like having a cook who makes you dinner, but then forgets to turn off the stove, almost burning the house down (61, 62).

Leukotrienes are your immune system's emergency flare, summoning white blood cells to fight infection or clean up damaged tissue. In moderation, they're essential for wound healing and fighting pathogens. But when overproduced, primarily from excessive Omega-6 intake, they can constrict airways (as in asthma), cause swelling, mucus overproduction, and worsen allergies or autoimmune flares (63).

The problem isn't that eicosanoids exist, they *must* exist. The trouble starts when your metabolic environment is primed to make too many. A high-PUFA diet loads your cell membranes with arachidonic acid, while inflammation and estrogen amplify the effect by upregulating enzymes like phospholipase A_2 (PLA_2) and cyclooxygenase (COX-1 and COX-2). The result is a steady overproduction of eicosanoids, keeping your body locked in inflammatory overdrive (64, 65).

Worse, excess eicosanoids don't just act locally. They can circulate through the bloodstream, triggering inflammation in distant tissues, suppressing mitochondrial energy production, impairing thyroid function, and reinforcing the stressed, adaptive state instead of the healthy, energetic one you want.

FUN FACT: Most traditional NSAIDS (ibuprofen, naproxen, aspirin) are COX-1 and COX-2 inhibitors, which means they work by reducing prostaglandin production everywhere. That is how they work to lower inflammation, fever, and pain.

As you can see, polyunsaturated fats can sabotage energy production from almost every angle. In the mitochondria, their fragile double bonds make them prone to oxidation, producing toxic aldehydes that punch holes in membranes, jam up the machinery, and stir up oxidative stress. In the thyroid, PUFAs disrupt hormone transport, slow the conversion from T4 to active T3, and may even dampen secretion at the gland. In the pancreas, PUFA byproducts damage insulin-producing beta cells, messing with blood sugar control and pushing the body into a stress-driven, low-energy mode. And, as if that wasn't enough, PUFAs fuel the overproduction of inflammatory eicosanoids, chemical messengers that keep the body stuck in a cycle of chronic inflammation and throttled energy output. The result isn't simply "less energy," it's a whole-body shift toward a slower, more fragile, stress-adapted metabolism.

The good news is that none of this happens overnight. PUFA damage is more like a slow drip than a sudden flood. Years, even decades, of dietary exposure build up quietly, and the effects can creep in so gradually you might not notice them until they're entrenched. But that slow build also means you can reverse course. Even after years of high-PUFA eating, strategic changes can shift your metabolism toward more resilience, better energy, and lower inflammation.

This comes from a two-step process of minimizing PUFA exposure and mitigating against the effects of PUFA.

How to Minimize PUFA Exposure

If PUFA damage is a slow drip, the easiest way to protect yourself is to turn off the tap. While you can't (and don't need to) remove every trace of polyunsaturated fat from your diet, you can dramatically lower your exposure by being strategic about your food choices.

1. Cut back on processed foods
The single biggest PUFA source in modern diets isn't nuts or seeds, it's ultra-processed, packaged foods. Crackers, cookies, chips, pastries, granola bars, protein bars, frozen dinners, and most packaged snacks are loaded with industrial seed oils. These oils are cheap, shelf-stable, and make food crispy, which is why manufacturers love them. Unfortunately, that crispness comes at a metabolic cost.

2. Dump the high-PUFA cooking oils
Skip oils made from seeds, nuts, and vegetables like safflower, sunflower, canola, vegetable (soy), sesame, corn, peanut, and cottonseed oil. These are some of the most concentrated sources of unsaturated fats and heating them during cooking accelerates their oxidation. Instead, use more stable fats like coconut oil, tallow, ghee, butter, and olive oil for dressings.

3. Limit eating out, especially fast food
Restaurants, particularly fast-food chains, almost always cook in cheap, PUFA-rich oils. Even "healthy" options like salads may be drenched in seed-oil-heavy dressings. If you do eat out, use apps like *Seed Oil Scout* to find restaurants that minimize or avoid seed oils altogether.

4. Choose better animal products
When possible, opt for grass-fed and pasture-raised meats over grain, soy, and corn-fed. Grain, soy, and corn-fed animals tend to

accumulate more PUFA in their fat. Leaner cuts of meat can also help lower your PUFA load without sacrificing protein.

5. Pick the right fish

Low-fat fish, like cod, haddock, white fish, and sole, provide protein and micronutrients without the high PUFA content of fatty fish, like salmon, mackerel, or sardines. Fatty fish can be beneficial in moderation, but daily consumption can tip your balance toward excess PUFA.

6. Moderate egg intake

Eggs are nutrient-rich and can be part of a healthy diet, but they do contain PUFA, especially if the hens are fed soy or corn. Enjoy them, but don't make them your main protein source at every meal. Limit eggs to 1-3 a day.

7. Be careful with nuts and seeds

If you eat nuts, choose lightly or dry roasted over raw, which are more prone to oxidation. Seeds like flax, chia, pumpkin, and sunflower are extremely PUFA-dense and easy to overeat. Best lower-PUFA nut choices: macadamia, hazelnut, and cashew.

8. Use stable fats for cooking

For high-heat cooking, stick with stable, saturated fats like coconut oil, butter, ghee, and beef tallow. These are less prone to oxidation, making them safer for frying or sautéing.

9. Check your condiments

Most store-bought salad dressings, mayonnaise, and sauces are made with PUFA-heavy oils. Read labels, or better yet, make your own dressings using extra virgin olive oil. While olive oil is mostly monounsaturated and much more stable, quality matters, look for brands that are certified pure, since adulteration with cheaper oils is far too common.

10. Be wary of avocado oil

While avocado oil is marketed as a "healthy" option, studies have found many brands are adulterated with cheaper, high-PUFA oils.

Unless you have a verified source, it's safer to stick with olive oil for cold uses and saturated fats for cooking (66).

One thing I want to mention, reducing PUFA is not a license to binge on saturated fat. Calories still count, especially in the early stages of healing. Overeating butter, coconut oil, or any fat can still cause weight gain if you surpass your body's needs. Track your intake with a food logging app, like Cronometer, to stay within your calorie budget, which is the number of calories you can consume and maintain weight.

How to Mitigate the Effects of PUFA (When You Can't Avoid Them)

Sometimes PUFA-rich foods are unavoidable, whether you're traveling, at a family gathering, or stuck with limited options. When that happens, do not worry or stress, no single food or meal is going to create poor health. To be honest, stressing about eating PUFAs can be far worse than just eating the food.

At the same time, you want to do your best to minimize PUFA consumption or at the very least, minimize the effects of dietary and stored PUFA (PUFA stored in your fat tissue). Thus, here are a few strategies you can do to help your body handle PUFA exposure.

1. Vitamin E — Your PUFA Protector

Vitamin E is a fat-soluble vitamin that comes in eight forms: four tocopherols and four tocotrienols (alpha, beta, gamma, and delta). Both groups act as antioxidants, meaning they help neutralize free radicals. Among them, alpha-tocopherol is the most biologically active form and the one our bodies use most efficiently. As an antioxidant, vitamin E helps protect cells from damage caused by free radicals and oxidative stress (67).

Think of vitamin E as a security guard stationed in your cell membranes, keeping delicate, double-bonded PUFAs from being junked-up by free radicals. Without enough of this guard, unstable fats can spiral into a chain reaction that produces harmful compounds like lipid peroxides and aldehydes (68). Vitamin E can stop these reactions before they damage your cells.

What type of vitamin E? Your body prefers alpha-tocopherol, which sits in cell membranes and stops PUFA from spiraling into lipid peroxides and nasty aldehydes. Choose natural d-alpha-tocopherol or mixed tocopherols over synthetic dl-alpha. I suggest taking it with food.

How much vitamin E? Well, the more PUFA you eat, the more protection you need. Research suggests aiming for about 0.5 mg ($\approx$2 IU) of α-tocopherol per gram of PUFA (69). For example, if you're eating a high-PUFA meal with 50 g of PUFA, supplementing with around 100 IU of vitamin E near the meal may help offset the oxidative load. That's because vitamin E gets "used up" as it neutralizes damage.

Studies also show that taking vitamin E before stressful events, like intense exercise, can reduce free radicals and lower lipid peroxidation in both young and older adults (70). This is especially relevant during fat loss, since stored PUFAs are released into the bloodstream when body fat is burned. Whether it's exercise, calorie restriction, or stress doing the burning, vitamin E can help keep that PUFA release from turning into an oxidative mess.

Bottom line? If you're about to dive into PUFA-heavy foods (fried restaurant fare, fatty fish, nut-laden desserts), a dose of vitamin E beforehand can help limit the fallout. And if you're losing body fat, consider it a buffer against oxidative stress. I personally don't recommend more than 100 IU/day without professional guidance. Higher dosages (normally above 200IUS) can impact blood clotting, create GI issues, and even impact thyroid hormone conversion.

2. Niacinamide (B3) — Supporting Glucose Oxidation

Niacinamide works by boosting your cell's levels of NAD^+. If you remember from the "Supportive Fuel" chapter, we talked about NADH. Think of NADH as a fully loaded delivery truck, packed with electrons. NAD^+, on the other hand, is the empty truck, ready to be sent out to pick up more electrons.

When you have more NAD^+ "trucks" on the road, your mitochondria can work at full speed, collecting more electrons and converting them into ATP. This efficient oxidative metabolism reduces your body's reliance on stress hormones like adrenaline and cortisol, keeping you out of the stressed adaptive state.

Better oxidative metabolism shifts your cells toward burning glucose instead of fat. That's important, because burning less fat, especially polyunsaturated fats, means fewer harmful byproducts like lipid peroxides and aldehydes are generated. Think of it like choosing premium, clean-burning fuel for your engine instead of dirty, unstable fuel that gums up the entire system (71, 72).

How much? Research suggests that therapeutic doses of niacinamide for reducing oxidative stress, improving mitochondrial respiration, and suppressing excessive free fatty acid release generally range from 200–500 mg/day, split into multiple doses (73, 74). While B3 is found in food, these therapeutic levels usually require supplementation. (You can check my preferred brands at the back of this book and at www.KateDeering.com.)

It should be noted, if you want to lose fat, you will eventually have to release stored fat into the bloodstream, and unless you've been eating low-PUFA for years, some of that stored fat is unsaturated. The safest approach is to release it gradually. Your body handles fat oxidation more easily at rest, producing less oxidative stress, which is why sleeping is one of the best times to burn fat safely.

For a deeper dive into why glucose is often the cleaner, safer fuel, return to Chapter 2. And to take a deeper dive into fat burning, jump to the next chapter.

3. The Magical Effects of Aspirin

One of the simplest (and cheapest) ways to blunt the damage from PUFA is plain old aspirin. Aspirin works by shutting off the enzymes

(COX-1 and COX-2) that normally turn PUFA into prostaglandins and thromboxane. Remember, these are the chemical messengers that trigger pain, blood clotting, and stress in the body.

Unlike other pain relievers, aspirin doesn't just block these enzymes for a short time, it permanently switches them off in platelets, giving a longer-lasting effect. Even better, aspirin helps the body make special compounds called "aspirin-triggered lipoxins" that calm and resolve inflammation, instead of just covering it up (75, 76).

Aspirin also has some surprising effects on blood sugar. Chronic inflammation is a key driver of insulin resistance, blocking insulin's ability to move glucose into cells. Inflammation from PUFA oxidation activates the NF-kB pathway, driving cytokine release and worsening beta-cell stress. An enzyme called IKKB activates the NF-kB pathway. Aspirin helps by blocking IKKB, keeping NF-kB from triggering an inflammatory "attack" on the beta cells. This restores insulin signaling, improving glucose uptake, which will suppress excess glucose output from the liver (77).

In both human and animal studies, high-dose aspirin (about 7grams/day) improved insulin sensitivity and lowered fasting blood sugar (78), while even low-dose aspirin (100mg/day) use has been associated with a reduced risk of developing type 2 diabetes (79). Now, I am not suggesting you should down 7 grams of aspirin/day to help with blood sugar (at least without medical supervision), but I am making the point that this simple, cheap medication can decrease PUFAs inflammatory effects, shifting the body away from relying on stress hormones (which happens when the cells cannot use glucose), and back toward clean, efficient glucose metabolism.

Aspirin's anti-inflammatory reach also extends into cancer prevention. Long-term studies show that regular aspirin use can lower the risk of several cancers, with the strongest evidence for colorectal cancer. In a 20-year follow-up of five randomized trials, daily aspirin use reduced colorectal cancer incidence by about 24% and mortality by 35%. The doses studied ranged from 75 mg to 1200 mg per day, but anything above 300 mg did not seem to add extra benefit—meaning even a baby aspirin was protective (80). Observational research further suggests a 20–30% reduction in overall cancer risk with extended use, as well as decreased recurrence of precancerous colon polyps (81). By limiting prostaglandin-driven inflammation, reducing platelet activation, and supporting normal cell turnover, aspirin appears to create a less favorable environment for tumor growth.

Typical doses depend on the goal: 75–100 mg/day is the "baby aspirin" cardiology dose, while 162–325 mg taken with food can help blunt PUFA-driven prostaglandin release after a heavy PUFA-filled meal. Most people can tolerate daily low-dose daily aspirin or even moderate dosages without issues.

That said, aspirin, like everything else on this planet, is not without risks. By lowering the protective prostaglandins that normally shield the stomach lining, it can raise the chance of gastritis or ulcers, especially in people with a history of GI issues, alcohol use, or who take other NSAIDs or blood thinners. To reduce this risk, aspirin should always be taken with food, and many people find it easier on the stomach if it's crushed and dissolved in water.

4. Minimize Fat Burning (Wait, What?)

If you've eaten a high-PUFA diet for years (vegetable oils, fried foods, packaged snacks, nuts and seed oils), chances are much of the fat stored in your body is PUFA. When you burn body fat, you're not just releasing calories, you're also releasing those unstable fatty acids back into circulation. Once released, just like dietary PUFA, your body ridden-PUFAs can oxidize into toxic byproducts like 4-HNE, which block energy production, suppress thyroid function, and promote inflammation.

This is why minimizing fat burning can be a logical and easy way to hinder PUFAs negative effects. If your body fat is PUFA-rich, mobilizing large amounts of it will flood your system with unstable fuel. Instead, support your metabolism with regular meals, emphasizing carbohydrates, protein, and saturated fats. This will allow your body to run on a "cleaner" fuel, all the while gradually turning your PUFA stores over, with healthier and safer saturated fats.

You see, your stored PUFA doesn't disappear overnight. Human fat tissue doesn't flip over all at once, it's constantly being remodeled. Studies show that about 10% of triglycerides in a fat cell are replaced each year, and the average age of a fat molecule is 1–2 years (82, 83). The key is that turnover is slow and gradual—not in a single sweep— so it takes years for most of it to change over.

That's why Ray Peat often said it can take up to four years to clear PUFA from tissues. In 1–2 years, some of the fat pool has been replaced, but plenty of old PUFA is still hanging around. By four years, most of your fat stores have cycled through, so the tissue finally reflects your new diet more than your old one. It's not an overnight process; it's a slow but steady replacement.

Interestingly, the body handles PUFA and saturated fats very differently. In the short term, PUFA (like linoleic acid) is often released from fat cells quickly when you burn body fat. But just because it enters the bloodstream doesn't mean it's fully used as fuel. A significant portion of PUFA is re-captured and recycled back into storage, whereas saturated fats are more likely to be burned completely for energy.

Over the long term, this recycling bias means PUFA gradually builds up in adipose tissue, while saturated fats are depleted. One likely reason is that burning PUFA produces more toxic byproducts, so the body shuttles much of it back into storage as a protective strategy. The tradeoff is that decades of high PUFA intake leave you with a toxic reservoir in your fat that can leak back into circulation whenever you fast, follow a restrictive diet, or push rapid fat loss (hello GLP-1) (84, 85).

What does this all mean?

1. Don't crash diet or force rapid fat loss, it just dumps more PUFA into your bloodstream.

2. Support metabolism with regular meals, plenty of carbs, and adequate protein.

3. Focus on improving thyroid and metabolic health first, rather than obsessing over the scale.

4. Over time, with steady nutrition and lower PUFA intake, adipose tissue will slowly remodel itself toward a more stable composition.

By minimizing PUFA release during fat loss, you give your body a chance to restore safer, more efficient energy metabolism without constantly battling the oxidative stress that comes from burning unstable fat.

5. Support a Healthy Metabolism Daily

One of the most powerful ways to defend yourself from PUFA, whether it's coming in through today's meal or being released from your own fat stores, is by running a high, thyroid-driven metabolism. (You know, everything I discussed in the first part of this book.)

A strong metabolism keeps your cells burning glucose as their primary fuel instead of relying on excessive fat oxidation. This matters because, as discussed in Chapter 2, glucose oxidation supports thyroid hormone production, produces more CO_2, is more efficient, and is cleaner, while fat oxidation, especially PUFA oxidation, creates far more toxic byproducts like lipid peroxides and aldehydes (86, 87). In other words, glucose is the premium fuel, while PUFA is the dirty diesel that gums up your engine.

When metabolism is sluggish, the body slips into those adaptive stress pathways. Stress hormones like adrenaline and cortisol rise, free fatty acids are dumped into the blood, and you end up oxidizing more PUFA exactly when your system is least equipped to handle it. This is the cycle that drives inflammation, thyroid suppression, and mitochondrial dysfunction (88).

By contrast, when your thyroid is active and your metabolic rate is high:

- Glucose oxidation takes priority. Your cells don't need to over-rely on excessive fat for energy, so PUFA (dietary or stored) stays in the background.

- Stress pathways stay quiet. You avoid chronic adrenaline- and cortisol-driven fat release, meaning fewer waves of PUFA flooding your bloodstream.

- PUFA oxidation is buffered by CO_2. Even when PUFA does get burned, a high metabolic rate increases CO_2 production. CO_2 itself buffers oxidative stress, it improves oxygen delivery and reacts with damaging radicals, helping neutralize some of the damage (89).

- Turnover improves. Over time, a fast metabolism cycles out old fat stores more smoothly, replacing unstable PUFA with more stable, saturated fats without overwhelming the system (90).

Essentially, a high metabolism is like a built-in PUFA buffer. You can't erase decades of past intake, and you can't avoid small amounts in otherwise healthy foods, but with thyroid and energy production running strong, your body can handle the exposure. The key to managing PUFA-ridden foods is to not avoid them completely, but to create a cellular powerhouse that can manage exposure and build up resilience.

In summary, polyunsaturated fatty acids (PUFAs) are everywhere, vegetable oils, packaged snacks, nuts and seeds, fast foods, and even in animal products fed soy and corn. Mainstream nutrition casts them as "heart-healthy" essentials, but through the lens of cellular energy production, they look more like intrusive vandals, damaging your cells. Their multiple double bonds make them fragile, easily oxidized, and prone to generating toxic byproducts like lipid peroxides and aldehydes. Instead of supporting your metabolism, they suppress thyroid function, impair mitochondrial efficiency, and push your body into stress-driven fuel modes.

That doesn't mean a single meal of fried food will wreck you. What matters is the long-term pattern. Over time, high-PUFA diets leave you with fat stores that act as a reservoir of instability, creating oxidative stress whenever those fats are mobilized.

The good news is there are some simple things you can do to support yourself. By limiting dietary PUFA, supporting thyroid health, and favoring clean fuels like carbs and saturated fats, you can shift the balance toward increased energy production and resilience. Nutrients like vitamin E, niacinamide, and aspirin offer additional buffering, while steady, nutrient-rich meals keep PUFA in the background instead of front and center.

Ultimately, protecting yourself from PUFA is less about fear and more about building a robust, glucose-driven metabolism. A body running on strong thyroid function, high CO_2 production, and ample ATP is a huge shield to the negative effects of PUFA. It doesn't erase decades of past intake, but it can protect against much of the fallout. This combination of minimizing exposure, supporting turnover, and strengthening metabolic defenses allows you to live in the modern food environment without fearing every nut, seed, or restaurant meal.

And that brings us to the next chapter of this book. Because I know what many of you are thinking: *If I should minimize PUFA exposure and increase glucose oxidation, how can I lose body fat safely?* In the next chapter, we'll tackle exactly that; how to mobilize and metabolize stored fat without negatively affecting your metabolism, so your journey toward a healthy body weight also supports long-term thyroid function, energy production, and overall health.

CHAPTER 12

THE BOTTOM LINE

The Polyunsaturated Fats: Heart Healthy Or Energy Killer?

PUFAs are fragile fats. They oxidize easily, creating byproducts that can damage mitochondria, gum up the ETC, and suppress thyroid-driven energy production.

5. Short-term wins do not equal long-term health. Swapping in PUFAs may lower LDL and some inflammation markers in the near term, but it can miss (or mask) slow-burn damage to cellular energy over years.

6. Tiny amounts of omega-6/omega-3 are sufficient; the modern diet supplies many times more than needed, especially from seed/vegetable oils and ultra-processed foods.

7. Excess PUFA stresses many systems. Think mitochondrial oxidation and aldehydes, impaired T4→T3 conversion, beta-cell strain, leaky-gut/endotoxin synergy, and eicosanoid overdrive.

8. Minimize high-PUFA oils/processed foods, cook with stable fats, favor whole-food sources, and support thyroid/glucose oxidation (sleep, carbs, protein, micronutrients).

9. To mitigate exposure; go slow on fat loss, consider protective buffers (e.g., vitamin E within limits), and build a resilient, glucose-driven metabolism, so PUFA stays in the background where it belongs.

PART 3

BETTER ENERGY IN ACTION

In Part 1, we built the foundation by understanding how the body actually creates energy. This includes what fuels your cells, the nutrients they crave, why oxygen and CO_2 matter more than you've ever been told, and why optimal thyroid function is essential for optimizing energy production.

In Part 2, we explored the "Energy Blocks." These included stress physiology gone wild, gut dysfunction, endotoxins, nutrient deficiencies, excess estrogen and iron, and of course, those annoying polyunsaturated fats that seem to sneak into everything.

In Part 3, we bring it all together.

This is where we move from understanding to implementation. From theory to practice. From "Okay, I get it," to "Okay, I can actually do this." It's also where we talk honestly about healthy fat loss, not through starvation, fear, or control, but as a natural result of restoring function, calming stress physiology, improving thyroid efficiency, and helping the body feel safe again.

Here we'll explore:

- What healthy fat loss looks like in a metabolically supported body

- Why a healthy body is needed for healthy fat loss

- Fat loss tools to make your fat loss count

- and most importantly... how to take everything you've learned so far and use it in real life

This isn't about forcing your body to change.

This is about creating *Better Energy*—so your cells work for you, not against you. When energy improves, health improves. Stability improves. Confidence improves. Strength improves. And yes, very often... fat loss follows.

Better Energy isn't just a concept.

It's a way of living—one that supports sustainable fat loss, healthier aging, clearer thinking, steadier moods, and a body that feels like home again.

CHAPTER 13

UNDERSTANDING HEALTHY FAT LOSS
AND WHY METABOLISM COMES FIRST

Raise your hand if you've ever jumped on a quick weight-loss program.

I'm going to guess nearly 100% of hands went up—including mine. Over my lifetime, I've tried at least 25 of them.

Now raise your hand if you gained back all (or most) of the weight within months or years. Hand still up? Mine too. Before I learned how to eat to support my metabolism, I lost and regained the same 20 pounds about 25 different times.

Here is the unfortunate truth, most people can't sustain their weight loss on quick-fix programs. A meta-analysis of 29 long-term weight-loss studies found that people regained about 50% of lost weight within 2 years and 80% within 5 years (1).

If the standard model of "calories in vs. calories out" worked long term, we'd all be thinner, healthier, and less diseased. Instead, the opposite is happening. Globally, we spend $333 billion every year on weight-loss programs, diets, and supplements (2). Yet, obesity rates and illness keep climbing at an alarming pace.

Now, this isn't solely the fault of the weight-loss industry. Our modern lifestyle doesn't do us any favors: working from home, food delivery at the push of a button, 24-hour streaming, and endless ultra-processed foods all play a role. But it's hard to ignore the irony when the industry built to help us lose weight is failing at its very purpose, at least when it comes to sustainable, long-term results.

Now, I want to be clear, eating fewer calories than you burn will lead to weight loss. We've all experienced that. The problem isn't losing weight; it's keeping it off. Restrictive, low-calorie diets simply aren't sustainable. And a diet you can't stick to is a diet that won't work long term.

As I've explained throughout this book (and in *How to Heal Your Metabolism*), the foods most restrictive diets encourage, low-calorie processed meals filled with PUFA oils, hard-to-digest ingredients, additives, and preservatives, are terrible for long-term health and metabolic stability. Another issue is most diets focus on weight loss at any cost, rather than true fat loss.

By chasing quick numbers on the scale, these diets ignore the deeper metabolic adaptations that occur, many of which set you up for rebound weight gain and worse health down the road. However, if you restore metabolic health (and do the other things I'll go over in this chapter) you can avoid the chaos of yo-yo dieting.

And let's not forget, the weight-loss industry profits more from your repeated failures than your long-term success. It's far more lucrative to sell you 20 different programs than to help you find one approach that works for life.

In this chapter, I'll shift the focus away from nourishing and fixing the body, to dropping pounds. You'll learn the difference between weight loss and healthy fat loss, how to know if your body is even ready to lose fat, and what really happens during the metabolic process of fat burning (yes, more science is coming!). Then we'll wrap with proven strategies to lose fat in a way that lasts.

Healthy Fat Loss 101

When done properly, healthy fat loss is not about chasing a number, but rather building a better body that naturally carries less body fat. We first support the metabolism, then the fat loss follows—slow, steady, and sustainable.

Here's the first thing you need to know: *weight loss is not the same thing as fat loss.*

When the scale goes down, that drop can come from many places: water, glycogen (your stored glucose), intestinal waste, muscle, and yes, some fat. Quick weight loss programs usually drain water and glycogen first, sometimes muscle too. True fat loss is slower, steadier, and more sustainable.

Think about this.

When you lose weight quickly, you lose water and glycogen first. For every gram of glycogen, you store (about 600 grams in total), you hold on to three grams of water (3). That means if you fast for 24 hours, you'll dump glycogen and water, and the scale may drop five pounds almost overnight. Add in the "bathroom factor" (losing a couple pounds of waste), and voilà, seven pounds gone in a day.

The next morning you beam with pride; "Wow, that wasn't so bad. I just didn't eat, and I lost seven pounds!" But by the end of the week, as soon as you eat normally again, the scale climbs right back up. That's not failure, that is basic biology.

Now let me introduce you to Julie.

Client Story: Julie

Julie, my 48-year-old perimenopausal client, went on a 1,200-calorie diet two years ago, and lost 20 pounds in three months. Fast forward to today and she had gained it all back. Sadly, Julie was the same weight as before but looked heavier and felt worse. Why? Because, due to Julie's low-calorie diet, with not enough protein, Julie had lost muscle and added back some fat—changing her body composition in a negative fashion.

Some critics will say Julie's program "worked," due to her losing weight. They may claim it was her lack of discipline that failed, as she stopped eating low calorie, thus putting the weight back on. I disagree. Talking to Julie, after her low-calorie diet, stress increased, and her eating was no longer sustainable. Essentially, if your plan cannot ebb and flow with life, it's not sustainable. And if it's not sustainable, it's doomed to fail.

In fact, according to the same 2019 Meta-analysis from above, if a weight loss program is not sustainable, you have a 100% chance of putting at least 80% of the weight back on in 5 years (1, 4).

So, here's the bottom line: quick fixes usually equal quick rebounds. If you want long-term fat loss, the focus must be on health first—because a healthy metabolism is what makes fat loss sustainable.

Healthy Fat Loss Comes from a Healthy Body

Here's the truth: *a healthy body produces healthy fat loss.*

When your metabolism is running well, your body efficiently turns fuel—especially carbs and fats (and a little protein)—into energy. That energy powers your brain, hormones, muscles, digestion, sleep, and mood. When all systems are supported, you can eat a generous amount of food without gaining excess fat because your body is actually using that fuel to live, move, and repair itself.

For most people reading this, the first step isn't fat loss—it's healing. If you've been under-eating, yo-yo dieting, avoiding nutrient-dense foods, or living with a laundry list of symptoms (low energy, poor sleep, digestive issues, hormone problems), you need to rebuild your metabolism (improve energy production) before even thinking about a fat loss phase.

That doesn't mean you won't lose *any* weight while healing. Many people naturally lean out once inflammation drops and energy production improves. But the *goal* of this phase is restoration, not fat loss.

How long does this take? Anywhere from a few months to a few years, depending on your current health and your history of restriction or stress.

Client Story: Jane

Jane, age 53 and postmenopausal, came to me wanting better sleep and energy—and eventually, fat loss. When we first met, she was eating about 1,600 calories per day and struggling with insomnia, fatigue, and sugar cravings.

Over six months, we gradually increased her intake to 2,300 calories per day—adding only about 50 calories per week. We focused on easy-to-digest carbs (fruit, low-fat milk) and nutrient-rich foods (liver, oysters).

Jane shifted her eating pattern, too. Instead of "saving" her biggest meal for dinner, she began eating more during the active part of her day and less when she was winding down. She also started strength training twice per week and walking 8–10k steps on non-training days.

The interesting part? The more carbs we added, the better Jane slept. At 2,300 calories she finally had enough energy to support deeper sleep, which in turn improved her daytime energy. We held her at that level for three months to confirm she was symptom-free and thriving.

With her metabolism finally supporting her internal and external demands, it was far easier to place Jane in a small deficit. For three months we lowered her total intake to 1,800 calories per day, about a 500-calorie drop. I closely monitored her energy and sleep to make sure the deficit didn't trigger symptoms. She lost about 10 pounds (mostly fat), gained strength, and could now maintain her weight on 2,000 calories per day, 400 calories higher than where she started.

Jane's story shows the order that works, build first, trim second. By slowly raising calories, prioritizing easy-to-digest carbs and nutrient-dense foods, shifting meals earlier in the day, and adding simple strength + walking, she fixed sleep and energy before touching a deficit. Then a small, well-monitored cut delivered steady fat loss without the usual crash, and she finished with a higher maintenance intake (2,000 vs. 1,600) and a stronger, leaner body. The lesson is simple, when you support the metabolism first, fat loss becomes easier, calmer, and far more sustainable.

I'll repeat this because it matters: if you're still cold all the time, waking up at night, battling fatigue, mood swings, anxiety, hair loss, skin issues, or hormone imbalances, you are not ready for fat loss. Those are red flags that your metabolism needs more support. Remember Jane? She didn't dive straight into a calorie deficit. She spent months healing first, eating more, sleeping better, and getting her energy back. Only after that foundation was solid did fat loss become both possible and sustainable.

The good news is that as you improve your metabolic rate by adding nutrients and removing blocks, your body naturally starts to burn more calories and fat. For some, that alone is enough to get leaner. For others, additional fat loss strategies will help once the foundation is in place.

And yes, there are exceptions. If you're already eating at or above your total daily energy expenditure (TDEE), your pulse and temperature are healthy, and you have minimal symptoms, you may be ready to start a fat loss phase now.

Which brings about the question: Is your body ready for fat loss?

The answer depends on how you have been doing with supporting your energy production ingredients and removing your energy blocks. Once you're consistently eating enough to cover your energy demands (remember: calorie maintenance = your total daily energy needs), your temperature and pulse are optimized (waking temp 97.5–98°F, midday temp 98–98.6°F, pulse 75–90 bpm), and your digestion, hormones, and stress levels have improved, then and only then, are you possibly ready to enter a fat loss phase.

Here's what readiness looks like in real life:

- Waking temperature 97.5–98°F
- Midday temperature 98–98.6°F
- Daily bowel movements (smooth, sausage-like stools)
- Pain-free, regular periods (for menstruating women)
- Reduced hot flashes (for peri- and postmenopausal women)
- Sleeping through the night
- Waking rested, with a healthy appetite
- Stable energy and mood throughout the day
- No new hair loss; new hair growth or improved quality

Because you're becoming your own health detective, you'll need to pay attention to these markers yourself. But remember, there is no need to rush. Jumping into fat loss before you're metabolically ready is the fastest way to repeat the diet–regain cycle.

If you've been dieting restrictively for years, dealing with chronic stress, or carrying multiple long-term health issues, your body will need time to recover. Sometimes that means months, sometimes years. And once your markers improve, it's wise to stay in a healing phase for another 3–6 months before dropping calories—this gives your body a chance to stabilize and truly adjust.

Yes, that feels like a long wait. But compare it to your alternatives: restrictive eating, carb avoidance, fad diets, binge–restrict cycles, processed "low-calorie" foods, or skipping meals. You already know where those paths lead.

Healing means letting your health metrics give you insight about how you feel, let them be your guide, not the number on the scale.

Why Understanding Different Fuels Matter for Fat Loss

Before we get into specific strategies, it's important to understand *how* fat is burned and why the state of your metabolism determines whether you lose fat efficiently, or whether your body digs itself into a deeper energy hole.

You already learned in Chapter 2 that glucose is your most efficient fuel source: it supports thyroid hormone conversion (T4 → T3), produces more carbon dioxide (which helps oxygen enter your cells), powers your nervous system directly, and creates a higher NADH-to-$FADH_2$ ratio—meaning more ATP, faster, with fewer damaging byproducts.

Fat can also be a great fuel, especially at rest or during sleep when energy demands are lower. But when you *force* fat oxidation (through starvation, over-exercise, or low-carb dieting), you pay a price: lower CO_2 production, slower ATP turnover, higher stress hormones (cortisol, adrenaline, glucagon), and reduced thyroid hormone conversion. Over time, this "forced" fat burning makes your body less efficient and more stressed, not leaner and healthier.

That's why readiness matters. If you push into a fat loss phase while your metabolism is sluggish, you're just stacking stress on stress. The result is often short-term weight loss followed by rebound gain, fatigue, and symptoms. But when your metabolism is strong—when glucose oxidation is working, your thyroid hormone is converting well, and your energy blocks are removed—then your body can dip into fat stores *without* trashing your systems in the process.

So, before we dive into strategies, let's walk through the metabolic process of fat burning itself. Once you understand that, you'll see why timing, readiness, and context matter so much.

Understanding Fat Burning (Oxidation)

First, let's clear something up: "burning fat" isn't literal. You're not tossing fat onto a fire inside your body. What's really happening is a series of metabolic processes that break fat down and convert it into usable energy (ATP). Scientists call this fat oxidation.

Here's how it works. Yes, more science—bear with me.

Step 1: Mobilization – Lipolysis

Fat stored in your tissues (adipose tissue) sits in the form of triglycerides—each made of three fatty acids attached to a glycerol backbone. When your body needs extra energy, it signals these triglycerides to break apart in a process called lipolysis, catalyzed by the enzyme lipase. This frees the fatty acids from glycerol, creating free fatty acids (FFA) that can now travel through your blood to the cells that need fuel (5).

- The glycerol part isn't wasted, it can be converted into glucose (via gluconeogenesis), turned into ATP directly, or recycled into new triglycerides.

- Lipolysis is often triggered by stress hormones like adrenaline, cortisol, and glucagon. That means while fat mobilization can feel exciting ("I'm burning fat!"), it's often a stress-driven response.

Step 2: Transport & Beta-Oxidation

Once the free fatty acids reach your cells, they're ushered into the mitochondria, the "power plants" of your cells, where the real energy conversion happens. Here's where beta oxidation comes in (6).

Imagine a fatty acid as a long loaf of bread with anywhere from 2–26 slices (carbon atoms). Beta oxidation slices off two carbons at a time, turning each "sandwich" into acetyl-CoA, the universal currency of metabolism. With every two-carbon slice, your body also produces one NADH and one $FADH_2$, electron carriers that will later power the electron transport chain.

- Glucose vs. fat difference: Glucose-derived acetyl-CoA produces more NADH (high-value "delivery trucks" that drop off at Complex I of the ETC). Fat-derived acetyl-CoA makes more $FADH_2$ (lower-value trucks that drop off at Complex II). More NADH = more ATP per run. More $FADH_2$ = less efficiency and more oxidative stress.

Step 3: Aerobic Respiration – The Power Plant

Now acetyl-CoA enters the Krebs (TCA) cycle inside the mitochondria. As the cycle turns, it makes NADH and $FADH_2$. These carry electrons to the electron transport chain (ETC), where oxygen, at Complex IV, acts as the final electron acceptor. That lets the ETC keep running and powers ATP synthase (Complex V) to make ATP (oxidative phosphorylation).

- The byproducts? Carbon dioxide (CO_2) and water.
- The ATP yield? Lots of ATP, but less per oxygen molecule compared to glucose.

FUN FACT: Fat oxidation requires more oxygen (almost double) per unit of energy than glucose. That's why you burn a higher percentage of fat at rest (when breathing is easy) and shift toward glucose during exercise (when oxygen is harder to spare).

Step 4: Why This Matters

At rest or while sleeping, your heart and muscles prefer fat because it's a slow, steady fuel. But when energy demand spikes (exercise, stress, even heavy thinking), your nervous system and tissues rely more heavily on glucose. Why? Because:

- Fat produces less CO_2 than glucose, which reduces oxygen delivery into tissues (the Bohr effect).

- Fat produces more $FADH_2$ relative to NADH, slowing energy production and increasing oxidative stress (ROS).

- Fat oxidation is tightly linked to stress hormones, glucagon, cortisol, and adrenaline, which, over time, can suppress thyroid function and lower active T3.

So, while fat is always being used in the background, forcing fat oxidation as your main fuel (low-carb diets, excessive fasting, over-exercising, or chronic stress) eventually comes at a metabolic cost.

In Summary:

1. Lipolysis frees fatty acids from triglycerides.
2. Beta oxidation slices fatty acids into acetyl-CoA, NADH, and $FADH_2$.
3. Aerobic respiration uses those molecules to generate ATP, CO_2, and water.
4. Fat oxidation requires more oxygen and produces less CO_2 than glucose—making it less efficient under stress or high demand.

When it comes to powering your metabolism, what's better—fat oxidation or carb oxidation? Well, as you learned from Chapter 2, it is a little bit of both.

Fat Oxidation vs. Carb (Glucose) Oxidation

By now, you know both carbs and fats are used daily for energy. The real question isn't *which one is "better,"* but *what balance of each helps your metabolism thrive?*

Here's the quick refresher:

- **Carbs (glucose):** Quick, efficient, and critical during stress, exercise, and for your nervous system.

- **Fat:** Slower burning, preferred at rest and overnight, always running in the background.

- **Protein:** Not a primary fuel, your body only leans on it (via gluconeogenesis) when carbs are too restricted.

At rest or sleep, you burn mostly fat. During activity or stress, carbs become your primary fuel. That's why a healthy metabolism doesn't just "burn fat" or just "burn carbs," it moves flexibly between both.

Ultimately, a strong metabolism = metabolic flexibility. Your body can easily switch fuels, burn stored fat between meals, and still have quick energy when life demands it.

Now that you understand the basics, the real question is: how do you tap into stored fat consistently, without crashing your metabolism?

How to Lose Fat Successfully (And Keep It Off)

Before we jump into strategies, let's be crystal clear: fat loss comes *after* healing and maintenance.

You need to:

- Improve your metabolic rate—Eating enough food with nutrition

- Minimize stress—Sleep, sun, and recovery

- Improve energy blocks. Improve digestion and adsorption, support estrogen excess, support iron levels, and reduce PUFA

- Stay at maintenance calories for 3–6 months

Only then is your body ready for sustainable fat loss.

Why does this matter? Because the more energy your cells produce, the more energy is available for every system in your body—digestion, hormones, sleep, skin, mood, metabolism. A warm body, steady energy, balanced hormones, strong hair and skin, and healthy weight maintenance all depend on this foundation.

Skip the healing and maintenance phase, and you'll end up frustrated. You might lose some weight, but you'll fight to keep it off. Think of it like building a house with twigs and leaves. You can throw up walls quickly with twigs and leaves, but when the first storm (stress) comes blowing, everything gets knocked down. A strong metabolism is the concrete foundation, the solid walls, and the strong roof, that makes fat loss last.

Once you've done the healing work and you're producing an abundance of energy, *then* it's time to tweak your nutrition, workouts, and habits to release excess fat.

Here are eight powerful strategies that support fat loss while keeping your metabolism strong.

Work on Quality Sleep

Sleep is one of the most underrated fat-loss tools. When you sleep, your heart and large muscles run primarily on fat oxidation, making nighttime a prime window for fat use.

Research is clear: people who consistently get 7+ hours of quality sleep each night lose more fat and keep it off more successfully than those who don't (7, 8). In one study, participants following the same controlled diet lost significantly less weight when restricted to just 4 hours in bed compared with those allowed 9 hours (9).

The problem? Up to 70 million Americans struggle with chronic sleep issues (10, 11), and poor sleep is linked to obesity worldwide. If you're not sleeping, it's much harder to regulate appetite, hormones, and metabolism.

So how do you improve both the length and quality of your sleep? Here are some proven strategies:

1. **Eat enough fuel** → Extremely low-calorie intake will disrupt sleep.

2. **Morning light** → Watch the sunrise, no sunglasses, to set your circadian rhythm.

3. **Grounding** → Walk outside barefoot to help regulate your nervous system.

4. **Ample sun exposure** → Natural light exposure supports sleep at night.

5. **Limit blue light** → Turn off screens 2–3 hours before bed.

6. **Blue light glasses** → If you do use devices, wear glasses that block blue light (12).

7. **Create a sleep-friendly environment** → Cool (<68°F), dark, distraction-free room.

8. **Calcium-rich snack** → Warm milk with a dash of salt and honey can promote sleep.

9. **Glycine-rich snack** → Gelatin-based gummies or bone broth can help you relax.

10. **Red light exposure** → 1–2 hours before bed, red light therapy has been shown to improve sleep (13).

11. **Targeted supplements** → Magnesium (14), L-theanine (15), Taurine, or even ⅛ tsp sea salt in orange juice may help.

The good news is as your metabolism heals, sleep usually improves on its own. But using some of these strategies can give you that extra nudge into longer, deeper sleep, and better fat loss.

Increase Energy Expenditure with Resistance Training

As you age, often from being less active and more stressed, you naturally start to lose muscle mass. Less muscle means a slower metabolism. A slower metabolism means fewer calories burned each day and less fuel converted into usable energy.

Did you know that muscle burns about three times more energy at rest than fat? Which means the more muscle you have, the more energy you will make and use. Increasing your metabolic rate means you will naturally burn more fat, even when you're resting or sleeping.

Yes, the truth is muscles also prefer to use fat as fuel at rest. This means building and maintaining muscle doesn't just make you stronger, it literally helps you oxidize more fat throughout the day and night. The good news is you can prevent muscle loss and even build more, at any age, with the right training program and by following the metabolic principles in this book.

Why This Matters for Fat Loss

Muscle is metabolically active tissue. It acts like an engine that keeps your body burning fuel at a higher rate. More muscle = more energy burned at rest, and more fat-oxidation during downtime. In addition, more muscle protects against the natural slowing of metabolism that happens with age.

What Real Weight Training Looks Like

Now, when I say, "weight training," I don't mean casually curling the 5 lb. weights that came with your Peloton. I'm talking about lifting weights that challenge your body enough to stimulate muscle growth.

If you stick with the same 5–10 lb. weights and crank out 20 reps without breaking a sweat, you won't build strength or muscle. For growth, your muscles need:

- Adequate stimulation → real internal stress on the muscle (aka mechanical tension).

- Progression → consistently making things harder so your muscles can't just adapt and plateau.

- Fuel + rest → nutrients and recovery to repair and grow.

In the strength world, this process of making training harder over time is called progressive overload. It means gradually increasing your weights, reps, sets, range of motion, or even tempo, anything that forces your muscles to keep adapting (16, 17).

Weight Training Basics

1. Start simple → 1–2 full-body workouts/week that hit all major muscle groups.

2. Use challenging weights → Push to near-muscular failure by the end of a set.

3. Target weak spots → Mix compound moves (squats, presses, deadlifts) with isolation work (hamstring curls, biceps, etc.).

4. Progress consistently → Add weight, reps, sets, or range of motion over time.

5. Get guidance → A trainer or solid program helps ensure form and progression.

6. Fuel properly → Aim for 1.6–2.2 g protein/kg (0.75–1 g/lb.) plus carbs to support recovery (18).

7. Recover well → Eat 20–40 g protein + 30–80 g carbs post-workout and allow 48 hours before hitting the same muscle again.

8. Rest strategically → Know when to push hard and when to back off if stress, poor sleep, or under-fueling stack up.

Just a quick note, Pilates, HIIT, yoga, and spin are great for conditioning and flexibility, but they don't usually provide the mechanical tension or progressive overload needed for real muscle growth.

Beyond fat loss, resistance training is also beneficial for bone density (19), heart health (20), blood sugar levels (21), flexibility and mobility (22), is great for brain health (23), and supports longevity (24).

So go lift some heavy sh#t!

Low to Moderate Intensity Aerobic Training

If you read my first book, you already know I'm not a big fan of long-duration cardio—at least not if your goal is sustainable fat loss. Back in the day, I trained for endurance events like a marathon and a 100-

mile bike ride. Sure, I got "endurance fit," but my body adapted by lowering my pulse and body temperature. Translation: I became more efficient at the activity but less metabolically active overall.

That's what aerobic fitness does, it teaches your body to do more while burning fewer calories per hour. Great if you're running 26 miles and don't want to eat every 30 minutes, but not so great if your long-term goal is a higher metabolism.

But here is the deal, while you burn tons of calories during those long training sessions, your basal metabolic rate usually drops afterward. This explains why many people lose some weight while training for a race, only to gain it all back (and then some) once the race is over. I learned this firsthand after my one and only marathon.

But I want to be clear: not all cardio is bad. In fact, low to moderate cardio, what's often called Zone 1 and Zone 2 training, is very supportive for long term, sustainable fat loss.

- Zone 1 = 50–60% of max heart rate
- Zone 2 = 60–70% of max heart rate

(Your max heart rate = 220 – age. At 54, mine is 168 BPM, which means my Zone 2 range is roughly 100–116 BPM.)

What the research says

- A 2014 study in the *Journal of Obesity* found that obese subjects doing low to moderate cardio (108–144 min/ week) lost more body fat than those doing HIIT (60–72 min/week) (25).

- A 2002 study in the *Journal of Applied Physiology* showed obese men doing 60 minutes of low-intensity cardio 3x/ week increased fat oxidation by 40%, while those doing HIIT had no increase (26).

What This Means for You

Go for a walk. A leisurely or brisk walk both support fat oxidation, and 20–60 minutes is plenty. Occasional longer sessions are fine, just fuel beforehand if you go over an hour.

Oh, and for all my fasting lovers out there. Here is what the research says about fasted vs. fueled workouts: While fasted training burns a higher percentage of fat during the workout, studies show total fat oxidation over 24 hours is the same whether you're fasted or fueled (27). So, eat if you want, you'll likely perform and feel better.

Walking is one of the most underrated exercises for fat loss (28), bone density, cardiovascular health (29), and even brain cognition (30). In today's world of remote work, food delivery, and constant convenience, we need walking more than ever.

Increasing Your NEAT (Non-Exercise Activity)

If you remember from the beginning of this book, I talked about NEAT or non-exercise activity thermogenesis. NEAT is everything you do during the day that isn't structured exercise: walking to the store, standing while you cook, fidgeting, cleaning, gardening, even laughing or singing.

Here's a big problem today, on average, Americans are moving less than ever. Since 2020 (when the world stopped for 2 years), we're walking about 600 fewer steps per day (31). With remote work, delivery services, streaming, and remote controls, modern life makes it far too easy to stay glued to a chair.

Client Story: Stacy

Stacy, one of my clients, had been eating a metabolically supportive diet for years and doing three workouts per week. Yet, during the pandemic, she put on about 10 pounds in two years, even though she hadn't changed her diet or exercise routine.

What happened? She stopped moving.

Stacy went from working in an office (averaging 6,000–8,000 steps per day just moving around) to working from home. When we tracked her, she was walking less than 2,000 steps a day on non-gym days, basically just shuffling between the bedroom, kitchen, and office. That added up to nearly 30,000 fewer steps per week.

Without realizing it, Stacy had slashed her daily energy expenditure. She was eating the same amount of food, just with far less movement. Her healthy metabolism was still running, but the math didn't work, so the weight crept on.

I set Stacy a daily step goal of 3,000, then increased it by 1,000 steps per week until she averaged 10,000 steps per day. Over six months, she dropped the 10 pounds she'd gained, all without changing her food or workouts.

If your metabolism is strong, tools like NEAT and exercise can help you tap into stored fuel (body fat) by raising your total daily energy expenditure. I think it's also important to see that even if you have a well running metabolic rate, if you eat more than your body is burning, you can still gain weight.

Dietary Changes

Once you've maximized your energy production and fuel intake, meaning you feel warm, have steady energy all day, sleep through the night, enjoy pain-free cycles, and crush your workouts, yet still want to lose a little extra fat, dietary tweaks can be the next lever.

These changes are meant to be temporary tools, not a permanent way of eating. Your goal should always be to return to a sustainable, pro-metabolic diet. But if you need an extra nudge for fat loss, here are two effective strategies:

1. Increase Protein Intake

Protein has the highest thermic effect of all the macronutrients. The thermic effect of food (TEF) is how much energy is required to digest and metabolize food. Protein uses 20–30% of its own calories just to be digested (32, 33). That means by increasing protein (while lowering fat to balance calories), you can burn more energy without cutting total calories.

I generally suggest increasing protein up to 1 gram per pound of bodyweight (2.2 g/kg) during a fat loss phase. Higher protein does more than just raise TEF—it also:

- Improves satiety (you'll feel fuller longer).
- Slows glucose release into the bloodstream, helping stabilize blood sugar.

For healthy individuals, these higher intakes are safe and effective short-term. But I wouldn't recommend this approach if you're still in a low metabolic state, sick, or already at your ideal weight. Once you're back to maintenance, you can reduce protein slightly if desired.

2. Reduce Dietary Fat Intake

Let me be clear: I love fat. I healed my hormones, skin, and sleep with a higher-fat (mostly saturated) diet over a decade ago. But when I later wanted to lean out, lowering dietary fat was one of the most effective levers.

Why? Because if you're eating in a calorie surplus, dietary fat is stored as body fat the fastest. Saturated fats are still more metabolically supportive than PUFA, but they're calorie dense.

- TEF of fat: ~5%
- TEF of carbs: ~10%
- TEF of protein: ~20–30% (31, 32).

Here's an example: If you swap 20 g of fat for 40 g of protein, calories stay nearly the same, but your daily thermogenesis improves by ~40 kcal/day. That adds up to roughly 4+ pounds of fat loss per year, without eating less food.

How to lower fat easily:

- Choose low-fat dairy options. Low fat milk, over whole fat and cream.
- Pick leaner cuts of meat. Fish over steak.
- Cut back on added cooking fats (butter, cream, oils).
- Minimize ice cream—yes, I love it too, but it is high in fat.
- Reduce processed foods—normally all high in fat.

One caveat: Some people genuinely feel better on higher fat diets. If lowering fat tanks your energy, wrecks your sleep, or destabilizes your blood sugar, then keep fat higher and focus on other fat-loss tools. Individuality matters.

3. Create a Strategic Calorie Deficit

I know what you're thinking; *"Wait, Kate...you've been telling us to eat MORE food to heal my metabolism, and now you're telling me to eat LESS?"*

It sounds contradictory, but it's not. Healing your metabolism and losing fat are two different dietary phases. During healing, you focus on restoring energy production, improving sleep, balancing hormones, and fueling your body generously. Once your metabolism is strong and robust, *then* you can safely shift into fat loss, and that requires a calorie deficit.

To lose body fat, you must use more fuel than you consume. Your resting metabolism (BMR) is the biggest driver of this, which is why I had you eat more at the start, to teach your body how to burn more. But now that you've built a strong foundation, we can ask your body to dip into stored fat for fuel by creating a deficit.

A deficit can come from multiple places:

- Increasing lean mass (muscle burns more fuel at rest).

- Moving more (exercise + NEAT).

- Increasing protein (higher thermic effect).

- Reducing dietary fat or carbs.

- Or simply eating fewer calories overall.

For most people, a 10–20% calorie deficit works best. For example, if you're eating 2,500 kcal/day, dropping by 250–500 kcal/day can yield about 0.5–1 pound of fat loss per week. Slow, steady, and sustainable.

How you create that deficit depends on your body. Some people do best by lowering dietary fat; others feel better by lowering carbs (though I recommend keeping at least 150 g/day for thyroid and nervous system support). If you go the fat-reduction route, you can drop as low as ~10% of total calories from fat (around 20 g fat for someone eating 2,000 kcal/day).

Important: fat loss should never be an endless deficit. A typical cycle lasts 4–12 weeks, followed by a "diet break," bringing calories back up to maintenance to give your body (and mind) a reset. Then you can re-enter another cycle if needed.

Hacks to Make a Deficit Easier

Feeling hungrier is normal at first. As your body taps into fat stores, that often eases up, but if hunger persists, these strategies can help:

1. Add a second raw carrot salad for satiety and detox support.

2. Choose whole fruit over juice for more fiber and fullness.

3. Aim for 25–35 g of complete protein at each meal.

4. Eat slowly, away from distractions.

5. Replace late-night starches with cooked fruit/veggies.

6. Use fat strategically—sometimes a little extra keeps hunger down.

7. Limit liquid meals if they leave you hungrier.

8. Don't wait until you're starving to eat.

9. Plan your meals ahead of time.

10. Have a piece of fruit before meals if your blood sugar feels low.

Client Story: Michele

Michele, 46, was a retired police officer who came to me exhausted, hormonally imbalanced, and stuck. Years of stress and low-carb dieting had left her with poor sleep, painful periods, and low energy.

Over 18 months, we worked on healing, raising her calories from 1,200 to over 2,000, adding strength training, and improving food quality. She gained about 15 lbs during this phase, but importantly, about a third of it was muscle. She also began sleeping deeply, had more energy, and, best of all, her periods became normal and pain-free.

When Michele was ready, we created a 15% calorie deficit (down to 1,700 kcal/day). She lost 8 lbs. in 12 weeks, then took a 2-week diet break at maintenance (1,900 kcal/day). After another 12 weeks at 1,700 kcal, she dropped the remaining 6 lbs.

In total, Michele lost 15 lbs. of fat over 26 weeks, but with more muscle and less fat than when she started. Today, she eats 1,800 kcal/day and maintains her weight effortlessly, which is 30% more food than her starting point.

Yes, it took 2.5 years from start to finish. But ask yourself: how many diets let you eat more food than when you started, while keeping the fat off? Sustainable fat loss takes patience, but it's worth it.

Supplements for Fat Loss

The reason I don't spend much time on fat-loss supplements is simple: 99% of healthy, sustainable fat loss comes from the basics, eating a metabolically supportive diet, building lean muscle, moving more, and creating a small, strategic calorie deficit.

That said, there are two supplements that deserve a mention: Caffeine and Vitamin E.

Let's start with caffeine, as it has the biggest impact on actual fat loss.

Good ole' caffeine is one of the safest and most effective tools to help move the fat-loss needle. Caffeine acts as a thermogenic, it increases heat production and raises metabolic rate in part by accelerating how quickly your body uptakes glucose.

Dr. Ray Peat once wrote, *"Caffeine has remarkable parallels to both progesterone and thyroid hormone, and the use of coffee or tea can help maintain their function or compensate for their deficiency."* Since both progesterone and thyroid support metabolism, it makes sense that caffeine, by mimicking their effects, can give metabolism a boost too.

And yes, there is research that backs this up. In a Harvard study on overweight men, those who consumed up to 4 cups of coffee per day lost about 4% of their body weight, compared with a placebo group (34). Another study found that ingesting 3 mg/kg of caffeine (roughly one strong cup of coffee) before low-to-moderate exercise significantly increased fat oxidation (35).

Of course, caffeine alone won't replace the fundamentals. Drinking multiple cups of coffee without addressing diet, movement, and sleep won't get you far. But when combined with everything else I've covered, caffeine can be that extra nudge in the right direction. And the best part? It often comes in the form of coffee, and who doesn't love coffee?

I usually recommend 1–4 cups of coffee per day as a reasonable range. But just like everything else in this book, it's about individuality. If caffeine makes you jittery, anxious, or disrupts your sleep, then scale back, or cut it entirely.

The second supplement and one I have already touched on earlier in this book—Vitamin E.

As discussed earlier, vitamin E is a family of fat-soluble antioxidants (tocopherols and tocotrienols) that protect against PUFA oxidation. This matters during fat loss because you're not just burning calories, you're mobilizing stored PUFA from adipose. That surge can raise oxidative stress, clog up mitochondria, and nudge thyroid function down. Vitamin E helps buffer that load while fat is being released and oxidized.

How much? We don't have a human RCT that sets a dose to "cover PUFA released during fat loss," so I use the same metric that ties vitamin E to PUFA exposure. If you're losing 1–2 lb/week and adipose is ~12–20% PUFA, you'll mobilize roughly 54–181 g PUFA/week. Using ~0.5 mg vitamin E per gram of PUFA, that's an extra ~4–13 mg/day ($\approx$ 6–19 IU/day). In practice, I like a modest, temporary bump during cuts, so 25–100 IU/day of natural d-alpha-tocopherol is my general suggestion (36).

What about food sources? Many vitamin E rich foods are also high in PUFA (wheat-germ oil, most nuts/seeds). If you're intentionally lowering PUFA, and you want to use food, lean on quality extra-virgin olive oil, avocado, eggs, and shrimp. If you want to avoid adding more PUFA, use a quality alpha-tocopherol supplement to hit your target.

The truth is Vitamin E won't melt fat, but it can keep the engine clean while you do the real work—sleep, protein, carbs, micronutrients, a sane deficit, and strength training. Think of it as PUFA insurance so your cut feels smoother, and your mitochondria stay happier.

At this point, you understand that healthy weight loss begins with a healthy metabolism.

A healthy body, warm, energized, hormonally balanced, and sleeping deeply, sets the foundation for sustainable fat loss. Only once you've healed and maintained your metabolic rate should you consider a fat-loss phase.

From there, fat loss becomes about layering in smart strategies:

- Improving sleep quality and duration
- Strength training to build lean muscle
- Incorporating Zone 1–2 cardio
- Increasing NEAT (daily movement)
- Making short-term dietary tweaks (protein up, fat down)
- Using strategic calorie deficits (with breaks)
- Leveraging caffeine to give your metabolism a little push

For some, improving metabolic health alone is enough to shed excess fat. For others, these tools, applied at the right time, will help unlock further fat loss.

The big takeaway: *fat loss is not the starting line; it's the finish line.* First you build health, then you layer in fat loss.

Now that you've learned about the key pieces of energy production—supportive fuel, nutrients, oxygen, thyroid, and all the common blocks that get in the way—along with practical fat loss strategies, it's time to bring it all together.

In the next and final chapter, "How to Use This Information", I'll show you how to take everything you've just learned and incorporate it into your life. Think of it as a general road map for understanding and improving energy production.

Almost there, just one more chapter to go.

CHAPTER 13

THE BOTTOM LINE

Understanding Healthy Fat Loss—Why Metabolism Comes First

1. Weight loss does not equal fat loss. The scale reflects water, glycogen, digestive contents, muscle, *and* fat, not just fat.

2. Healthy fat loss comes from a healthy body. Focus on healing and raising your metabolic rate first. Use your health markers (warmth, energy, sleep, digestion, hormones) to know when you're ready.

3. Fat burning is complex. It involves lipolysis, beta-oxidation, and aerobic respiration, all working together to convert stored fat into ATP.

4. Fat and glucose are always burning together. At rest you'll oxidize more fat, while during activity (and stress) you'll rely more on glucose.

5. Once your foundation is solid, layer in fat-loss tools. These include optimizing sleep, progressive resistance training, Zone 1–2 cardio, increasing NEAT, strategic dietary tweaks, caffeine, and, if needed, a temporary calorie deficit.

CHAPTER 14

HOW TO USE THIS INFORMATION

By now, you've discovered more about your body than most people ever will in their lifetime. You've seen how energy connects everything—your hormones, your digestion, your breath, your mood, even the way you think and deal with stress.

You've learned that fixing your health isn't about following another rigid plan or restricting yourself into exhaustion. It's about learning how your cells make energy and understanding that energy is the foundation of all health. Once you see your body through this lens, everything changes.

You stop asking, *"What foods will heal me?"* and start asking, *"What does my body need right now to make energy—so that energy can heal me?"*

When you begin viewing health through creating energy, your choices start to align naturally with what your body needs—not what's trendy, not what worked for your friend, not what the random TikTok health influencer said, but what supports your unique physiology in this moment.

As Ray Peat often said, energy isn't just something your body uses—it's what holds your structure together. "Energy itself is a structural element," he wrote. "When energy falters, the very architecture of your cells begins to change, and with it, function declines."

In laymen terms, energy is needed for you to function, but also for you to maintain your structure. As Forrest Gump would say, the two go together like peas and carrots.

Energy Equals Health

Every chapter in this book has pointed back to one simple truth: Energy equals health.

When your cells produce energy efficiently, every system—hormonal, immune, digestive, detox, and nervous begins to function better. When energy falters, everything struggles.

This is why people who "eat right" and "exercise" can still feel exhausted, anxious, or cold. They have an energy balance issue—too many demands for their current level of energy production. As you have continued to learn, health is not about pushing your body to the max but about creating enough energy to meet your body's demands. True healing happens when your cells have the energy to repair, regenerate, and restore balance.

If you take one thing from this book, let it be this: *Support your energy production, and your energy will support you.*

I don't want you to think of this book as a new plan or program. It's a reference point—something to return to when you feel tired, run down, or confused. Revisiting physiology helps you reconnect with the "why" behind the "what." That understanding will always guide your next step better than any diet trend or supplement stack ever could.

With that said, I want to give you a framework on how to use this information—as I know, it can feel like a lot. Use this framework as a general guide about how you can apply this information so that you become your own health detective.

So how do you take this information and use it in your daily life? Let's walk through it step by step.

Find Your Starting Point

Every journey begins with awareness.

If you don't know where you are, it's nearly impossible to find your way forward. The first step in improving your body's energy is identifying your starting point.

When I begin working with clients, I ask them a series of simple but revealing questions. Not to judge or label them, but to help them see clearly where they're starting from. Because once you know your baseline, you can create a realistic path toward change.

Just like you can't give driving directions without knowing the starting address, you can't improve your health without first understanding where you are right now.

Here's where to begin:

- Write down everything you eat for at least 14 days. Use a food logging app like Cronometer or MyFitnessPal to get insight into calories, protein, fat, and carbohydrates.

- Track how you feel after meals. Do you feel energized or sleepy? Calm or jittery?

- Note your body temperature and pulse a few times each day (morning, midday, evening).

- Observe your sleep, digestion, and mood.

- Record your body weight and a few key measurements (chest, waist, hips, arm, thigh).

This isn't about analyzing your every waking moment but rather creating awareness and a clear starting point.

Most of my clients are stunned when they first see the data. Some discover they're eating far less or far more than they thought. Others realize they're consuming large amounts of fat and not enough protein or carbohydrates to fuel proper metabolism. Food logging can reveal how your diet affects everything: your weight, mood, digestion, sleep, energy, and even your hormones.

Awareness is the beginning of change. You can't shift what you refuse to see.

Find Your Maintenance Calories

Once you've logged your food for a couple of weeks, the next step is identifying your maintenance calories—the amount your body currently needs to maintain its weight.

This step isn't about dieting. It's about understanding your metabolic reality so you can move from where you are to where you want to be, without shocking your system.

Many people transitioning to a bioenergetic way of eating skip this step. They dive straight in, loading up on milk, cheese, ice cream, and juice. While those foods can be wonderfully supportive, if you suddenly consume far more fuel than your body can currently use, you'll likely gain weight.

To be clear, it's not because these foods are "bad." It's because your energy production hasn't caught up yet. Not all supportive foods are supportive to everyone all the time—a lot depends on your current state of health.

To find your calorie maintenance:

1. Track your intake for 14 days while taking your morning weight.

2. Find your average daily calories and average weekly weight each week. Compare week one with week two.

3. If your weight stays stable, you've found maintenance. If it goes up, you're in surplus. If it drops, you're in deficit.

Once you know your maintenance level, you can begin to make gradual, informed changes. If you've been under-eating, don't suddenly double your intake. Move slowly and give your body time to adapt.

Improving energy production is like rekindling a fire. You don't dump huge logs on a tiny fire; you could overwhelm it. However, if you fuel it slowly, allowing the fire to adapt to the increased wood, it will eventually increase in size burning the bigger logs—just like your body will learn to utilize the bigger meals.

Track Objective and Subjective Markers

As you start making changes, track both objective and subjective feedback. This is where science meets intuition—where numbers meet the felt experience of your body.

Objective markers

These are measurable signals that tell you how your body is producing energy:

- Waking temperature (aim for around 97.8 F (36.5), rising to 98.6 F (37 C) after meals).

- Pulse rate (70–90 bpm is often ideal for an active metabolism).

- Sleep length and depth: How often do you wake? How long does it take to fall asleep? How much deep and REM sleep?

- Digestive rhythm: How often do you have bowel movements? Stool—lose or constipated?

- Weight and body measurements. Scale weight, and circumference measure of waist, chest, hips, biceps and mid-leg.

- Blood sugar markers: Upon waking and after meals—if needed.

- Possible lab markers.

Subjective markers

These are the subtle sensations that tell you how you feel:

- Warmth in your hands and feet.

- Calmness after eating.

- Mental focus and emotional steadiness.

- Restful sleep and a stable mood.

- Consistent hunger and satiation cues.

When you combine both sets of information, patterns emerge, and those patterns are your roadmap.

For example, if your temperature rises after breakfast and your mood improves, that's a sign you have good energy production. If your digestion stalls after a stressful day, that is a sign you didn't eat enough, or the stressed state is overriding peristalsis.

This is what I mean by becoming your own health detective, using real clues instead of random guesses.

But numbers and feelings can give insight into your progress.

Focus on Energy Production

Now that you've established your baseline with data, the real work begins: supporting energy production itself.

Food is your foundation; it is the fuel that drives every metabolic process. But rather than thinking in terms of restriction, think in terms of replacement.

Food First—Replace, Don't Restrict

While staying near your calorie maintenance, start improving food quality. Replace foods that drain you and are unsupportive with foods that fuel you.

Some examples:

- Swap seed oils for saturated fats like butter or coconut oil.
- Add fruit, honey, or juice for quick, digestible carbohydrates instead of processed desserts or heavy starches.
- Choose animal proteins (eggs, dairy, shellfish, gelatin) over plant-based ones like beans, tofu, and nuts.
- Add nutrient-dense foods like oysters, liver, and dairy before reaching for synthetic supplements.

As I wrote in *How to Heal Your Metabolism*, the food you eat is a huge part of healing. Understanding what foods are best and why helps you make better choices for your health—as you were never meant to starve, you were meant to be nourished.

If you haven't revisited that book in a while, this is a good time. It goes deeper into the "why" and the "what" in the context of specific carbs, proteins, and fats.

In practice, this often means getting 40–60% of calories from carbohydrates, 15–30% from fat, and 20–25% from protein—but remember, these are frameworks, not laws.

Energy production happens when the fuel is easy-to-digest, nutrient rich, and enjoyable.

Check Your Breathing

Energy isn't just about what you eat, it's about how well oxygen and carbon dioxide are exchanged in your body. Every breath affects energy production. When you're anxious or under-fueled, you tend to breathe quickly and shallowly, losing CO_2 and triggering a stress response. This makes it harder for oxygen to enter your cells and produce energy efficiently.

Slow, nasal breathing and relaxed posture help restore that balance. Breathing is the simplest way to support mitochondrial function, because oxygen is the final acceptor in the electron transport chain—the last step in ATP production.

If you suspect anemia or poor oxygen delivery, ask your doctor for a full iron panel and thyroid test. Support red blood cell production with foods rich in iron, copper, and B vitamins, this includes beef liver, shellfish, eggs, and dairy. And remember breathing calmly isn't just about "feeling" relaxed. It's about optimizing cellular metabolism.

Oxygen and carbon dioxide work together to keep your cells producing energy efficiently.

Your Thyroid Matters

Your thyroid is your body's internal thermostat, the gland that regulates how well your cells produce energy. If thyroid function is sluggish, you'll struggle to make energy efficiently no matter how well you eat.

Support your thyroid by focusing on:

- Adequate calories and carbohydrates: under-eating or low-carb diets suppress thyroid function.
- Thyroid-supportive foods: shellfish, beef liver, eggs, dairy, and easily digested carbs like fruit or juice.
- Managing stress: cortisol and adrenaline directly suppress thyroid hormone conversion.
- Supporting liver health: your liver converts inactive T_4 to active T_3, the form your cells use.

If you've been eating well but still feel cold, sluggish, or have low pulse and temperature, it's worth getting a full thyroid panel. Discuss the possibility of thyroid support with your practitioner. Sometimes, your system simply needs a nudge to restart efficient energy production, while other times it might need exogenous thyroid support.

When thyroid function improves, every system in your body can improve.

Work on One Energy Block at a Time

You may have several "energy blocks"—those sneaky little energy drains that keep your body from producing energy efficiently. These could include poor digestion, endotoxins, stress hormones, excess iron or estrogen, or high polyunsaturated fat (PUFA) intake.

But here's the deal, don't try to fix them all at once.

Healing requires slow and steady steps. It is best to identify one weak link, work on it, observe results, and only then move to the next.

A few examples:

- If digestion is weak: focus on easily digested foods, reducing endotoxins, and lowering stress around meals.

- If stress hormones are high: prioritize sleep, take walks after meals, and reduce overall demands on your system.

- If estrogen is running amuck: add a daily raw carrot salad, support bile flow, improve thyroid function, and balance blood sugar.

- If energy is low: increase carbohydrates and mineral-rich foods gradually while managing stress.

When I was trying to fix my nervous system and improve energy production, I wanted results yesterday. The more I pushed, the slower I progressed—and sometimes I even regressed. Healing only started when I met my body where it was instead of trying to drag it to where I wished it would be. Once your body takes one small step, it will be ready for the next.

You can't force healing—you can only take steps, allow for the body to follow, and then step again.

Reassess Every Few Weeks

Improving energy production isn't linear, instead, it's an up and down roller coaster with a few twists and spins. Some weeks you might feel amazing, while others, your body will be giving you the middle finger while it's rebuilding and recalibrating. This is normal. Your life is not a vacuum, and things will continue to stress you and challenge you. These little bumps can throw you off sometimes—but, instead of throwing in the towel, take note.

Every 2–4 weeks, review your data and reflections:

- Are your temps and pulse improving?
- Are you sleeping better or feeling calmer after meals?
- Is your digestion smoother?
- Has your cycle or libido changed?
- Are your hair, nails, and skin stronger?

If the answer is yes, keep going. If not, pause and re-evaluate. Sometimes your body isn't ready for the next step, it might need more time in safety and nourishment before it can take another leap forward.

Improving energy production isn't about doing more; it's about doing what your body can handle.

Never Stop Learning

The process of improving energy production doesn't end. You'll continue to learn, experiment, and refine. You will go through life's ups and downs. And in some situations, you will fall back—but, this doesn't mean failure, it just means it is time to ask more questions.

We all need to remember that health isn't a destination; it's a never-ending journey. You're learning to trust your body again after years of beating it up—repeatedly.

When something feels off, ask questions instead of reacting.

- If you're cold, maybe you need more fuel.
- If you're anxious, maybe your blood sugar has dropped.
- If you're bloated, maybe you're eating too fast or you're too stressed.
- If you're having hot flashes, maybe you're stressed.
- If you're exhausted, maybe you have a sluggish thyroid, high iron, or are under fueled.

Every symptom is feedback. None of them mean you are "broken," but rather that your cells are struggling to produce enough energy.

Personally, my own journey hasn't been smooth. I've had setbacks, frustrations, and moments of doubt. But each one taught me something new. And with everything I have learned, my on-going goal is to make learning about health and healing easier for all of you. The truth is we learn the most in our struggles, not in the things that are easy.

My Final Thoughts

Don't let this book become another rulebook. Let it be a guide, a resource, a reference point you return to when you feel off, tired, or uncertain. The physiology you've learned here gives you a map, but your application, experimentation, and desire to keep learning Is what will make it work for you.

Improving energy production is a never-ending lesson. And as long as you keep living, it will be a lesson you will keep learning, again and again, each time with a deeper understanding and wisdom.

My own health story doesn't have a clear beginning or end. It's an ongoing journey of ups and downs, learning and observing, failures and wins. And with each chapter of life, I'm reminded of one humbling truth: the more I learn, the less I know.

My health has improved dramatically since those dark days of nervous system chaos—the sleepless nights, the anxiety, the constant state of fight-or-flight that drove me to study all this in the first place. You see life never stops when the sh#t hits the fan. Challenges still come, new lessons still appear, and my body continues to teach me.

That's what I want for you, not perfection, not control, but curiosity. A lifelong relationship with your own physiology that deepens over time. Because when you understand your body, you trust it. And when you trust it, healing stops being a destination and becomes a way of living.

Remember if you ever feel lost, go back to the foundation. Revisit *How to Heal Your Metabolism* to remind yourself of the foods that build you. Then come back to this book to understand the physiology that they work in. Between the two, you have everything you need to navigate your health, metabolism, and body composition—with *Better Energy* production as your ultimate guide.

CHAPTER 14

THE BOTTOM LINE

How to Use This Information

1. Energy equals health. Optimal energy production supports every cell's structure and function. When energy production is compromised, everything in the body begins to struggle.

2. Find your starting point. Collect data to understand where you're starting from—without knowing your current state, it's impossible to chart a clear direction forward.

3. Know your maintenance calories. Understanding how many calories your body needs to maintain its weight helps you adjust your diet thoughtfully, without over-restricting or gaining unnecessary weight.

4. Track key health markers. Monitor body temperature, pulse, sleep, body measurements, mood, focus, energy, and hunger. These markers reveal whether your choices are truly moving you in the right direction.

5. Focus on energy production. Prioritize high-quality, nutrient-dense foods, balanced macronutrients, proper breathing, and thyroid support—all of which are essential for efficient energy metabolism.

6. Address one energy block at a time. Don't try to fix everything at once. Work on one area at a time to avoid overwhelm. Slow, steady progress is more sustainable than quick, scattered changes.

7. Reassess every 2–4 weeks. Healing and energy improvement aren't linear. Expect fluctuations. Reassess regularly, make small adjustments, and stay consistent—progress comes with patience and persistence.

APPENDIX A

Ray Peat's Carrot Salad

In recent years, Ray Peat's carrot salad has become a viral sensation, with nearly every TikTok "health" influencer making a video about it. The reason for its popularity is simple—it works.

The recipe consists of one medium raw carrot, 1-2 tsp. coconut oil, 1 tsp. vinegar (commonly white vinegar), and salt.

Dr. Peat explained that the fibers in raw carrots produce natural fungicides and bacteriostats, which act as a natural antibiotic and antiseptic for the bowel. When combined with coconut oil and vinegar, both known for their antibacterial, antifungal, and antimicrobial properties—the carrot salad becomes a natural gut cleanser. It functions like a scrub brush for the intestines, removing toxins, binding to endotoxins, and supporting hormone detoxification.

Beyond gut cleansing, the carrot salad may help remove broken-down estrogens, excess cholesterol, and endotoxins. After over a decade of recommending daily carrot salad to my clients, I've seen incredible results, including improved bowel transit time, reduced bloating, relief from both constipation and diarrhea, fewer hot flashes, better sleep, clearer skin, lower cholesterol levels, and even weight loss in some cases.

This simple addition to your diet can be beneficial for anyone struggling with bloating, constipation, diarrhea, PMS, hot flashes, skin issues, SIBO, or IBS.

Carrot Salad FAQ

Can I just eat a whole carrot and still get the benefits?
Yes, eating a raw carrot alone can still be beneficial, but the full carrot salad recipe enhances its effects. The added coconut oil and vinegar provide additional antimicrobial, antibacterial and antifungal support.

Does it matter how I cut the carrot?
Not really. Peeling the carrot into long strips creates the most surface area for binding toxins, but shredding works just as well.

Can I drink carrot juice instead?
No. The beneficial fibers are removed in the juicing process, and they are essential for binding toxins and cleansing the gut.

What size should the carrot be?
A medium to large carrot, about 75-100 grams, is ideal for the salad.

Do I need to eat the carrot salad every day?
Most people see the best results when they eat it daily.

Can I add other ingredients to the carrot salad?
Yes, you can add raisins, cheese, raw beets, jicama, or onions for extra flavor—do what helps you eat the carrot most consistently.

When should I eat the carrot salad?
It should be eaten 20-60 minutes before a meal. Since the carrot binds to toxins, eating it with meals may reduce nutrient absorption.

Does the carrot need to be organic?
No, but organic is preferred. If using non-organic carrots, be sure to wash and peel them before eating.

What if I don't like carrots? Are there alternatives?
Yes! If carrots don't work for you, there are other gut-cleansing options—keep reading.

Boiled White Button Mushrooms

If carrot salad isn't appealing, well-cooked white button mushrooms offer a similar gut-cleansing effect while acting as a natural antibiotic for the bowel. Unlike pharmaceutical antibiotics, which can disrupt gut flora, white button mushrooms can be used safely every day.

These mushrooms have additional benefits beyond gut health. They act as aromatase inhibitors, which reduce estrogen production by blocking the aromatase enzyme. They are also natural antihistamines and anti-serotonin agents, helping to regulate inflammation, allergies, and excess serotonin levels in the gut. Research has even shown that white button mushrooms may help slow the progression of breast and prostate cancers.

White button mushrooms are also surprisingly nutritious. They provide about eight grams of protein per 250-gram serving and contain vitamin D, B vitamins, copper, and selenium.

Proper preparation is important. White button mushrooms contain hydrazine, a natural carcinogen, which must be removed through cooking. Boiling the mushrooms for at least an hour allows the hydrazine to be released in the steam. This is why boiling, rather than sautéing, is the preferred cooking method. Some people worry that excessive cooking will reduce the nutritional value of the mushrooms, but any nutrients lost can be retained by consuming the broth as a soup.

This doesn't mean that raw mushrooms should never be eaten. However, if you are consuming them daily for gut health, they must be fully cooked to ensure safety.

If you get tired of carrot salad or find it irritates your gut, boiled white button mushrooms can serve as an excellent alternative.

Boiled Bamboo Shoots

Another natural gut-cleansing option is boiled bamboo shoots, which, like carrots and white button mushrooms, have antibacterial, antimicrobial, and antibiotic properties that benefit gut health.

In a 2009 study published in the *Nutrition Journal*, eight healthy young women consumed 350 grams of cooked bamboo shoots daily. After just six days, researchers observed improvements in lipid profiles, more frequent bowel movements, and increased stool size.

Like white button mushrooms, bamboo shoots contain toxins that must be properly prepared before consumption. Slicing the bamboo shoots into thin strips helps release hydrogen cyanide, a natural plant toxin. Once cut, the bamboo shoots should be boiled for at least an hour to fully remove the cyanide. Canned bamboo shoots have already been pre-cooked and are safe to eat without further preparation.

Which Gut Cleanser Should You Choose?

All three of these foods offer natural, daily-use alternatives to pharmaceutical antibiotics and gut-disrupting medications. Each has its own unique benefits.

Carrot salad is the best option for hormonal detoxification, particularly for those dealing with excess estrogen. White button mushrooms are ideal for histamine and serotonin regulation due to their antihistamine and anti-serotonin properties. Bamboo shoots are particularly effective at improving gut motility and stool bulk, making them useful for constipation and sluggish digestion.

If one option doesn't work for you, try another. The key is consistency—adding one of these gut cleansers into your routine daily can significantly improve digestion, hormone regulation, and overall gut health.

APPENDIX B

LOW FODMAP FOODS

What foods to avoid and eat if you have SIBO—Low FODMAP. FODMAP stands for Fermentable Oligosaccharides, Disaccharides, Monosaccharides, and Polyols. These are short-chain fermentable carbohydrates that are poorly absorbed in the small intestine and can cause bloating, gas, diarrhea, and other digestive issues, especially in people with SIBO or IBS.

Vegetables

Avoid onions, garlic, cauliflower, asparagus, Brussels sprouts, leeks, cabbage, mushrooms, and artichokes, as these vegetables are highly fermentable and can trigger bloating and gas.

Fruits

Limit apples, pears, cherries, watermelon, peaches, mangoes, nectarines, blackberries, and plums, as they contain high amounts of fermentable sugars like fructose and polyols.

Legumes & Beans

Stay away from lentils, chickpeas, black beans, kidney beans, soybeans, and split peas, since they contain galacto-oligosaccharides (GOS) that are difficult to digest and fuel bacterial overgrowth.

Grains & Starches

Reduce or eliminate wheat, rye, barley, couscous, bran, whole grain cereals, high-fiber bread, and pasta, as these contain fructans that ferment quickly in the small intestine.

Dairy Products

Avoid milk, soft cheeses, yogurt, cream, sour cream, ice cream, and buttermilk, since they contain lactose, which can contribute to fermentation and bloating in those with SIBO.

Beverages

Limit beer, wine, soda, and kombucha as they either contain fermentable sugars, carbonation, or alcohol, all of which could worsen symptoms.

Sweeteners

Avoid honey, agave, high-fructose corn syrup, and sugar alcohols like sorbitol, xylitol, and maltitol, since these can rapidly ferment and cause digestive distress.

Miscellaneous

Watch out for processed foods containing inulin, chicory root, artificial sweeteners, and thickeners like carrageenan, as they can promote bacterial overgrowth and increase gut irritation.

List of SIBO-Friendly Foods that are low in FODMAPs, easy to digest, and less likely to contribute to bacterial overgrowth.

Vegetables

Stick to zucchini, carrots, bell peppers, cucumber, and green beans. These are lower in fermentable fibers and gentler on digestion compared to high-FODMAP vegetables like onions and cauliflower.

Fruits

Choose organic bananas, blueberries, kiwi, grapes, pineapple, cantaloupe, oranges, orange juice, coconut water.

Proteins

All animal proteins are naturally low in FODMAPs, so feel free to eat beef, chicken, turkey, fish (cod, sole, and tuna), shellfish, and eggs. These provide essential nutrients without feeding bacterial overgrowth.

Grains & Starches

Opt for white rice, peeled and well-cooked potatoes, small portions of sweet potatoes, gluten-free oats, and traditional sourdough bread (gluten-free or fermented properly).

Dairy & Dairy Alternatives

Stick to hard cheeses like cheddar, parmesan, and Swiss, as they contain little to no lactose. Butter, lactose-free yogurt, coconut milk, are also good alternatives.

Sweeteners

Safe choices include maple syrup, dextrose, beet sugar, white sugar, and coconut sugar.

Fats & Oils

These include olive oil, coconut oil, ghee, butter, and beef tallow in your meals.

REFERENCES AND RESEARCH

The concepts and perspectives presented in this book are grounded in decades of scientific research, clinical observation, and independent inquiry. In order to keep this book accessible, readable, and physically manageable, the full list of research references has not been included in print.

A comprehensive reference list—spanning over 550 peer-reviewed studies, articles, and source materials—is available as a free download on my website.

To access the full reference library, visit:
www.KateDeering.com/Better-Energy

These materials are provided for readers who wish to explore the science more deeply, verify sources, or continue their own research beyond the pages of this book.

In addition, for a complete list of products, books, and supplements I support, please visit: **www.KateDeering.com/products-1**

REMEMBER TO GET YOUR FREE MONTHLY NEWSLETTER

Continued education matters when it comes to your health, metabolism, and energy. Join Kate's community of thousands of curious, independent thinkers and receive a FREE monthly newsletter featuring up-to-date, science-based insights on nutrition, hormones, and energy production.

You'll find information on:

- Why carbohydrates are essential for optimal energy production
- Why estrogen is not a "female hormone," but a stress hormone
- Why fat burning is not always a good thing
- What most health practitioners are missing when it comes to true healing
- How to improve menopause symptoms without hormone therapy

To join the community of out-of-the-box, nutritionally minded readers, visit **www.KateDeering.com** and enter your name and email.

For daily insights on metabolism, hormones, and energy, please follow Kate on social media: Instagram & Facebook: @KateDeeringFitness

INDEX

Ray Peat 11, 19-20, 98, 138, 145, 209,
220-225, 241, 278, 282, 290, 337,
376, 395, 425, 429, 442
Ray Peat Carrot Salad 222, 290
Reactive oxygen species (ROS) 46, 52-54,
81, 85, 197, 246, 287, 345-348, 371,
381, 412
Recovery 19-21, 25, 155-156, 160, 183, 205,
283, 305, 342, 357, 413-417
Rectum 235, 252, 264
Red light therapy 415
Regulatory Proteins 66-69
Resistance training 415-417, 428
Reticuloendothelial System (RES) 21, 109,
339-342, 351-355, 364
Retinoic acid 130
Retinol 132
Reverse T3 (rT3) 124-128, 140-143, 149,
173, 280
Riboflavin (B2) 29, 39, 71-72, 92, 211, 237,
313, 342
Ribose 83
Rice 41, 47, 90-92, 178-179, 219, 257, 290,
448
Rice Diet 179

S

Saccharomyces boulardii 223, 257, 261
Safflower oil 56
Salad dressings 389
Salmon 71-73, 131, 317, 369, 379, 389
Salt 129, 166, 184-187, 219-223, 230, 260,
286, 316, 336, 415, 442
Saponins 88-89
Saturated fats 54-55, 62, 226, 230, 260,
330, 365-374, 379-380, 389-390,
394-398, 421, 435
Sea salt 415
Seed oils 23, 249, 365-371, 376-378, 388,
394, 435
Selenium 128-130, 140-143, 149, 211, 215,
287, 322, 382, 444
Serotonin 211-213, 222, 230, 252-256,
261-262, 277-278, 285, 291, 296,
444-445
Shellfish 29, 70, 92, 119, 130, 143, 219,
314-317, 336, 435-436, 448
Short-chain fatty acids 241
Sigmoid Colon 235, 264

Sleep 9, 19, 25-37, 41, 48-51, 61-62, 79-80,
93, 113-120, 139, 143-149, 153-160,
170, 176, 184-186, 191, 206,
217-218, 226-230, 241, 257, 262,
268, 273-274, 284, 291, 300-301,
306-310, 322, 331, 343, 361, 386,
399, 405-409, 413-437, 441-443
SOD1 80-81, 85
SOD2 85
Soil-Based Probiotic 223
Sourdough 29, 47, 89, 219, 257, 448
Sprouting 89
Steroid sulfatase (STS) 311, 319-324, 336
Stress response 42, 46, 50-52, 61-62, 131,
142, 153, 157-166, 170-173, 177,
185-189, 222, 226, 274, 279-280,
288-291, 307, 336, 436
Stroke 135, 239, 295-299, 386
Structural Proteins 44, 67-68, 296
Sucrase 66, 210
Sugar (sucrose) 41-43, 47-50, 59-62, 83, 159,
167-189, 210, 216, 223-230, 237,
246, 250, 259-261, 273-274, 280,
288, 307-308, 330-332, 352-356,
384-387, 393, 406, 417, 421-424,
433, 437-439, 447-448
Sulfation 313-315, 320-321, 333
Sun exposure 207-208, 322-323, 415
Sunflower oil 56
Sympathetic nervous system 163, 194
Symptoms of estrogen excess 266, 289, 297,
326
Symptoms of iron overload 352
Sydney Diet Heart Study 374

T

Taurine 184-186, 207, 223, 260, 314-317,
336, 415
Tannins 88-89, 340
TEF 32-35, 421
Testosterone 52, 60, 164-165, 267-268, 284,
315, 319-320, 333, 370
Theca cells 267
Thermic effect of food (TEF) 32-35, 421
Thiamine (B1) 29, 39, 71-76, 92, 104,
111-114, 119, 199-201, 207-209,
214, 223, 237, 287, 314
Thromboxanes 386
Thyroid 12, 16, 22-25, 29-31, 35-37, 41-42,
46, 50-52, 57-62, 76-80, 87, 94, 104,